Mastering The Boards and Clinical Examinations in Internal Medicine

Neurology

A.B.R. Thomson

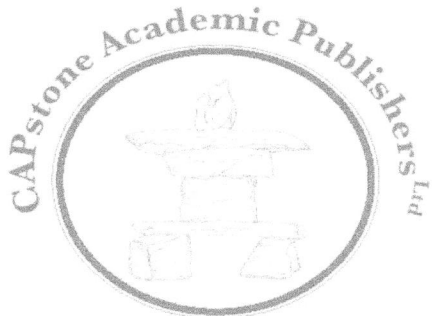

CAPstone (Canadian Academic Publishers Ltd) is a not-for-profit company dedicated to the use of the power of education for the betterment of all persons everywhere.

"The Democratization of Knowledge"

Medical drawings by S. Lee and E. Howell

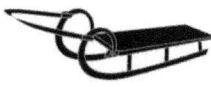

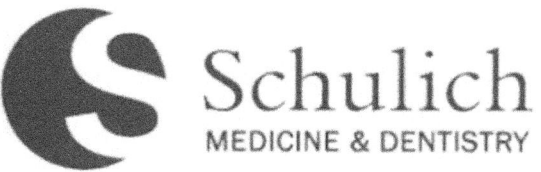 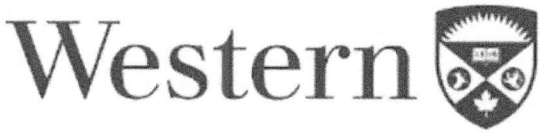

THE WESTERN WAY

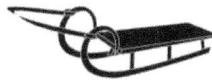

Mastering the Boards: Neurology   A.B.R. Thomson

Table of Contents

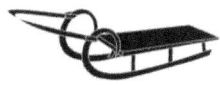

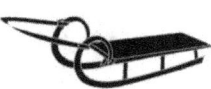

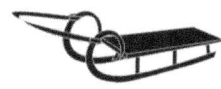

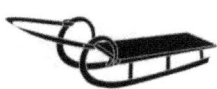

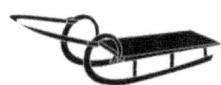

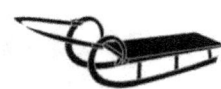

DISCLAIMER

The primary purpose of this publication is education. The author, editor and publisher acknowledge that the development of new material opens to way for possible errors – what is correct today might not be the standard of care tomorrow. Readers are advised to ensure that the doses of drugs which they use are in compliance with their country's product information, and that the use of any therapeutic agent, be it a pharmaceutical or a technology, should be guided by local guidelines. There is often a wide diversity of professional opinion, and guidelines from one country are not always congruent with another.

The author, editor and publisher do not guarantee the safety, reliability, accuracy, completeness or usefulness of this material.

They disclaim any and all liability for damage and claims that may result from the use of information, publications, technologies, products, and for series provided in this publication.

I have made every attempt to trace the holders of copyright for material reproduced in this book. If by some oversight I have omitted a copyright holder, please contact me to correct this.

Thank you.

Alan Thomson

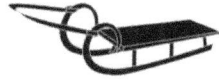

Mastering the Boards: Neurology   A.B.R. Thomson

MASTERING THE BOARDS AND THE CANMED OBJECTIVES

Medical Expert
The discussion of complex cases provides the participants with an opportunity to comment on additional focused history and physical examination. They would provide a complete and organized assessment. Participants are encouraged to identify key features, and they develop an approach to problem-solving.

The case discussions, as well as the discussion of cases around a diagnostic imaging, pathological or endoscopic base provides the means for the candidate to establish an appropriate management plan based on the best available evidence to clinical practice. Throughout, an attempt is made to develop strategies for diagnosis and development of clinical reasoning skills.

Communicator
The participants demonstrate their ability to communicate their knowledge, clinical findings, and management plan in a respectful, concise and interactive manner. When the participants play the role of examiners, they demonstrate their ability to listen actively and effectively, to ask questions in an open-ended manner, and to provide constructive, helpful feedback in a professional and non-intimidating manner.

Collaborator
The participants use the "you have a green consult card" technique of answering questions as fast as they are able, and then to interact with another health professional participant to move forward the discussion and problem solving. This helps the participants to build upon what they have already learned about the importance of collegial interaction.

Manager
The participants are provided with assignments in advance of the three day GI Practice Review. There is much work for them to complete before as well as afterwards, so they learn to manage their time effectively, and to complete the assigned tasks proficiently and on time. They learn to work in teams to achieve answers from small group participation, and then to share this with other small group participants through effective delegation of work. Some of the material they must access demands that they use information technology effectively to access information that will help to facilitate the delineation of adequately broad differential diagnoses, as well as rational and cost effective management plans.

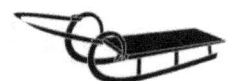

Health Advocate
In the answering of the questions and case discussions, the participants are required to consider the risks, benefits, and costs and impacts of investigations and therapeutic alliances upon the patient and their loved ones.

Scholar
By committing to the pre- and post-study requirements, plus the intense three day active learning Practice Review with colleagues is a demonstration of commitment to personal education. Through the interactive nature of the discussions and the use of the "green consult card", they reinforce their previous learning of the importance of collaborating and helping one another to learn.

Professional
The participants are coached on how to interact verbally in a professional setting, being straightforward, clear and helpful. They learn to be honest when they cannot answer questions, make a diagnosis, or advance a management plan. They learn how to deal with aggressive or demotivated colleagues, how to deal with knowledge deficits, how to speculate on a missing knowledge byte by using first principals and deductive reasoning. In a safe and supportive setting they learn to seek and accept advice, to acknowledge awareness of personal limitations, and to give and take 360° feedback.

Knowledge
The basic science aspects of gastroenterology are considered in adequate detail to understand the mechanisms of disease, and the basis of investigations and treatment. In this way, the participants respect the importance of an adequate foundation in basic sciences, the designing of clinical research studies to provide an evidence-based approach, the relevance of their management plans being patient-focused, and the need to add "compassionate" to the Three C's of Medical Practice: competent, caring and compassionate.

"They may forget what you said, but they will never forget how you made them feel."

Carl W. Buechner, on teaching.

"With competence, care for the patient. With compassion, care about the person."

Alan B. R. Thomson, on being a physician.
PROLOGUE

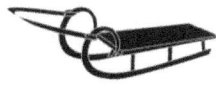

HREs, better known as, High Risk Examinations. After what is often two decades of study, sacrifice, long hours, dedication, ambition and drive, we who have chosen Internal Medicine, and possibly through this a subspecialty, have a HRE, the [Boards] Royal College Examinations. We have been evaluated almost daily by the sadly subjective preceptor based assessments, and now we face the fierce, competitive, winner-take-all objective testing through multiple choice questions (MCQs), and for some the equally challenging OSCE, the objective standardized clinical examination. Well we know that in the real life of providing competent, caring and compassionate care as physicians, as internists, that a patient is neither a MCQ or an OSCE. These examinations are to be passed, a process with which we may not necessarily agree. Yet this is the game in which we have thus far invested over half of our youthful lives. So let us know the rules, follow the rules, work with the rules, and succeed. So that we may move on to do what we have been trained to do, do what we may long to do, care for our patients.

The process by which we study for clinical examinations is so different than for the MCQs: not trivia, but an approach to the big picture, with thoughtful and reasoned deduction towards a diagnosis. Not looking for the answer before us, but understanding the subtle aspects of the directed history and focused physical examination, yielding an informed series of hypotheses, a differential diagnosis to direct investigations of the highly sophisticated laboratory and imaging procedures now available to those who can wait, or pay.

This book provides clinically relevant questions of the process of taking a history and performing a physical examination, with sections on Useful background, and where available, evidence-based performance characteristics of the rendering of our clinical skills. Just for fun are included "So you want to be a such-and-such specialist!" to remind us that one if the greatest strengths we can possess to survive in these times, is to smile and even to laugh at ourselves.

Sincerely,

Alan Thomson

Emeritus Distinguished University Professor, University of Alberta

Adjunct Professor, Western University

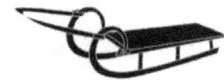

ACKNOWLEDGEMENTS

Patience and patients go hand in hand. So also does the interlocking of young and old, love and justice, equality and fairness. No author can have thoughts transformed into words, no teacher can make ideas become behaviour and wisdom and art, without those special people who turn our minds to the practical – of getting the job done!

Thank you, Naiyana and Duen for translating those terrible scribbles, called my handwriting, into the still magical legibility of the electronic age. Thank you, Sarah, for your creativity and hard work.

My most sincere and heartfelt thanks go to the excellent persons at JP Consulting, and CapStone Academic Publishers. Jessica, you are brilliant, dedicated and caring. Thank you.

When Rebecca, Maxwell, Megan Grace, Henry, Felix, Toby and Grady ask about their Grandad, I will depend on James and Anne, Matthew and Allison, Jessica and Matt, and Benjamin to be understanding and kind. For what I was trying to say and to do was to make my professional life focused on the three C's - competence, caring, and compassion – and to make my very private personal life dedicated to family – to you all.

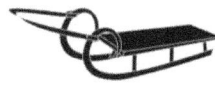

Mastering the Boards: Neurology   A.B.R. Thomson

DEDICATION

To Matante Hélène

In Memory of Uncle Donald

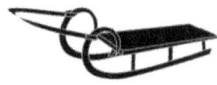

ARE YOU PREPARING FOR EXAMS IN GASTROENTEROLOGY AND HEPATOLOGY?

See the full range of examination preparation and review publications from CAPstone on Amazon.com

Gastroenterology and Hepatology

First Principles of Gastroenterology and Hepatology in Adults and Children - Volume I – Gastroenterology (ISBN: 978-1494345624)

First Principles of Gastroenterology and Hepatology in Adults and Children - Volume II - Hepatology and Paediatrics (ISBN: 978-1494345501)

Medical Mini Review Series in Gastroenterology and Hepatology: Efficient Refresher for the Busy Clinical Gastroenterologist (ISBN: 978-1502472199)

Medical Mini Review Series in Gastroenterology and Hepatology: Efficient Refresher for the Busy Clinical Gastroenterologist (ISBN: 978-1502472199)

Guideline-Based Management in Gastroenterology (ISBN: 978-1515078623)

Guideline-Based Management in Hepatology (ISBN: 978-1502928078)

Endoscopy and Diagnostic Imaging - Part I: Skin, Nail and Mouth Changes in GI Disease; Esophagus; Stomach; Small intestine; Pancreas (ISBN: 978-1477400579)

Endoscopy and Diagnostic Imaging - Part II: Colon and Hepatobiliary (ISBN: 978-1477400654)

Scientific Basis for Clinical Practice in Gastroenterology and Hepatology (ISBN: 978-1475226645)

The Physiology and Pathophysiology of Gastrointestinal and Hepatopancreaticobiliary Disorders: Preparing for Professional Competence. (ISBN: 978-1500298265)

General Internal Medicine

Achieving Excellence in the OSCE - Part One: Cardiology to Nephrology (ISBN: 978-1475283037)

Achieving Excellence in the OSCE - Part Two: Neurology to Rheumatolgy (ISBN: 978-1475276978)

Mastering the Boards and Clinical Examinations in Internal Medicine, Part I: Cardiology, Endocrinology, Gastroenterology, Hepatology and Nephrology (ISBN: 978-1461024842)

Mastering The Boards and Clinical Examinations In Internal Medicine, part II: Neurology, Respirology and Rheumatology (ISBN: 978-1478392736)

Bits and Bytes: Surviving Morning Rounds (ISBN: 978-1478295365)

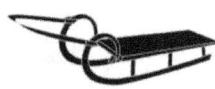

Mastering the Boards: Neurology   A.B.R. Thomson

GENERAL NEUROLOGICAL HISTORY AND PHYSICAL EXAMINATION

➢ Neurologic examination

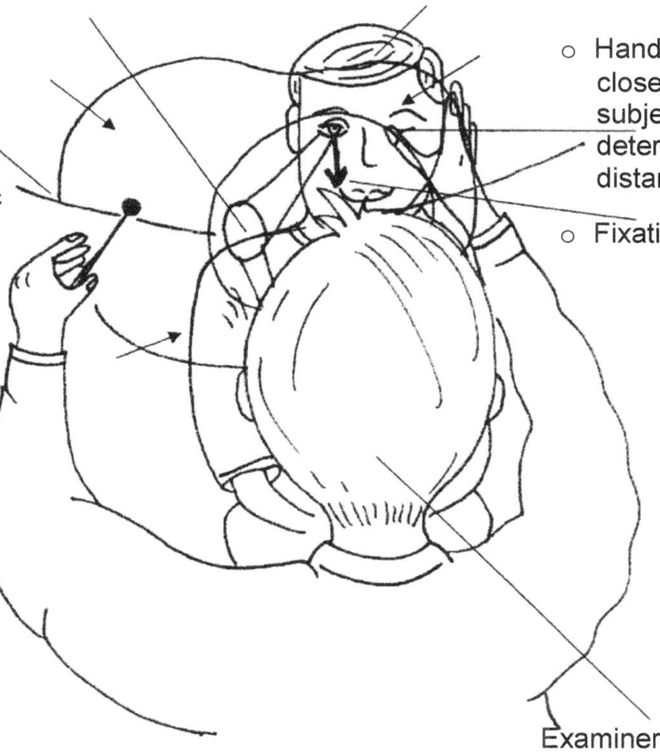

- ○ Subject co-operation may be checked by comparison of blind spots

- ○ Subject

- ○ Hand holds eye closed, steadies subject's head and determines distance

- ○ Bring object in from this position in an arc and on same arc from the nasal side as shown

- ○ Fixation point

Examiner

Adapted from: Mangione S. *Hanley & Belfus* 2000, page 409.

Useful terms

➢ Odds that a given symptom or sign is present in a person without the targeted disorder.

- ○ Sensitivity (SENS)
    - Likelihood of finding a sign or symptom when the target disorder is present (pid – positive in disease)
- ○ Specificity (SPEC)
    - Likelihood of not finding a sign or symptom when the target disorder is not present (nih- negative in health)

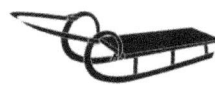

Mastering the Boards: Neurology   A.B.R. Thomson

➢ Odds that a given symptom or sign is present in person with the target disorder (likelihood ratio)

   o LR (>1) = SENS/ 1-SPEC of a present finding in a person with the target disorder

   o LR (<1) of an absent finding in a person with the target disorder = 1-SENS/SPEC

<table>
<tr><td colspan="7" align="center">Probability</td></tr>
<tr><td colspan="3" align="center">Decrease</td><td colspan="4" align="center">Increase</td></tr>
<tr><td>-45%</td><td>-30%</td><td>-15%</td><td>+15%</td><td>+30%</td><td>+45%</td><td></td></tr>
<tr><td>0.1</td><td>0.2</td><td>0.5</td><td>1</td><td>2</td><td>5</td><td>10</td></tr>
</table>

NLR   PLR

➢ Sen N out – <u>Sen</u>sitive test; when negative, rules <u>out</u> disease

➢ Sp P in – <u>Sp</u>ecific test; when positive, rules <u>in</u> disease

Abbreviation: NLR, negative likelihood ratio; PLR, positive likelihood ratio

Source: Filate W, et al. *The Medical Society, Faculty of Medicine, University of Toronto* 2005, page 25.

The Language of Neurology

➢ Agnosia

   o Failure to recognize, whether visual, auditory or tactile; related to receptive dysphagia.

➢ Apraxia

   o Inability to carry out purposive movements in absence of motor paralysis, sensory loss or ataxia; related to expressive dysplagia.

➢ Dysarthria

   o Difficulty with articulation

   o Causes
      - UMN lesion of the cranial nerves – pseudobulbar or bulbar
      - Extra pyramidial disease – monotonous speech
      - Cerebellar disease – altered rhythm of speech
      - Mouth ulcerations
      - Hearing
      - Alcohol intoxication

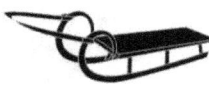

➢ Dysphasia
   o Disorder in use of symbols for communication, whether spoken, heard, written or read.
      - Expressive – Lesion of post. inf. 3rd frontal convolution
      - Receptive – Lesion of post. sup. temporal cortex, an angidengyrus of parietal lobe
   o Dominant higher centre disorder of the use of language (handedness: 94% of right-handed people and 50% of left-handed people have a dominant left hemisphere for language and math)
   o Screening flowing speech "Describe the room"
   o Comprehension "Touch your chin", "Is this your right hand?"
      - Ask patient to name two objects you point to
      - Say "British constitution"
   o Writing
      - Conductive aphasic patients have impaired writing (dysgraphia) while receptive aphasic patients have abnormal content of writing.
      - Patients with dominant frontal lobe lesions may also have dysgraphia.
   o Receptive
      - No understanding for spoken (auditory dysphasia) or written words in absence of deafness or blindness
      - Cannot follow verbal or written commands ('touch your nose, then your chin, then your ear')
      - Cannot repeat "No ifs, ands or buts"
      - Lesion in posterior part of first temporal gyrus of the dominant hemisphere (Wernicke's arga)
   o Expressive dysphasia
      - Motor apraxia – the patient understands spoken or written words, but cannot answer correctly
      - Automatic (recite a list, such as days of the week); emotional speech, maybe preserved
      - Lesion in posterior part of the third frontal gyrus (Broca's area) of the dominant hemisphere
   o Nominal dysphasia
      - Specific objects cannot be named, but person may give a long answer to try to explain what the object is (circumlocution)
      - Lesion of posterior temporoparietal area of dominant hemisphere; encephalopathy; increased intracranial pressure (poor localizing value, and may occur in the recovery phase of receptive, expressive or conductive dysphasia)

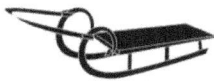

- o Conductive dysphasia
    - - Poor naming, poor repetition of statements, good following of commands
    - - Lesion of fibres joining Wernicke's and Broca's areas, or lesion in arcuate fasciculus

➢ Dysphonia
- o Decreased volume and altered tone of speech.
    - - Damage to larynx or recurrent laryngeal nerve palsy

➢ Echolalia
- o Parrot-like repetition by the subject of statements or acts made before them.

➢ Epilepsy
- o A paroxysmal transitory disturbance of brain function, ceasing spontaneously, with a tendency to recurrence.

➢ Myoclonus
- o A brief shock-like contraction of a number of muscle fibres, a whole muscle or several muscles, either simultaneously or successively.

➢ Perseveration
- o Meaningless repetition of an activity.

➢ Verbigeration
- o Meaningless repetition of words or sentences.

"A lot of things in medicine that make sense, don't work out;

You need data as evidence, not opinion."

Grandad

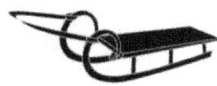

- Neuroanatomy refresher

CNS lesion localization

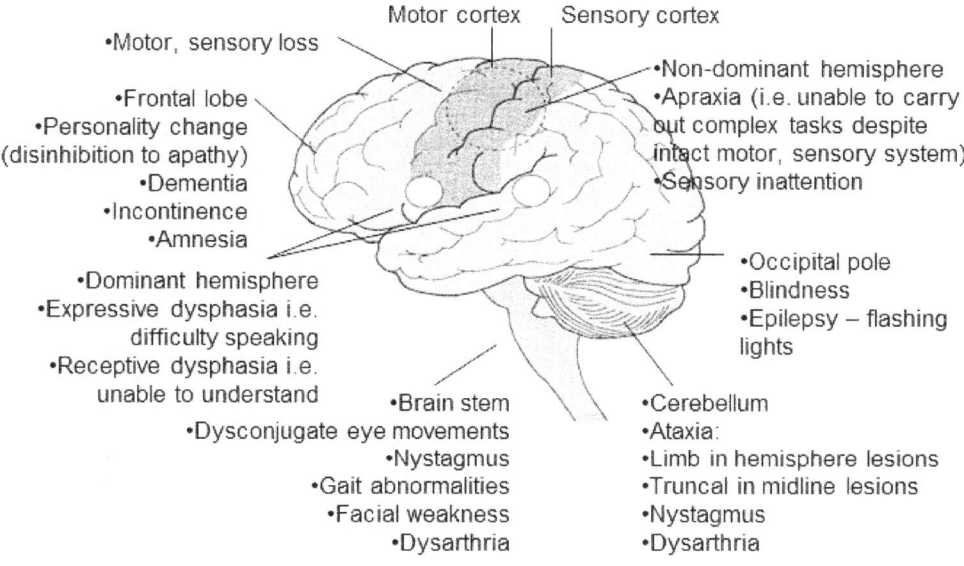

•Motor cortex   Sensory cortex

•Motor, sensory loss

•Frontal lobe
•Personality change
(disinhibition to apathy)
•Dementia
•Incontinence
•Amnesia

•Non-dominant hemisphere
•Apraxia (i.e. unable to carry
out complex tasks despite
intact motor, sensory system)
•Sensory inattention

•Dominant hemisphere
•Expressive dysphasia i.e.
difficulty speaking
•Receptive dysphasia i.e.
unable to understand

•Occipital pole
•Blindness
•Epilepsy – flashing
lights

•Brain stem
•Dysconjugate eye movements
•Nystagmus
•Gait abnormalities
•Facial weakness
•Dysarthria

•Cerebellum
•Ataxia:
•Limb in hemisphere lesions
•Truncal in midline lesions
•Nystagmus
•Dysarthria

Adapted from: Davey P. *Wiley-Blackwell* 2006, page 88.

- Spinal cord section

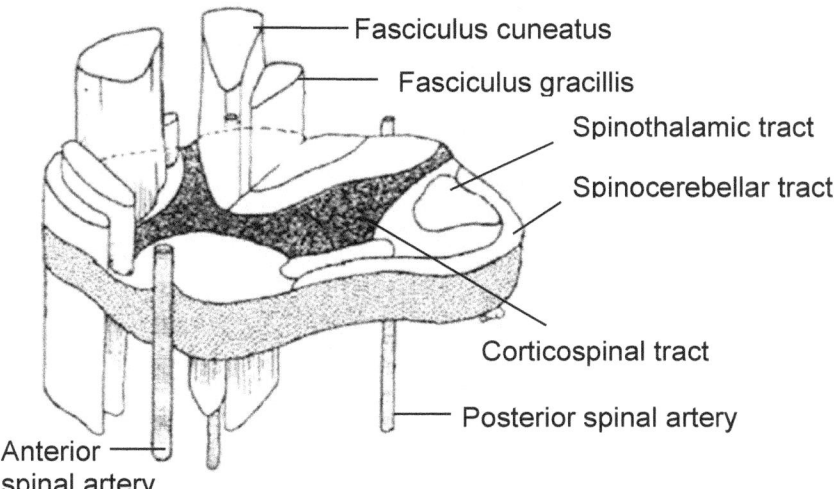

Fasciculus cuneatus

Fasciculus gracillis

Spinothalamic tract

Spinocerebellar tract

Corticospinal tract

Posterior spinal artery

Anterior
spinal artery

Adapted from: Filate W., et al. *The Medical Society, Faculty of Medicine,
University of Toronto* 2005, page 155.

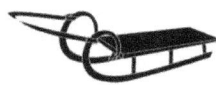

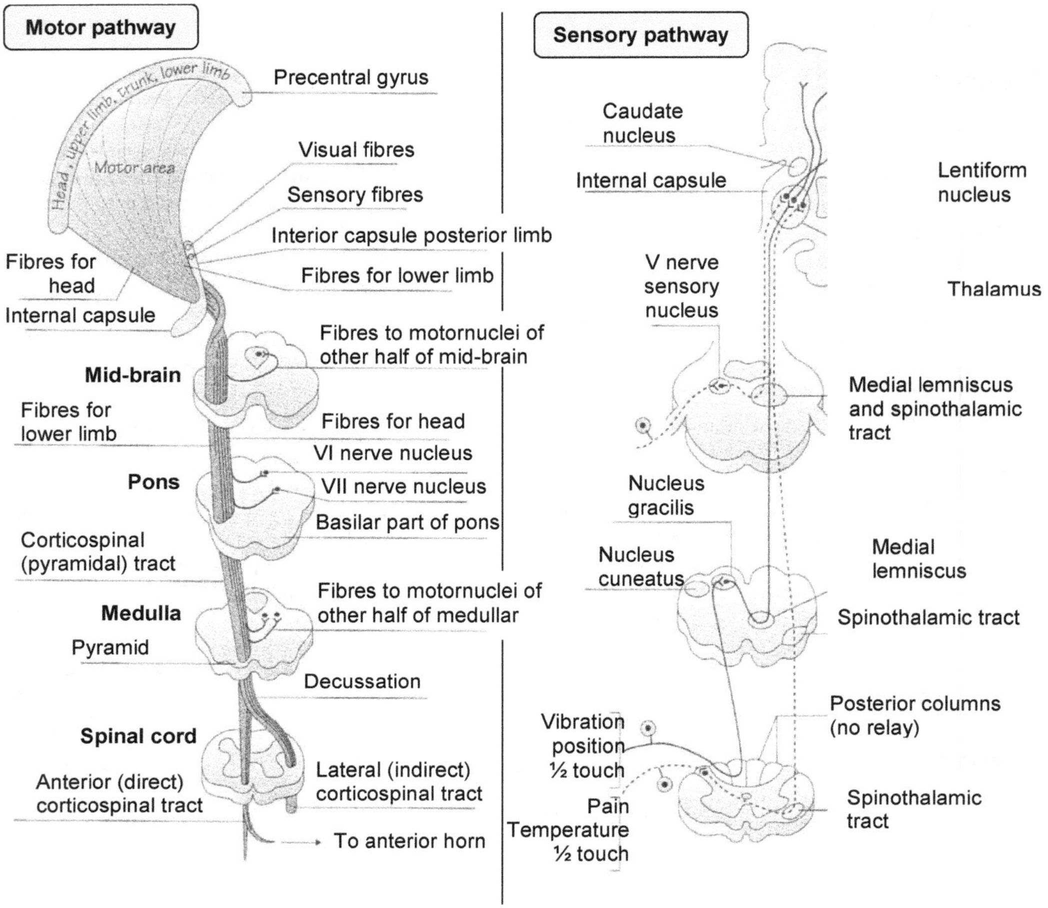

Motor pathway

Precentral gyrus

Head, upper limb, trunk, lower limb

Motor area

Visual fibres

Sensory fibres

Interior capsule posterior limb

Fibres for head

Fibres for lower limb

Internal capsule

Mid-brain

Fibres to motornuclei of other half of mid-brain

Fibres for lower limb

Fibres for head

VI nerve nucleus

Pons

VII nerve nucleus

Basilar part of pons

Corticospinal (pyramidal) tract

Medulla

Fibres to motornuclei of other half of medullar

Pyramid

Decussation

Spinal cord

Anterior (direct) corticospinal tract

Lateral (indirect) corticospinal tract

→ To anterior horn

Sensory pathway

Caudate nucleus

Internal capsule

Lentiform nucleus

V nerve sensory nucleus

Thalamus

Medial lemniscus and spinothalamic tract

Nucleus gracilis

Nucleus cuneatus

Medial lemniscus

Spinothalamic tract

Vibration position ½ touch

Posterior columns (no relay)

Pain Temperature ½ touch

Spinothalamic tract

Adapted from: Davey P. *Wiley-Blackwell* 2006, page 88.

"The best way to predict the future is to create it."
Unknown

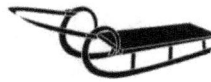

Mastering the Boards: Neurology   A.B.R. Thomson

Useful background: Muscle weakness may be caused by disorders at several sites of the nervous system:

- o UMN
- o LMN
- o Cerebellum
- o Extrapyramidal tracts
- o Muscle diseases
- o Malingering
- o Sensory disturbance (the patient may describe their disability as "weakness").

- Perform a focused physical examination of the nervous system to determine the site of the disorder causing the muscle weakness, altered tone as well as deep tendon reflexes.

	LMN*	UMN
o Weakness	+	+
o Wasting	+	-
o Fasciculations	+	-
o Tone	↓	↑ ("clasp knife" rigidity)
o Affected muscle groups	Involves only a few muscles	Affects muscles of entire limb
o Reflexes deep	↓ / Absent	↑
o Superficial	↓	↓
o Extensor plantars	-	+ (up-going toe)
o Clonus	-	+

*Caused by involvement of motor pathway anywhere from anterior horn cell to nucleus (unlikely to be in spinal cord).

➤ Distinguish the hypotonicity of a LMN lesion from other lesion sites
  - o Cerebellar
  - o Posterior column
  - o Sensory nerve tract
  - o Transient after acute lesions of hemispheres or spinal cord

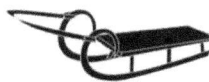

➤ Hypertonicity of an UMN lesion for extrapyramidal lesions

➤ ↓ deep tendon reflexes (DTR) of a LMN lesion from
  o A lesion of first sensory neurons (posterior nerve root or posterior column)
  o Decreased reflexes in absence of wasting, suggests a peripheral lesion

➤ ↑ DTR of an UMN lesion from
  o Pain
  o Emotion
  o Anxiety
  o Hysteria

➤ LMN
  o Weakness
  o Wasting
  o Fasciculation
  o Decreased tone
  o Decreased or absent reflexes (Reflexes present until late in the course of the muscle disease)
  o LMN wasting involves only a few muscles, whereas disuse affects muscles of an entire limb

➤ UMN
  o Weakness
  o Increased tone clasp knife rigidity
  o Extensor plantars
  o Sustained true clonus
  o Increased deep tendon reflexes
  o Decreased superficial reflexes

Localizing Signs in UMN Weakness

Anatomic location	Associated finding
➤ Cerebral hemisphere	o Seizures o Hemianopia o Aphasia (right hemiparesis) o Inattention to left body, apraxia (left hemiparesis) o Cortical sensory loss* o Hyperactive jaw jerk

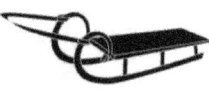

Anatomic Location	Associated Finding
➢ Brainstem	○ Crossed motor findings unilateral cranial nerve palsy opposite the side of limb weakness) ○ Contralateral third nerve palsy (midbrain) ○ Contralateral sixth nerve palsy (pons) ○ Sensory loss on contralateral face
➢ Spinal cord	○ No sensory or motor findings in face ○ Specific sensory level ○ Pain and temperature sensory loss on contralateral arm and leg ○ Additional LMN findings (e.g., atrophy, fasciculations)

Printed with permission: McGee SR. *Saunders/Elsevier* 2007, page 720.

➢ Muscle stretch reflex scale

Grade	Finding
0	Reflex absent
1	Reflex small, less than normal; includes a trace response or a response brought out only with reinforcement
2	Reflex in lower half of normal range
3	Reflex in upper half of normal range
4	Reflex enhanced, more than normal; includes clonus if present, which optionally can be noted in an added verbal description of the reflex

Source: McGee SR. *Saunders/Elsevier* 2007, Table 59-2, page 757.

- Perform a focused physical examination of the nervous system.
  - ○ Handedness and conscious level
  - ○ Neck stiffness and Kernig sign
  - ○ Cranial nerves

I	Smell
II	Visual acuity and fields Fundoscopy
III, IV, VI	Pupils and eye movements
V	Corneal reflexes Facial sensation
VII	Facial muscles
VIII	Hearing
IX X	Palate and gag
XI	Trapezius and sternomastoids
XII	Tongue

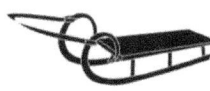

- o Upper limbs
- o Lower limbs
  - – Motor system (Tone, power, reflexes)
  - – Co-ordination
  - – Sensation
- o Saddle region
- o Back
- o Gait

Adapted from: Talley NJ, et al. *Maclennan & Petty Pty Limited* 2003, page 441.

Useful background: Take a neurological history (mnemonic "**SHOVE**")

- o **S**yncope, speech defect, swallowing difficulty
- o **H**eadache
- o **O**cular disturbances; diplopia, field defects
- o **V**ertigo
- o **E**pilepsy; seizures
- o History pertaining to motor and sensory components of the cranial nerves and limbs, e.g. pain paraesthesia, weakness, inco-ordination

Source: Baliga RR. *Saunders/Elsevier* 2007, page 107.

Neurological Examination

- ➤ Assessing level of mental status
  - o Alertness
  - o Lethargy
  - o Consciousness

- ➤ Orientation
  - o Time
  - o Place
  - o Person
  - o Memory
  - o Stuper
  - o Coma
  - o Language/speech

- ➤ Localization of Neurologic Disorders
  - o Level
    - – Cerebral hemisphere
    - – Cerebellum
    - – Brainstem
    - – Spinal cord
    - – Nerve root
    - – Peripheral nerve
    - – Neuromuscular junction
    - – Muscle
  - o Extent
    - – Focal
    - – Diffuse

Source: Mangione S. *Hanley & Belfus* 2000.

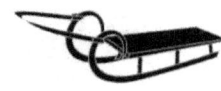

Useful background: Directed history for disorders of the central (CNS) and peripheral nervous system (PNS) (e.g. the Neurological system).

➢ **Where** is the lesion and **what** is the lesion? (example - loss of consciousness [LOC]/[syncope vs.. seizure])
  ○ Complete vs.. partial
  ○ Duration
  ○ Changes in body position (e.g., loss of balance, fetal position, prone)
  ○ Associated symptoms (e.g., tongue biting, body movements, incontinence)
  ○ Preceding symptoms (e.g., light-headedness)
  ○ Post attack symptoms (e.g., confusion, sleepiness)
  ○ Previous diagnosis of systemic disorders (e.g., cardiovascular problems)
  ○ Current medications
  ○ Collateral/corollary information (e.g., bystanders)

➢ Course
  ○ Onset (e.g., thunderclap)
  ○ Pattern (e.g., worse in the morning=increased ICP)
  ○ Differences from previous headaches (type/pattern)
  ○ Associated symptoms (e.g., nausea and/or vomiting, neck stiffness)
  ○ Preceding symptoms/aura
  ○ Systemic conditions (e.g., infections)
  ○ Current medications/addictions

Abbreviations: CNS, central nervous system; LOC, loss of consciousness; PNS, peripheral nervous system

Source: Filate W., et al. *The Medical Society, Faculty of Medicine, University of Toronto* 2005, Table 2, page 156 to 159; and Baliga RR. *Saunders/Elsevier* 2007, page 107.

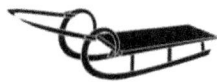

Mastering the Boards: Neurology   A.B.R. Thomson

CEREBRAL CORTEX

Position of the lobes and the motor and sensory areas

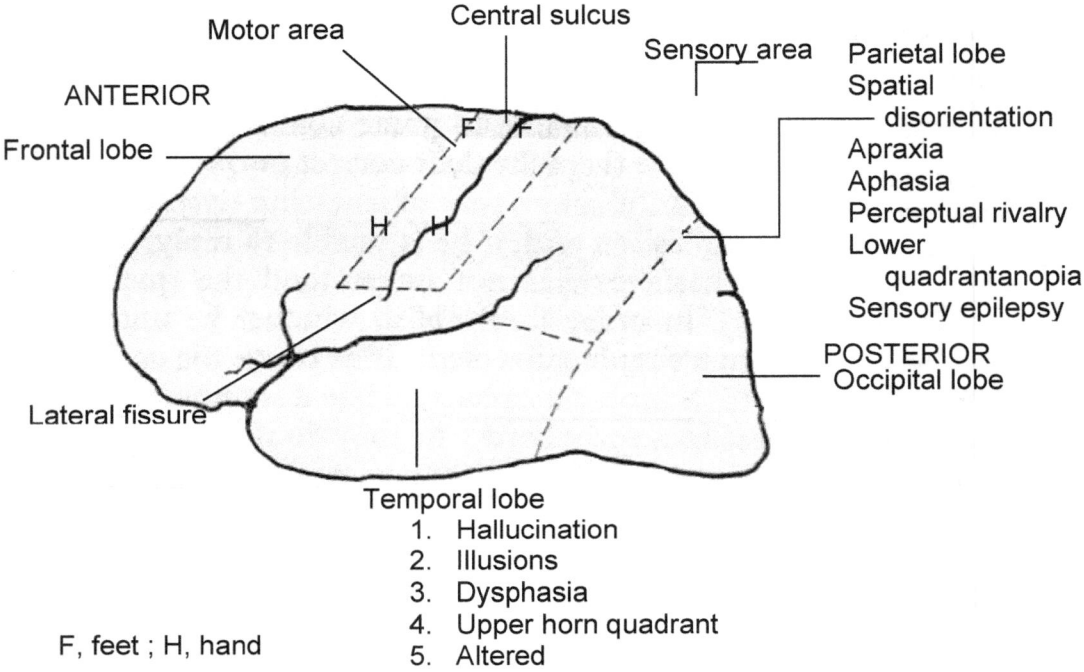

F, feet ; H, hand

Adapted from: Davey P. *Wiley-Blackwell* 2006.

- Take a directed history and perform a focused physical examination for disease of the cerebral hemispheres.

    o Mental status

    o Cortex
        - Seizures

    o Speech/language
        - E.g.,aphasia

    o Eyes
        - Visual field defects

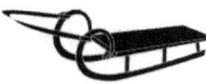

- Motor
  - Hemiparesis
  - Involuntary movements
    - Dystonia
    - Choria
    - Hemiballismus
- Sensory
  - Hemianesthesia

- Precentral gyrus
  - Anterior to central sulcus
  - Motor function
  - The top of the motor cortex (precentral gyrus) is involved with movements of the feet, whereas the bottm of the motor cortex is involved with movement of the face.

- Postcentral gyrus
  - Posterior to central sulcus
  - Sensory function
  - Just as with the presentral gyrus, with the post central gyrus, the top of the sensory cortex (post central gyrus) is involved with feet, and the bottom is involved with the face.

- Frontal lobe
  - Forethought
  - Consequences
  - Apathy
  - Dementia
  - Group reflex
  - Ataxia
  - Akinesia
  - Aspasia

- Motor cortex
  - UMN hemiplegia
  - Jacksonian-epilepsy
  - Expressive dysphasia

- Parietal lobe
  - Spatial disorientation
  - Apraxia
  - Agonesia
  - Perceptual
  - Receptive dysphasia
  - Homonynous hemianopin
  - Jacksonian sensory epilepsy

- Temporal lobe
  - Hallucinations
  - Illusions
  - Receptive dysphagia
  - Altered - memory, concentration, behaviour
  - Upper homonymous quadrant anopia

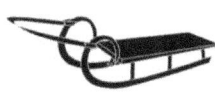

- Take a directed history to detect disease of the frontal, parietal or temporal lobe, or the motor cortex.

Frontal Lobe	Motor Cortex	Parietal Lobe	Temporal Lobe
o Forethought o Consequences o Apathy o Dementia o Grasp reflex o Ataxia o Akinesia o Aspasia	– UMN hemiplegia – Jacksonian epilepsy – Expressive dysphasia	▪ Spatial disorientation ▪ Aproxia ▪ Agnesia ▪ Perceptual rivalry ▪ Receptive dysphasia ▪ Homonymous hemianopia ▪ Jacksonian sensory epilepsy	– Hallucinations – Illusions – Receptive dysphasia – Altered memory, coma – Upper temoral quadrantanopia

Abbreviation: UMN, upper motor neuron
Adapted from: Talley NJ, et al. *Maclennan & Petty Pty Limited* 2003, Table 10.4, page 353.

- Perform a focused physical examination of the **motor cortex**.
  - o Expressive dysphasia
  - o Hemiplegia focal
  - o Jacksonian focal epilepsy
  - o Agnosia (sensory, receptive)
    - – Failure to recognize
      - ▪ Visual
      - ▪ Auditory
      - ▪ Tactile
  - o Apraxia (motor, expressive)
    - – Failure to carry out proposeful movements in the absence of motor, sensory

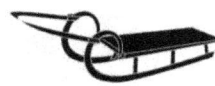

- Perform a focused physical examination for a **disorder of the frontal lobe cortex**.
  - o Intellectual function
    - – Dementia
    - – Indifference
    - – Incontinence
    - – Lack of forethought
    - – Failure to anticipate/recognize consequence of behaviour

  - o Precentral motor cortex
    - – Hemiplegia
    - – Jacksonian focal epilepsy
    - – Expressive dysphasia (only if the frontal lobe of the dominant hemisphere is affected)
    - – "grasp" reflex of limbs of the opposite side of the body

  - o Compression of olfactory tracts
    - – Anosmia

  - o Compression of optic nerves
    - – Optic atrophy of affected side
    - – Papiledema of opposite side

THIS IS FOR THE NEUROLOGY RESIDENT

In the context of the parietal lobe, give the meaning of Gerstmann syndrome.
  - o Confusion of the right and left side of the body
  - o Lack of ability to identify figures
  - o Acalculia

- Perform a focused physical examination for a disorder of the cortex of the parietal lobe.

  - o Eyes
    - – Lower homonymous quadrantanopia

  - o Post-central gyrus
    - – Cortical sensory loss to the same side of the body
    - – Tests of cortical sensory loss:
      - ▪ Stereognosis
      - ▪ Two point discrimination
      - ▪ Localization of stimulus to the correct part of the body
      - ▪ Correct recognition of letters or figures traced out on the skin

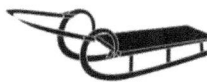

- o Dominant lobe, parietal lobe cortex
  - Sensory aphasia
  - Acalculia
  - Alexia
  - Agraphia

- o Non-dominant lobe
  - Inattention
  - Inability to recognize the left half of the body

- o Variation of signs from one day to another

- Perform a focused physical examination for a disorder of the **temporal lobe**.

  - o Eyes
    - Upper homonymous quadrant anopia

  - o Hallucinations
    - Taste and smell
    - Auditory (associated with temporal lobe epilepsy)
    - Dazed look

  - o Illusions
    - Excessive number of sensations of deja-vu phenomenon

  - o Receptive dysphasia

  - o Altered memory, consciousness, memory

- Take a directed history and perform a focused physical examination to determine the presence of disease of the parietal, temporal, frontal and occipital lobes.

- ❖ Parietal lobe
  - o Dysphasia (dominant)
  - o Dominant parietal lobe signs (Gerstmann syndrome)
    - Acalculia
    - Agraphia
    - Left – right disorientation
    - Finger gnosia
    - Sensory and visual inattention
    - Construction and dressing apraxia
    - Spatial neglect and inattention and non-dominant parietal lobe signs
  - o Non-dominant parietal lobe signs
    - Lower quadrantic hemianopia
    - Asterognosis

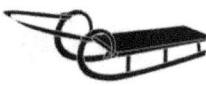

Mastering the Boards: Neurology   A.B.R. Thomson

❖ Temporal lobe
  o Memory loss
  o Upper quadrantic hemianopia
  o Dysphasia (receptive if dominant lobe)
  o Seizures

❖ Frontal lobe
  o Personality change
  o Primitive reflexes (e.g., grasp)
  o Anosmia
  o Optic nerve compression (optic atrophy)
  o Gait apraxia
  o Leg weakness (parasagittal)
  o Loss of micturition control
  o Dysphasia (expressive)
  o Seizures

❖ Occipital lobe
  o Homonymous hemianopia
  o Alexia
  o Seizures (flashing light aura)

Adapted from: Talley NJ, et al. *Maclennan & Petty Pty Limited* 2003, page 353.

Apraxia

➤ Definition
  o "..... the inability to perform a previously learned skilled motor task despite
    – Intact motor and sensory systems
    – Clear comprehension, and
    – Full co-operation

  o Ideomotor apraxia "....a subtype of apraxia ...... in which a patient
    has a clear concept of the proposed action but cannot execute it"
    (Source: MKSAP 16 2012, Neurology, page 132)

➤ Cause
  o A lesion of the dominant parietal lobe

➤ Implication
  o Defining feature
  o Presenting feature
    Parkinson-plus disease
    Corticobasal degeneration

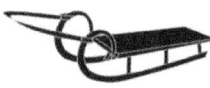

SEIZURES AND EPILEPSY

➢ Definition

- o Paroxysmal cerebral dysfunction due to sudden abnormal electrical discharge
- o Epilepsy – any brain disorder characterized by ≥ 2 unprovided seizures
- o Status epilepticas – continuous seizure for ≥ 30 mins
- o Pseudoseizure – on-off asymchronous movement of arms or legs, lasting 10-30 min

➢ Terms

- o Seizure
  - Abnormal, excessive or synchronous neuronal activity in cerebral cortex
  - Often generalized, synchronized involvement of cortical neurons
  - Less often focal involvement of discharge from cortical neurons
- o Epilepsy syndromes
  - ≥ 2 seizures experienced
  - Often present as partial (focal) seizures in adults

Seizure	Electrical discharge	Number of modalities	Responsive	Loss of consciousness
o Simple partial	Focal / localized site	1	/	No
o Complex partial		Automatism	No	No
o Generalized (primary)	Simultaneous discharge	Tonic (stiffening) Clonic (jerking) Myotonic (brief rapid jerking)		/

- o Secondary-focal discharge spreading to entire cerebral cortex

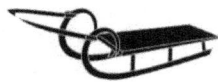

- ➤ Investigation
  - ○ EEG (electroencephalogram)
  - ○ MA/brain/CT head
  - ○ CSF
    - – Fever
    - – Postictal confusion
    - – Severe headache

- ➤ Treatment
- • Pharmaceutical
  - ○ Rationale for starting anticonvulsant therapy after unprovoked 2 seizures
  - ○ Principles
    - – One agent

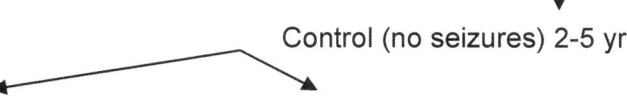

        dose until actienring;   cortisol, adverse effects
            (AEs)
                                        ↓
                                    ▼ failure of clinical
        response

    - – Stop first drug, start second (new) drug, ↑ dose with control, AEs

                        ↓

    Proceed until control of clinical response

                        ↓

    Control (no seizures) 2-5 yr

Stop maintenance   Do **not** stop maintenance
  - ○ Juvenile myoclonic epilepsy
  - ○ Difficult to achieve remission (frequent seizures before achieving remission)
  - ○ Mentally challenged
  - ○ Abnormal neurological examination
  - ○ Abnormal ECG before/during withdrawal of Rx

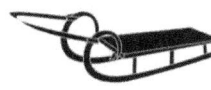

Δ   Simple/complex partial seizures- carbamozepine or lamotrigene valpac acid or lamotrigine

Δ   Primary generalized (tonic-clonic seizures or myelonic)

- o Unprovoked seizures
  - – Risk of recurrence
    - ▪ 50%
    - ▪ 80%

➢ Terminology

Epilepsy - localized (or partial) seizures
- Simple: normal conscious level
- Complex: altered conscious level

Focal motor seizures
= Jacksonian seizures

- Jerking of affected muscle
- Neighbouring muscle groups jerk as electrical discharge spreads ('marches') over motor cortex
- Post-ictal loss of motor function ('paralysis') for a few hours/day ('Todd's paresis)

Temporal lobe seizures
Often relate to structural abnormality e.g scarring from (prolonged) childhood febrile convulsions

Aura
- Over – under-familiarity with surroundings (déjà vu and jamals vu)
- Unpleasant taste or smell
- Epigastric discomfort

Seizure
- Facial grimacing
- Complex motor actions e.g undressing
- Bizarre behaviour

Post-ictal
- Usually rapid recovery
- Amnesia of seizure events

Typical epileptic seizure

Aura ⟶
Usually < 1 min
Depends on site

Seizure ⟶
Lasts < few minutes
Rarely continues for prolonged
Periods = status epilepticus

Post seizure phenomena
= post ictal
If generalized → very sleepy < few hours
If focal → temporary loss of function

Focal sensory seizures
- Unpleasant tingling 'marching' over body in < few seconds
- Differential diagnosis includes migraine sensory symptoms here 'march' over body in 10-15 min

Occipital seizures
- Produce 'flashing' lights
- Can produce complex distortion of vision

Generalized seizures
- Often involve diencephalic structures
- Typical childhood absences ('petit mal') - Occur in childhood, very rare to continue in adulthood, common
- Myoclonic epilepsy
- Akinetic epilepsy → sudden complete loss of postural tone → sudden collapse. Rare.
- Grand mal seizures (see text)

Adapted from: Davey P. *Wiley-Blackwell* 2006, page 327.

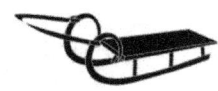

> **Clinical Features of Seizures**
>   o Simple partial seizures
>   – Motor, sensory, autonomic or cognitive/perceptual features
>   – No impairment of awareness
>   – Usually brief (<60 seconds)
>
>   o Complex partial seizures
>   – Focally originating seizures characterized by impaired awareness and a blank stare
>   – May begin with an aura (simple partial seizure), but may also have impaired awareness from onset
>   – Usual duration of 1-2 minutes
>   – Frequently accompanied by motor automatisms, such as lip smacking, chewing movements or fumbling/picking hand movements
>   – Brief postictal confusion or fatigue is common
>   – Commonly misdiagnosed as absence seizures, a much less common seizure type (please see below)
>
>   o Absence ("petit mal")
>   – Primarily generalized seizure type
>   – Usually last only 10-15 seconds
>   – Recur daily (sometimes > 100 times per day) in the untreated patient
>   – No warning signs or postictal confusion
>   – Onset in childhood or adolescence (almost never *begin* in adulthood)
>   – Do not confuse with complex partial seizures (please see above)
>
>   o Primarily or secondarily generalized tonic-clonic ("grand mal"):
>   – Fairly uniform sequence of motor feature (tonic and clonic phases)
>   – Impaired consciousness
>   – Duration of 1-2 minutes
>   – Postictal stupor, confusion and headache
>   – A careful history may reveal a partial seizure, e.g.,simple partial or complex partial, that secondarily evolves to a generalized tonic-clonic seizure
>
>   o Atonic seizures
>   – Abrupt loss of consciousness and muscle tone
>   – No other motor features
>   – Return to awareness within seconds
>   – Occur as part of a clinical scenario in patients with childhood onset epilepsy, significant intellectual disability and other seizure types
>   – Almost never occur in otherwise intellectually and physically normal adults

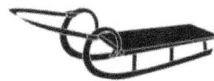

- o Myoclonic seizures
  - A generalized seizure type consisting of brief, bilateral "shock-like" jerks
  - Multifocal asynchronous myoclonic jerks most commonly occur in the setting of a metabolic encephalopathy
- o Consider whether the clinical features suggest one of the entities commonly mistaken for epileptic seizures, such as syncope or psychogenic nonepileptic seizures

Reproduced with permission: Therapeutics Choices. Sixth Edition. Ottawa, Canada: *Canadian Pharmacist Association* 2012, page 292-293.

- In the context of the frontal lobe of the cerebral cortex, give the meaning of the Foster Kennedy syndrome.
  - o Optic atrophy on the side of compression of the optic nerve by the frontal lobe, and papilledema of the opposite eye resulting from increased intracranial pressure.

- Take a directed history and perform a focused physical examination to determine the type of a seizure.

Grey J, Therapeutic Choices. 6th Edition, *Canadian Pharmacists Association*: Otttawa, ON, 2011, page 292-293.

- Give the clinical characteristics of the 3 major types of seizure, and their treatment.

Type	Level of Consciousness at Beginning	Postictal	Neurologic Modality	Region of Body	Rx
o Partial					
– Simple	Conscious	-	Single	Single	
– Complex	Unresponsive, or starting	Confusion	Automatism	-	Lamotrigine, or carbama-zepine
o Primary generalized	Unconscious	Confusion	Tonic-clonic myoclonic	Whole body	Lamotrigine, or Valproic acid

- – Status epilepticus (SE)
  - Continuous seizure ≥ 30 min
    - MR (mortality rate), 20%
  - Rx
    - IV lorazapam, then phenytoin

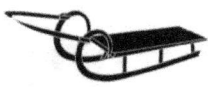

Mastering the Boards: Neurology   A.B.R. Thomson

Course	Risk of Recurrence
After 1 seizure	~ 50%
2 seizure	~ 85%

Clinical Alert

Status epilepticus may be nonconvulsive i.e., in the patient with coma but no clinical evidence of seizure activity, perform urgent EEG to exclude nonconvulsive status epilepticus.

Pearls and Gems

- o Use anti-convulsant therapy for epilepsy, i.e., ≥ 2 seizures

- o Use monotherapy; if one drug doesn't work, stop and start another

- o In pregnancy
  - Do not stop anti-convulsant therapy
  - Avoid valproic acid
  - Use lowest possible dose of other drug

➢ Causes

- o Idiopathic

- o Congentital   – Cerebral malformation
  - Lipidoses (Tay-Sachs disease)

- o Trauma   – Birth injury
  - Scar
  - Tumour

- o Infection   – Abscess
  - Cysticercosis
  - Encephalitis
  - GPI
  - Meningitis
  - Pyrexia (especially in children)

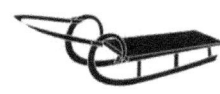

- o Metabolic
  - – Alkalosis
  - – Anoxia
  - – Hepatic coma
  - – Hypocalcemia
  - – Hypoglycemia
  - – Uremia
  - – Water intoxication

- o Drugs/toxins
  - – Barbiturate withdrawal
  - – Cocaine
  - – Ether
  - – Lead poisoning
  - – Nikethamide

- o Tumour
- o Vascular
  - – CVA
  - – Hypertension

- o Degenerative
  - – Presenile dementias

Adapted from: Burton JL. *Churchill Livingstone* 1971, page 70.

➢ Clinical

• Take a directed history for seizures.

  - o Age (at onset)
    - – Onset, offset, duration, fluctuation

  - o Type – "phase out", myoclonic, tonic, tonic clonk, atonic ("drop seizures"), partial (affecting only a part of the brain rather than a generalized seizure affecting all the brain; partial seizures may include OR not include awareness of events)
    - – Simple partial seizures
      - ▪ Motor, sensory or psychomotor phenomena without loss of consciousness
      - ▪ Seizures can begin in one part of the body and spread to other parts
    - – Complex partial seizures
      - ▪ May be preceded by an aura (sensory or psychic manifestations that represent seizure onset)
      - ▪ Staring, performing of automatic purposeless movements, uttering of unintelligible sounds, resisting aid
      - ▪ Motor, sensory or psychomotor phenomena
      - ▪ Post-ictal confusion

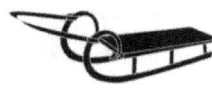

- Tonic-clonic seizures (formerly known as grand-mal)
  - Tonic phase – stiffening of limbs
  - Clonic phase – jerking of limbs
  - Respiration may decrease during tonic phase but usually returns during clonic phase, although it may be irregular
  - Incontinence may occur
  - Post-ictal confusion
- Atonic seizures
  - Brief, primarily generalized seizures in children
  - Complete loss of muscle tone, resulting in falling or pitching to the ground
  - Risk of serious trauma, particularly head injury
- Absence seizures
  - Brief, primarily generalized attacks manifested by a 10 to 30-second loss of consciousness
  - Eyelid flutterings at a rate of 3 Hz
  - No loss of axial muscle tone
  - No falling or convulsing
  - No post-ictal symptoms
- Status epilepticus – a medical emergency!
  - Repeated seizures with no intervening periods of normal neurologic function
  - Generalized convulsive status epilepticus may be fatal
  - With complex partial or absence seizures, an EEG may be needed to diagnose seizure activity

- o Jacksonian epilepsy
  - Clonic movements
  - Always start at same site
  - Always show same order of speed
  - Early on, may be followed by transient paralysis
  - Later on, may be followed by later paralysis
  - Sometimes, no causative lesion is found

- o Generalized seizures
  - Generalized tonic-clonic seizures.
  - Petit mal and atypical absences
  - Myoclonus
  - Akinetic seizures. Petit mal describes only 3 Hz seizures, rather than clinically similar absence attacks which are partial seizures

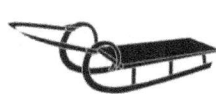

- o Partial or focal seizures (a partial seizure is epileptic activity confined to one area of cortex with a recognizable clinical patter)
  - Simple partial seizures (no impairment of consciousness)
  - Jacksonian epilepsy: it is a simple partial seizure which usually originates in one portion of the prefrontal motor cortex so that fits begin in one part of the body (e.g., thumb) and then proceed to involve that side of the body and then the whole body.
  - It suggests a space-occupying lesion
  - Complex partial seizures
  - Partial seizures evolving to tonic-clonic

- o Todd paralysis
  - Paresis of a limb or hemiplegia occurring after an epileptic attack, which may last up to 3 days.
- o No precipitating factor identified (e.g.,sleep deprivation, alcohol use)
- o Associations – aura, salivation, tongue biting, incontinence, chewing, lip smacking, Jacksonian march, onset during sleep or with fever
- o Other factors
  - Family history of seizures (in first degree relative)
  - History of febrile seizures or birth trauma
  - Postictal Todd paralysis
- o Abnormal electroencephalogram (spikes, or non-specific pattern)
- o Abnormal imaging study
- o Causes
  - Congenital – malformations – birth injury
  - Ideopathic
  - Trauma
  - Tumour
  - Infection
    - Meningitits
    - Encephalitis
    - Abscess
    - Syphilis
    - Cysticercosis
  - Vascular
    - CVA
    - NTN
    - Hypertermia, especially in children
    - Hypthermia
  - Degeneration – presenile dementia

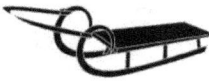

- Metabolic*
  - Anoxia
  - Hypoglycemia
  - Hypocalcemia
  - Renal failure
  - Hyponatremia
  - Alkalosis
  - Motor intoxication
- Drugs
  - Lead
  - Cocaine
  - Barbiturate, alcohol withdrawal

o Abnormal neurologic examination- CVA, trauma, meningism

*Metabolic causes may cause delirium.

Abbreviation: CVA, cerebral vascular accident; NTN

Adapted from: Jugovic PJ, et al. *Saunders/ Elsevier* 2004, page 84; Filate W, et al. *The Medical Society, Faculty of Medicine, University of Toronto* 2005, page 173; Burton JL. *Churchill Livingstone* 1971, page 70; Baliga RR. *Saunders/Elsevier* 2007, page 241.

Status Epilepticus (SE)

➢ Definition
  o "Convulsive SE was traditionally defined as recurrent primarily or secondarily generalized tonic-clonic seizures
    - Lasting > 30 minutes, or
    - Intermittent seizures lasting > 30 minutes, without return to baseline consciousness between events".
  o "….almost all, isolated tonic-clonic seizure last < 2 minutes"
  o "tonic-clonic seizure lasting > 5 minutes most likely suggests impending SE and should be treated aggressively"
  o "any seizure type CMN evolve to non-convulsive SE"
  o "non-convulsive SE should be considered in any patient with unexplained coma"
  o "brain injury begins at 30-45 minutes after onset of SE"

(Moeller JJ, et al. Chapter 24. In: Therapeutic Choices. Grey J, Ed. 6th Edition, *Canadian Pharmacists Association*: Otttawa, ON, 2011, page 298).

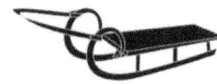

➤ Treatment

- Give the non-pharmaceutical therapy of epilepsy.
  - Stimulator for the vagus nerve
  - Surgical resection of mesial temporal lobe sclerotic lesion

Generalized Convulsive Status Epilepticus

➤ Definition: "........ continuous or repetitive seizure activity lasting longer than 30 minutes" (Source: MKSAP 16 2012, Neurology, page 22)
  - However,
    - Only person who has a seizure for > 5 min should have treatment initiated as if they has status epilepticus (i.e., do not wait 30 min to achieve the above definition)

➤ Cause
  - ½ have a history of previous seizure
  - ½ have no previous history, and may have status epilepticus because of
    - Hypoxic brain injury
    - Alcohol/drug intoxication/withdrawal
    - Metabolic disorders
    - Cerebrovascular disease
    - Suboptimal AED levels
  - Note:
    - Mortality rate 20% overall; from anoxic brain injury, ~ 70%

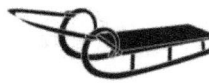

➢ Treatment
  o ABCs plus thiamine 100 mg IV plus 50 mL 50% dextrose IV, where indicated
  o Lorazepam
    - 2 mg IV q 5 min for up to 5 doses (avoid respiratory depression)
    - 2-4 mg IM q 5 min for up to 10 mg
    - Diazepam 20 mg PP, 1 dose, plus
    - Fosphenytoin IV or IM 18-20 PE/kg at 150 PE/min, or
    - Phenytoin 18-20 mg/kg IV, given at 50 mg per min, or
    - Valproate 30 mg / kg IV, given at 3 mg / kg per min, if convulsions continue beyond 20 to 60 min, either
  o Intubate plus IV anesthesia, and add
    - Valproate 30 mg/kg IV, given 3 mg/kg per min, or
    - Phenobarbital 20 mg/kg IV, given at 60 mg/min

Abbreviation: PE, phenytoin equivalent

  o Special considerations

- Phenytoin	▪	Take great care IV does not go interstitial, since extravasation may cause necrosis of skin
- Propofol	▪	High-dose for long intervals → Rhabdomyolysis plus multiorgan failure
- Valproic acid	▪	Avoid in woman of childbearing potential
	▪	Consider using in place of fosphenytoin or phenytoin for those patients were previously diagnosed as having idiopathic generalized epilepsy
- Critically ill patients (ICU)	▪	ICU patients may have Non-convulsive seizure Non-convulsive status epilepticus
	▪	Comatose ICU patients EEG shows seizures

EEG		
1 hr	12-24 hr	48 hr
50%	80%	96%

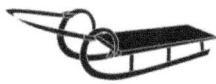

➤ Non-ICU patients, non-convulsive status epilepticus (SE)

Types	Past history of epilepsy
- Absence SE	▪ Generalized
- Complex partial	▪ Focal
- De novo absence SE ("spike-wave stupor")	▪ None (may occur in setting of benzodiazepine withdrawal)

- o Diagnosis of non-convulsive SE in / out of ICU
  - EEG plus video monitoring
  - response to low dose of benzodiazepine

Partial (Focal) Seizures

➤ Causes

- o Commonest form (~ ½) of epilepsy, aka temporal lobe epilepsy, with hippocampal atrophy (mesial temporal sclerosis) on brain MRI Tumour, CVA, vascular disease, abnormal development of cortex

➤ Types

- o Simple
- o Complex
  - Change in LOC (involvement of 1/both temporal lobes) for 1 to 2 min, followed by confusion for 5 to 10 min sartomatisma:
    - ▪ Eyes   - Blank stare
    - ▪ Lipo   - Smacking
    - ▪ Swallow   - Repetitive
    - ▪ Hands   - Fumbling

Note: May be progression from simple focal usual presentation of temporal lobe epilepsy → complex focal → secondary generalized.

- o Secondary generalized
  - Diffuse involvement of both hemispheres, leading to convulsions
  - Aura
  - Tonic/chronic contractions
  - Tongue biting
  - Incontinence
  - Post ictal
    - ▪ Confusion/agitation, 10 min
    - ▪ Fatigue

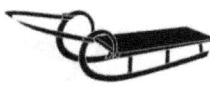

- A patient with temporal lobe epilepsy is refractory to pharmaceutical treatment. Give the findings on diagnostic imaging which would suggest that a temporal hemilobectomy would give > 50% likelihood of further seizures.

  o An identifiable lesion in the temporal lobe gives a high chance of success of surgery for example
    - Vascular malfunction
    - Tumour
    - Sclerosis (mesial temporal sclerosis)

- In the context of a seizure, give the meaning of **Todd paralysis**.

  o Focal deficit on side opposite to where the seizure began (a contralateral postical focal deficit)

- Give the meaning of "**absence seizure**".

  o Generalized seizure with LOC < 2 seconds

- Give the **distinction** between secondary generalized seizure versus primary generalized seizure.

	Primary	Secondary
o Aura	-	+
o Progression	-	+
o Todd paralysis	-	+
o Loss of consciousness (LOC)	< 5 sec	1 to 2 min

Idiopathic Generalized Epilepsy

Useful background

  o Represents 1/3 of population with seizures

  o May present after age 20, but usually earlier

  o After age 20, usually associated with use of alcohol, or sleep deprivation

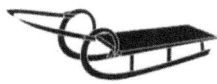

➤ Clinical
 ○ Variable combination of presentations
  - Generalized tonic-chronic
  - Absence
  - Myoclonic
   ▪ Family history is common
   ▪ AM jitteriness/myoclonus
   ▪ Diagnose and treat to prevent the development of convulsions
 ○ Complications (please see below)

- Give the **complications**/comorbidities of epilepsy.

 ○ Depressive (~50%)
  - Major
  - Bipolar
  - Suicidal ideation
 ○ Cognition
  - Cognitive decline
  - ↓ memory
   ▪ Visual
   ▪ Verbal
  - ↓ attention, especially with
   ▪ Frontal lobal syndromes
   ▪ Generalized

 ○ Osteoporosis
  - ↑ prevalence
  - May be related in part to enzyme-inducing AEDs
  - Perform screening after 5 yr AEs, and
  - Supplement with calcium / vitamin D
 ○ ↑ mortality rate
  - The disease, or its causes and treatment (AEDs)
  - Suicide
  - Sudden unexplained death

➤ Diagnosis
 ○ The order in which tests are obtained in the investigation of the patient with a history of seizures depends upon clinical features.
 ○ Electroencephalogram (EEG) may help about 1/3 of epileptic patients
 ○ Standard EEG is positive in only about 1/3 of epileptic patients
 ○ Prolonged (2 to 7 day) inpatient continuous and simultaneous monitoring of EEG and video may be necessary

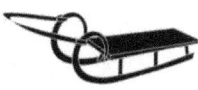

- About 1/5 of persons referred for this combined EEG / video monitoring are diagnosed with pseudoseizures (aka psychogenic non-epileptic seizures).

➢ Treatment
- Considerations
  - One unprovoked seizure in a patient normal EEG / MRI, risk of recurrence of seizure is ~ 1/3 in 2 yr
  - ≥ 2 unprovoken siezure, risk of recurrence is 60%
  - ↑ risk of recurrence of seizure in several conditions, which helps to make decision to use AEDs
  - AEDs ↓ risk of seizures by ~ 50% with 1 AED, ↓ risk by 13% co-administering 2 AEDs, so decisions needs to be balanced between risk, benefit, adverse effects

- Choice of drug(s)
  - Monotherapy → polytherapy, depending upon response and AEs (adverse effects)
  - Certain AEDs will worsen generalized epilepsy syndromes, and should not be used in such an individual
    - Carbamazepine
    - Gabapentin
    - Phenytoin
    - Pregabalin
  - The AED(s) selected depends upon AEs, and comorbidities

- CNS
  - Ataxia
  - Sedation

- Give the **common** adverse effects of anti-epileptic drugs (AEDs).
  - Liver failure
    - Carbamazepine
    - Felbamate
    - Lamotrigine
    - Phenobarbital
    - Valproic acid
  - Skin rash, SJS (Stevens Johnson Syndrome)
    - Carbamazepine
    - Lamotrigine
    - Oxcarbazepine
    - Phenobarbital
    - Phenytoin
    - Zonisamine

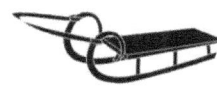

34

o	Blood dyscrasias	- Carbamazepine
		- Felbamate
		- Lamotrigine
		- Levetiracetam
		- Phenobarbital
		- Phenytoin
o	Hypersensitivity syndrome	- Lacosamide
		- Oxcarbazepine
		- Phenytoin

Some AEDs have unique AEs

- Give the **unique** adverse effects (AEs) of AEDs (anti-epileptic drugs).

o	Carbamazepine	- Severe hyponatremia
o	Gabapentin	- ↑ weight
o	Levetiracetam	- Depression/psychosis
o	Oxcarbazepine	- Severe hyponatremia
o	Phenytoin	- Gingival hyperplasia
		- Dysrhythmias
		- Lupus-like syndrome
o	Pregabain	- ↑ weight
o	Topiramate	- Renal calculi
		- Metabolic acidosis
o	↓ weight	- Headstroke
		- Acute angle closure glaucoma
o	Valproic acid	- Platelet dysfunction
		- Thrombocytopenia
		- ↑ weight
o	Vigabatrin	- Blindness (peripheral vision)
		- Peripheral neuropathy
o	Zonisamide	- Renal calculi
		- Skin rash
		- Depression
		- Psychosis
		- ↓ weight

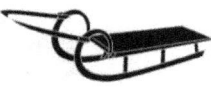

Metabolism of AEDs

Liver	Kidney
o Carbamazepine	- Gabapentin
o Lacosamide	- Lacosamide
o Lamotrigine	- Lamotrigine
o Oxcarbazapine	- Levetiracetum
o Phenytoin	- Oxcarbazepine
o Valproic acid	- Pregabalin
o Vigabatrin	- Topiramate
- Use with care in elderly	- Vigabatrin
▪ Carbamazepine	- Zonisamide
▪ Oxcarbaxepine	
▪ Phenytoin	

- Give the factors which ↑ risk of **recurrent seizure**.

  - Patient   - Age > 65 yr
  -                  - Head injury

  - Seizure   - Focal
  -                  - Todd paralysis

  - Investigation   - EEG / MRI (brain) →focal findings

  - When to start AEDs (anti-epileptic drugs)
    - After
      - 1 seizure if ≥ 1 of the above risk factors
      - 2 seizures, otherwise

The mortality rate of persons with epilepsy is increased, in part due to the condition itself and its causes, as well as the treatment with AEDs (anti-epileptic drugs, and partly because of associated sudden unexplained death.

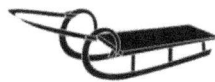

- Give the clinical features of the patient with epilepsy which **alerts the physician** to possible increased mortality rate.

  o Generalized tonic-clonic seizures

  o Refractory epilepsy

  o ↓ cognition

  o Mood disorder

  o Major depression

  o Suicidal ideation

  o ↓ adherence to AEDs

Failure of AEDs

  o Successful control
  - 1 AEDs ~ 50%
  - 2 AEDs ~ 63%
  o Remaining non-responders to 3 AEDs only 10% overall response with pharmacotherapy
  o Considerations for pharmacotherapy non-responders

  - Diet
    - Low carbohydrate (CHO; adults)
    - Low CHO, high fat (ketogenic; children)
  - Stimulation
    - Vagus nerve
    - Thalamus, anterior nucleus
  - Surgery
    - Removal of focal epileptogenic focus

AEDs, Fertility and Pregnancy

➤ Management of Epilepsy in Pregnancy
  o Plan pregnancy
    - Stop valproic acid
    - Achieve lowest level of single anticonvulsant for mother to be (lamotrigne) free of seizures

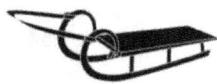

Mastering the Boards: Neurology   A.B.R. Thomson

- Give the AEDs which ↓ drug level of OCAs (oral contraceptive agents).

  - Carbamazepine
  - Felbamate
  - Lamotrigine
  - Oxcarbazepine

  - Phenobarbital
  - Phenytoin
  - Topiramate

  If contraception required, use alternate/additional method, rather than using above listed AEDs.

CLINICAL CAUTION

Do not use these AEDs in Pregnancy

- **Valproic acid**
  - Teratogenicity
  - ↑ POS (polycystic ovary syndrome)
  - ↓ development of cognitive function
- **Phenytoin**
  - ↑ fetal malformation
- **Phenobarbital**
  - ↑ fetal malformation
- **Topiramate**
  - ↑ cleft palate
- PS: Don't forget to give a folic acid supplement to all women during pregnancy (↓ risk of neural tube defects).

  - ↑ risk of pregnancy-associated seizures
    - Lamotrigine ⎤ → ↑ estrogen-associated metabolism → ↓ blood levels → ⎦
    - Oxcarbazepine ↑ seizure
  - "breastfeeding is considered generally safe with most AEDs" (Source: MKSAP 16 2012, Neurology, page 21)

➢ Dose adjustment
  - Begin low dose, target balance between benefits /adverse effects
  - Monitor patient's personal optimal drug dose
  - Consider weaning off AEDs when no seizures for 2 to 4 yr and EEG / MRI / CT of brain / head normal (risk of recurrence after stopping AEDs is ~ 1/3)

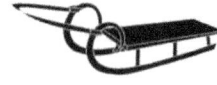

CEREBRAL ARTERIES

- **Anterior cerebral artery** (ACA)
  - o The medial straite artery (Heubner artery) provides blood to the anterior portion of the internal capsule, which carries fibres which supply the upper portion of the body.

- ➤ Occlusion of the ACA beyond the medial striated artery will cause the signs:
  - o Speech
    - Motor dysphasia
      - Involvement of dominant side
      - Results from damage to the precentral gyrus (motor cortex) of the frontal lobe

- ➤ Sensory
  - o Cortical sensory loss of contralateral leg (only if the superior surface of the cerebral cortex is affected)

- ➤ Motor
  - o Cortical flaccid weakness of contralateral leg

- ➤ Frontal lobe signs
  - o Grasp reflex
  - o Incontinence
  - o Intellectual decline
  - o Indifference

- **Middle cerebral artery** (MCA)
- ➤ This important artery supplies
  - o Most of the internal capsule by way of the lateral striated arteries
  - o Cortical receptive and expressive speech areas
  - o Superior part of the motor and sensory cortex (upper part of the body)
  - o Most of the frontal, temporal and parietal lobes

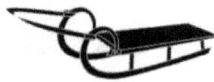

➤ Obstruction of the lateral striate branches causes:

  ○ Eyes
  - Hemianopia (visual fibres in the internal capsule)

  ○ Motor
  - Contralateral spastic paralysis, or
  - Flaccid paralysis (if frontal branches are blocked)

  ○ Sensory
  - Cortical sensory loss in the upper part of the body (frontal branches)

  ○ Parietal and temporal lobe signs (of branches to the parietal and temporal lobes are obstructed)

- **Posterior cerebral artery** (PCA)

➤ Flows to the occipital lobe, thalamus and midbrain

➤ Occlusion of PCA

  ○ Distal to the thalamic branch
  - Homonymous
  - Hemianopia with mucular sparing

  ○ Proximal to the thalamic branch
  - As above, plus the thalamic syndrome
  - Thalamic syndrome
    ▪ Enhanced sensory sensitivity of one half of body

  ○ Severe pain

➤ Occlusion of both PCAs

  ○ Cortical blindness
  - Blindness:
    ▪ Patient does not know when a light is shone in the eyes
    ▪ Patient may not realize that they are blind, or may even deny that they cannot see

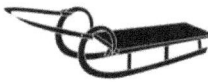

- Perform a focused physical examination to distinguish between an intramedullary from an extramedullary cord lesion.

	Intramedullary	Extramedullary
o Root pain	– Rare	▪ Common
o Corticospinal signs	– Late onset	▪ Early onset
o LMN signs	– Extend for several segments	▪ Localized
o Sensory loss	– Dissociated sensory loss (pain and temperature) may be present	▪ Brown-Sequard syndrome if lateral cord compression
o Sacral sparing	– May have sacral sparing	▪ No sacral sparing
o CSF fluid	– Normal or minimally altered	▪ Early, marked abnormalities

Abbreviations: CSF, cerebrospinal fluid; LMN; lower motor neuron

Adapted from: Talley NJ, et al. *Maclennan & Petty Pty Limited* 2003, Table 10.28, page 427.

- Perform a focused physical examination for the "dorsal midbrain syndrome".

(A hint: aka "Parinaud Syndrome", "Sylvian Aqueduct Syndrome", or "Pretectal Syndrome")

o Light-near dissociation

o Vertical gaze palsy

o Lid retraction

o Convergence-retraction nystagmus (a rhythmic inward movement of both eyes from co-contraction of the extraocular muscles, usually elicited during convergence or upward gaze)

o Causes
  - Pinealoma (in younger patients)
  - Multiple sclerosis and basilar artery stokes (in older patients)

Adapted from: McGee SR. *Saunders/Elsevier* 2007, page 216.

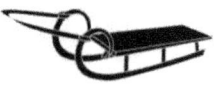

Cerebral Vascular Disease And Stroke

➢ Definition: "Stroke [is] recognized clinically as the sudden onset of a focal disturbance of central nervous system function" (Phillips SJ, et al. Chapter 41. In: Therapeutic Choices. Grey J, Ed. 6th Edition, *Canadian Pharmacists Association*: Otttawa, ON, 2011, page 559).

    o Stroke-sudden focal neurological deficit caused by ischemia or hemorrhage

    o TIA (transient ischemic attack)
      - Sudden focal neurological deficit cause by ischemia, lasting < 24 hr and not associated with infarction on diagnostic imaging.

➢ Types

• Give a classification of the types of CVA (cerebrovascular accidents; strokes injury).

    o Ischemic (85%)   - Obstruction
       (cerebral infarction)   ▪ Artherosclerosis (large artery)
                                      ▪ Cardioembolic
                                      ▪ Small-vessel disease

    o Hemorrhagic (15%)   - Rupture
                                        ▪ Intracerebral (10%)
                                        ▪ Subarachnoid (5%)

    o Stroke subtypes to be considered
      - Transient ischemic attack (TIA)
      - Ischemic
           ▪ Cardioembolic
           ▪ Large artery atherosclerosis
           ▪ Small subcortical infarcts
           ▪ Cryptogene
      - Hemorrhagic
           ▪ Intracerebral hemorrhage
           ▪ Subarachnoid hemorrhage

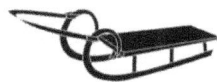

➤ Clinical
  o NIH prognostic score, based on
    - Level of consciousness
      - Eyes
        ▪ Gaze
        ▪ Visual fields

      - Face
      - Strength
        ▪ Strength
        ▪ Arms
        ▪ Legs

      - Ataxia
      - Sensation
      - Language
        ▪ Pinprick
        ▪ Aphasia (name objects)
        ▪ Dysarthria (speech)

Please see: www.ninds.nih.gov/doctors/NIH_Stroke_Scale.pdf
http://earn.heart.org/ihtml/application/student/extinction/inattention

NIH Stroke Scale correlates with
  ▪ Size of infarction
  ▪ Prognosis

Also please see Modern textbooks of Internal Medicine or Neurology,
UpToDate, or reviews such as MKSAP 16 2012, Neurology, Table 12, page 25.

• Take a directed history for **warning signs of a stroke**.

    o Sudden Pain
      – Severe headache

    o Eyes
      – Visual challenges

    o Speech
      – Difficulty speaking

    o Balance
      – Loss

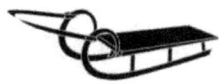

Useful background: The National Institutes of Health **Stroke Scale**[a]

Item	Response
1a. Level of consciousness	0=Alert 1= Not alert 2= Obtunded 3=Unresponsive
1b. Level of consciousness questions	0= Answers both correctly 1= Answers 1 correctly 2= Answers neither correctly
1c. Level of consciousness commands	0= performs both tasks correctly 1= Performs 1 task correctly 2= Performs neither task
2. Gaze	0= Normal 1= Partial gaze palsy 2= Total gaze palsy
3. Visual fields	0= No visual loss 1= Partial hemianopsia 2= Complete hemianopsia 3= Bilateral hemianopsia
4. Facial palsy	0= Normal 1= Minor paralysis 2= Partial paralysis 3= Complete paralysis

5. Motor arm
  a. Left
  b. Right
	0= No drift
	1= Drift before 5 s
	2= Falls before 10s
	3= No effort against gravity
	4= No movement

6. Motor leg
  a. Left
  b. Right
	0= No drift
	1= Drift before 5 s
	2= Falls before 5 s
	3= No effort against gravity
	4= No movement

7. Ataxia	0= Absent 1= One limb 2= Two limbs

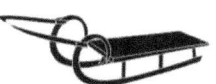

Mastering the Boards: Neurology   A.B.R. Thomson

Item	Response
8. Sensory	0= Normal 1= Mild loss 2= Severe loss
9. Language	0= Normal 1= Mild aphasia 2= Severe aphasia 3= Mute or global aphasia
10. Dysarthria	0=Normal 1= Mild 2= Severe
11. Extinction/inattention	0= Normal 1= Mild 2= Severe

[a]The actual form for recording the data contains detailed instructions for the use of the scale. This is avaliable at www.ninds.nih.gov/doctors/NIH_stroke_Scale.pdf .

An online course for provider education is available at www.ninds.nih.gov/doctors/stroke_scale_training.htm
b Score= sum of scores from each item.

The NIH stroke scale, as published in Simel D L, et al. *JAMA* 2009, Table 48-2, page 630.

- **Bamford clinical classification of stroke**

❖ Total anterior circulation syndrome

- o Unilateral motor deficit of face, arm and leg

- o Homonymous hemianopia

- o Higher cerebral dysfunction (e.g., aphasia, neglect)

❖ Parietal anterior circulation syndrome

Any two of the following features:

- o Unilateral motor and/or sensory deficit

- o Ipsilateral hemianopia or higher cerebra dysfunction

- o Higher cerebral dysfunction alone, or isolated motor and/or sensory deficit restricted to one limb or to the face

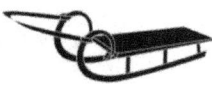

❖ Posterior circulation syndrome

One or more of the following features:

o Bilateral motor or sensory signs not secondary to brainstem compression by a large supratentorial lesion

o Cerebellar signs, unless accompanied by ipsilateral motor deficit (see ataxic hemiparesis)

o Unequivocal diplopia with or without external ocular muscle palsy

o Crossed signs, for example left facial and right limb weakness

o Hemianopia alone or with any of the four items above

❖ Lacunar syndrome

o Pure motor stroke:
  - Unilateral, pure motor deficit
  - Clearly involving two of three areas (face, arm and leg)
  - With the whole of any limb being involved

o Pure sensory stroke:
  - Unilateral pure sensory symptoms (with or without signs)
  - Involving at least two of three areas (face arm and leg)
  - With the whole of any limb being involved

o Ataxic hemiparesis
  - Ipsilateral cerebellar and corticospinal tract signs
  - With or without dysarthria
  - In the absence of higher cerebral dysfunction or a visual field defect

o Sensorimotor stroke:
  - Pure motor and pure sensory stroke combined (i.e., unilateral motor or sensory signs and symptoms)
  - In the absence of higher cerebral dysfunction or a visual field defect

Stroke is characterized by rapidly progressive clinical symptoms and signs of focal, and at times global, loss of cerebral function lasting more than 24 hours or leading to death, with no apparent cause other than that of vascular origin.

Bamford clinical classification of stroke, as published: Baliga RR. *Saunders/Elsevier* 2007, page 127.

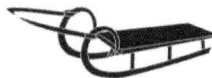

➢ Subtypes

- **Oxfordshire classification of subtypes of cerebral infarction**

    o Total anterior circulation infarction syndrome (TACS)

    o IC/MCA- A combination of new higher cerebral dysfunction (ie dysphasia, dyscalculia, visuospatial disorder); homonymous visual field defect; and ipsilateral motor or sensory deficit of at least 2 areas of the face, arm and leg.

    o Partial anterior circulation infarction syndrome (PACS)

    o MCA- Only 2 of the 3 components of the TACS syndrome are present with higher cerebral dysfunction alone or with a motor/sensory deficit more restricted than those classified as LACS (ie confined to 1 limb or to face and hand, but not to the whole arm).

    o Lacunar infarction syndrome (LACS)

    o Penetids- Pure motor stroke, pure sensory stroke, sensorimotor stroke, or ataxic hemiparesis.

    o Posterior circulation infarction syndrome (POCS)

    o Ventrilosis basilar- Any of the following
      - Ipsilateral cranial nerve palsy with contralateral motor or sensory deficit
      - Bilateral motor or sensory deficit
      - Disorder of conjugate eye movement
      - Cerebellar dysfunction without ipsilteral long tract deficit (ie ataxic hemiparesis)
      - Isolated homonymous visual field defect.

Oxfordshire classification, as published in Simel DL, et al. *JAMA* 2009, Box 48-1, page 634.

- Give the reason why the upper portions of the body are affected less than the lower body by a vascular lesion of the middle cerebral artery (which supplies the internal capsule).

    o The fibres which supply the lower portion of the body are in the posterior portion of the internal capsule, and are supplied by only one vessel, whereas the fibres which supply the upper portion of the body are in the anterior portion of the internal capsule, which has a dual blood supply.

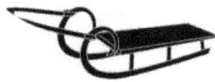

➢ Anatomy: The cerebral cortex showing the distribution of the cerebral arteries.

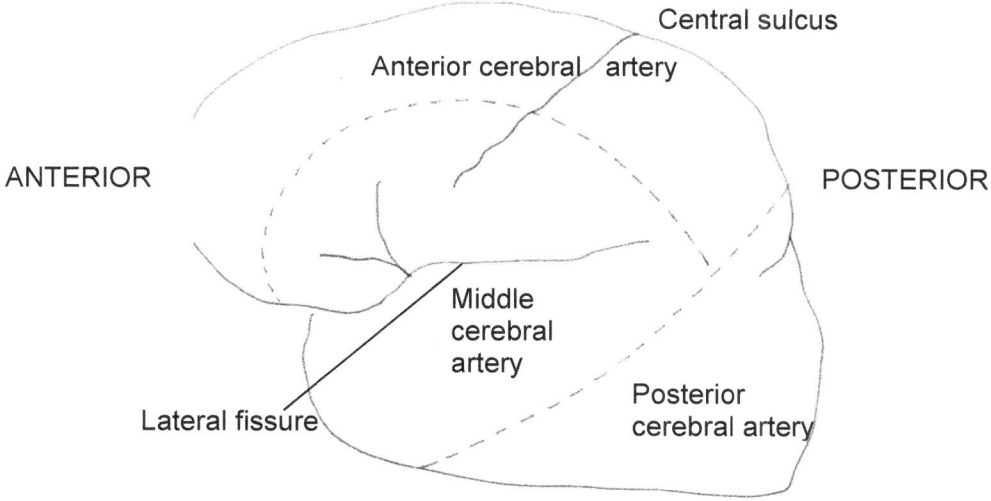

Adapted from: Davey P. *Wiley-Blackwell* 2006, Figure 17, page 256.

- Take a directed history and perform a physical examination for a cerebral vascular accident (**CVA**) or for transient ischemic attack (**TIA**).

- History
  - o Weakness
    - Location and extent
    - Time course (onset, duration, change with time)
    - Previous episodes (TIAs)
    - Quality of deficit (sensory, movement, power)

  - o Associated symptoms
    - Paresthesia
    - Pain
    - Dizziness
    - Level of consciousness
    - Amaurosis Fugax
    - Slurred speech
    - Skin changes (colour, swelling, warmth)
    - Injury or trauma
    - Infection (fever, chills, sweating)

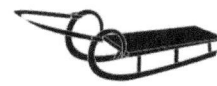

- o Risk factors
  - Family Hx of neurological Disease
  - Hx of stroke
  - Hx of MI, Murmur, Palpitations, Rheumatic heart disease
  - Atherosclerosis RF (hypertension, DM, FHx of CAD, hypercholesterolemia, smoking)
- o Impact on ADLs
  - Is the patient R or L handed?
  - Gross motor (reaching shelves, opening doors)
  - Fine motor (buttoning shirt, using keys, writing)
  - Impact on personal and family life

- Physical examination
  - o Inspection
    - Compares right arm to left arm for:
    - Atrophy
    - Fasciculation
    - Abnormal position
    - Abnormal movements
  - o Tone
    - Compares right arm to left arm for:
    - Rigidity
    - Spasticity (velocity dependant)
  - o Power
    - Compares and grades right arm to left arm power for:
    - Shoulder extension and abduction
    - Elbow flexion, extension, pronation and supination
    - Wrist flexion, extension, ulnar and radial deviation
    - Digit abduction, adduction, thumb extension and thumb opposition
    - Pronator Drift Test
  - o Reflexes
    - Compares and grades right arm to left arm reflexes for: Biceps (C5-6), Brachioradialis (C5,6) and triceps (C7,8)
  - o Co-ordination
    - Finger to nose test
    - Rapid alternating movement

Abbreviations: ADL, activities of daily living; AF, atrial fibrillation; CAD, coronary artery disease; CVA, cerebral vascular accident; HBP, hypertension; MI, myocardial infarction; TIA, transient ischemic attack

Source: Jugovic PJ, et al. *Saunders/ Elsevier* 2004, pages 149 and 150.

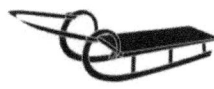

CLINICAL TIP

    o   Once it is established that the patient has suffered a CVA, be prepared for an OSCE question asking you to examine the patient to determine the likely blood supply of the involved area.

- Take a directed history and perform a focused physical examination for identification of persons with a **high risk of CVA** (cerebrovascular attack, aka "stroke")

    - o Nonmodifiable factors
        - Age > 60 years
        - Gender
        - Family history

    - o Modifiable factors
        - Habits
            - Smoking
        - Heart
            - Hypertension (≥ 140 / 90 mm Hg)
            - Atrial fibrillation
            - Carotid disease (a surrogate marker for associated coronary artery disease)
        - Metabolic
            - Diabetes
            - Dyslipidemia

  - o Possible factors

    - Rhythm
        - Atrial fibrillation
        - Paroxysmal atrial fibrillation
        - Sustained atrial fibrillation
        - Sick sinus syndrome
        - Spontaneous echocardiographic contrast

    - Valve defect
        - Mechanical valve
        - Rheumatic valve disease
        - Calcification of mitral annulus

    - Valve infection
        - Infectious endocarditis
        - Nonbacterial thrombotic endocarditis

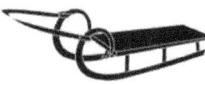

- Lumen
  - Intracardiac thrombus
- Wall
  - Intracardiac mass (eg. atrial myxoma, papillary fibroelastoma)
  - Dilated cardiomyopathy
  - Patent foramen ovale with or without atrial septal aneurysm
  - Hypokinetic or a kinetic left ventricular segment
- Vessels
  - Recent (within 1 month) myocardial infarction
  - Atherosclerotic debris in the thoracic aorta
  - Myocardial infarction 2-6 month earlier

Adapted from: Ghosh AK. *Mayo Clinic Scientific Press* 2008, page 773.

Note: The prognosis of TIA is worse with

  o Age ≥ 60 years

  o Hypertension ≥ 140 / 90 mm Hg

  o Diabetes

  o TIA duration of symptoms > 10 minutes

  o Speech and/or motor symptoms

Adapted from: Cote' R, et al. Chapter 40. In: Therapeutic Choices. Grey J, Ed. 6th Edition, *Canadian Pharmacists Association*: Otttawa, ON, 2011, page 550.

"Trustworthiness is a gating mechanism for social interactions."

Grandad

 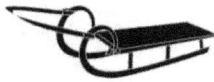

➢ Anatomy

    ○ The arteries at the base of the brain and the circle of Willis.

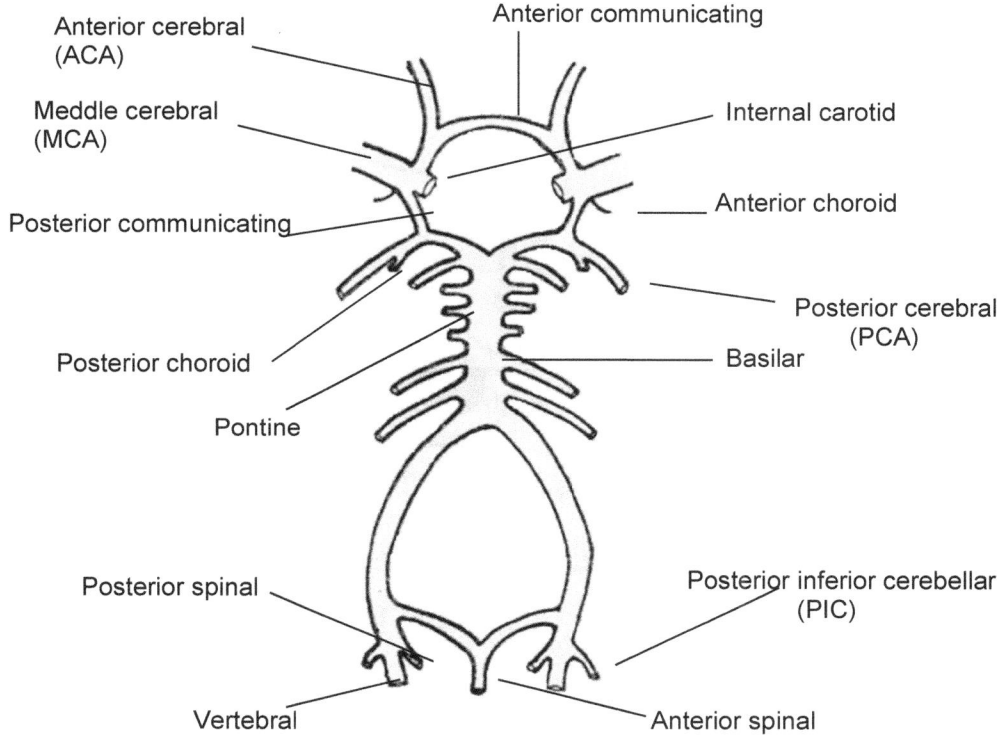

Useful background: Carotid artery stenosis

    ○ In patients with TIA, a carotid bruit indicates the presence of a > 50% stenosis of the carotid artery (confirmed by carotid angiography) with 29% sensitivity and 88% specificity.

Adapted from Sauve JS et al., *JAMA* 1993; 270: 2843-5.

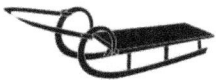

- Perform a focused physical examination to determine which vessel of the circle of Willis has been blocked by a thrombus or embolus and is responsible for a cerebrovascular "accident' (CVA).

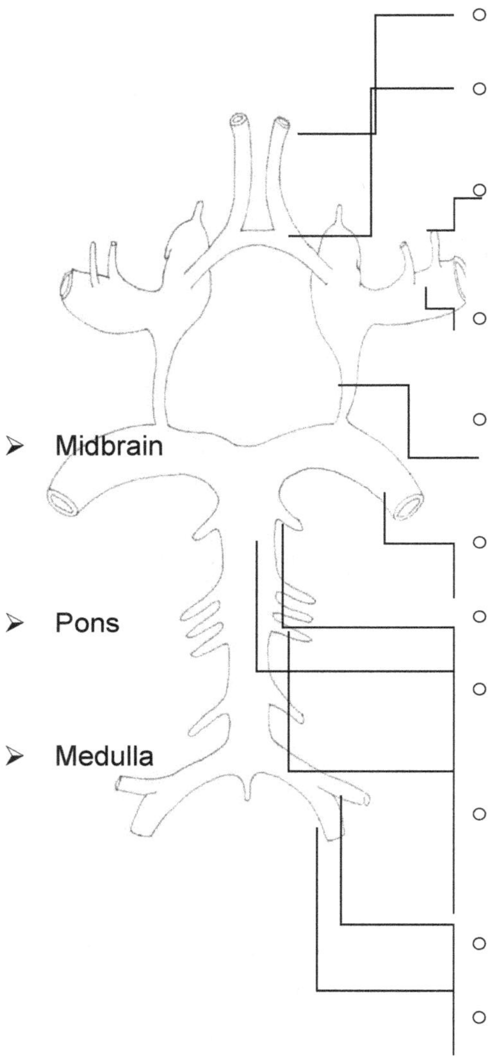

Artery	Functional Importance
o Anterior cerebral artery	-- Leg primarily involved
o Anterior communicating artery	-- Connects right and left internal carotid
o Penetrating, subcortical branches of middle cerebral artery	-- Subcortical lacunes No cortical deficit
o Internal carotid, middle cerebral artery	-- Aphasia, or nondominant hemisphere dysfunction
o Posterior communicating artery	-- May be large with posterior circulation getting significant supply from internal carotid
o Posterior cerebral artery	-- Field cut (supplies occipital lobe), no hemiplegia
o Superior cerebellar artery	-- Infrequently involved alone
o Basilar artery	-- Occlusion results in quadriplegia and death unless, there are god anterior collaterals
o Penetrating branches of the basilar artery to brainstem	-- Small brainstem infarcts, often classic lacunes
o Anterior inferior cerebellar artery	-- Infrequently involved alone
o Posterior inferior cerebellar artery	-- Lateral medullary syndrome, usually secondary to occlusion of the vertebral artery from which it arises

➤ Midbrain

➤ Pons

➤ Medulla

*Lacunes: Small infacts typically from atherothrombotic occlusive disease of the penetrating branches

Adapted from: Talley NJ, et al. *Maclennan & Petty Pty Limited* 2003, Figure 10.50, page 417; Davey P. *Wiley-Blackwell* 2006, page 248.

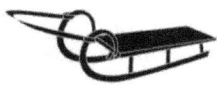

Areas supplied by the arteries at the base of the brain and the circle of Willis:

➢ Anterior cerebral artery (ACA) or anterior communicating artery
  o Optic atrophy (compression of optic nerves)
  o Frontal lobe symptoms (compression of frontal lobes)

➢ Middle cerebral artery (MCA)
  o Supplies the
    - Upper optic radiation
    - Optic radiation as it passes through the internal capsule
  o Occlusion of MCA
    - Defects of lower visual fields

➢ Posterior cerebral artery
  o Both cerebral peduncles
  o Ipsilteral III, IV
  o Conjugate eye movement
  o Thalamus
  o Supplies-lower optic radiation
    - Occipital visual cortex
    - Midbrain
  o All cerebral arteries are end anterior
  o Occlusion of even just one vessel supplying the circle of Willis may cause signs

➢ Anterior inferior cerebellar (AIC)
  o CN-V-VIII
  o Conjugate eye movement
  o Corticospinal, medial lemniscus
  o Anteriolateral spinothalamic
  o Pinpoint pupils
  o Hyperventilation

➢ Posterior inferior cerebellar (PIC)
  o Ipsilateral CN V to X; ipsilateral palsy
  o Ipsilateral spinocerebellar tract
  o Ipsilateral Horner syndrome
  o Contralateral pain and temperature
  o Contralateral hemiplegia

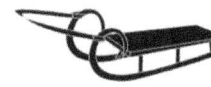

Mastering the Boards: Neurology   A.B.R. Thomson

- Perform a focused neurological examination to determine the location of an arterial cerebral occlusion.

Middle Cerebral Artery (MCA)	Posterior Cerebral Artery (PCA)	Anterior Cerebral Artery (ACA)	Internal Carotid Artery (ICA)
o Infarction middle third of hemisphere: UMN face, arm> leg	– Infarction of thalamus and occipital cortex	▪ Cortical sensory loss leg only	- Contralateral HCA and MCA signs
o Homonymous hemianopia; aphasia or non-dominant hemisphere signs (depends on side)	– Contralateral sensory loss – Contralateral hemianopia	▪ Contralateral weakness of leg and shoulder shrug ▪ Urinary incontinence	- Ipsilateral transient monocular blindness (amaurosis fugax)
o Cortical sensory loss			

- o Perforating artery

- o Internal capsule infarction: UMN face UMN arm> leg

- o Left-sided
  - – Aphasia

- o Right-sided
  - – Neglect of left space
  - – Lack of awareness of deficit
  - – Apathy
  - – Impersistence

- o Basilar artery
  - – Bilateral motor weakness
  - – Diplopia
  - – Opthalmoplegia

Abbreviation: ACA, anterior cerebral artery; ICA, internal carotid artery; MCA, middle cerebral artery; PCA , posterior cerebral artery; UMN, upper motor neuron lesion

Adapted from: Talley NJ, et al. *Maclennan & Petty Pty Limited*, 2003, Table 10.22, page 418; Filate W, et al. *The Medical Society, Faculty of Medicine, University of Toronto* 2005, Table 18, page 171.

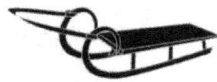

- Perform a focused physical examination to determine if a lesion affects functions of the **dominant cerebral hemisphere**.

  o Dominant hemisphere
    - Right-left orientation
    - Finger identification
    - Calculation

  o Non-dominant hemisphere
    - Facial recognition
    - Awareness of body and space
    - Drawing ability
    - Topographic ability
    - Construction
    - Dressing
    - Motor persistence

Source: Baliga RR. *Saunders/Elsevier* 2007, page 150.

- Perform a focused physical examination to determine the presence of **parietal lobe dysfunction**.
  o ↓ accurate localization (of touch, position, joint sense and temperature appreciation)
  o ↓ two-point discrimination
  o Astereognosis
  o Dysgraphethesia
  o ↓ Sensory attention
  o Attention hemianopia, homonymous hemianopia, or lower quadrantic hemianopia

Source: Baliga RR. *Saunders/Elsevier* 2007, page 150.

- Perform a focused physical examination of the patient's visual fields to determine the **site of an occlusion** of posterior cerebral artery (**PCA**).
  o Complete occlusion
    - Complete homonymous, with macular sparing
  o Partial occlusion
    - Upper homonymous quadrantanopia (as in vertebra-basilar insufficiency)
    - Aneurysm of PCA or posterior communicating artery
      ▪ Isolated CN III palsy

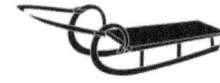

- Perform a focused physical examination of the patient's visual fields to determine the **site of an occlusion of the internal carotid artery**.

  o Occlusion of internal carotid
    - Findings of middle cerebral artery (MCA) occlusion (since MCA is a continuation of carotid artery)
  o Aneurysm of internal carotid artery
    - Nasal or homonymous heminopia (pressure of optic chiasm or optic tracts)
    - If aneurysm is in the cavernous sinus, the anterior choroidal arterymay be affected, causing-signs of CN III, IV, VI or CN V, ophthalmic division disorder
      - Homonymous congruous scotoma

Amaurosis fugax

➢ Definition

  o Transient monocular blindness due to episodic retinal ischemia, usually associated with ipsilateral carotid artery stenosis or embolism of the retinal arteries resulting in a sudden and frequently complete, loss of vision in one eye.

- Give the performance characteristics for unilateral cerebral hemispheric disease.

Finding	PLR	NLR
o Arm rolling test	21.7	NS
o Pronator drift	10.3	0.1
o Finger tapping test	6.6	0.3
o Babinski response	19.0	0.6
o Hyperreflexia	5.8	0.4

Abbreviation: NLR, negative likelihood ratio; PLR, positive likelihood ratio

Note that hemianopia and hemisensory disturvance are not included since had a PLR < 2.

Adapted from: McGee SR. *Saunders/Elsevier* 2007, Box 57-1, page 726

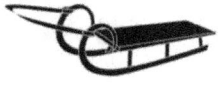

NORMAL   RIGHT CEREBRAL LESION
                          (Left-sided findings)

Upper limb drift (pronator drift)

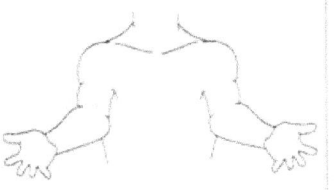 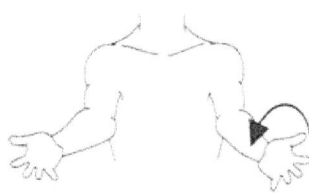

- For 45 sec stretche out both arms, with palms upright and eyes closed
- Positive test: the arm on the side opposite to the cerebellar lesion drifts downward and pronates

Forearm rolling test

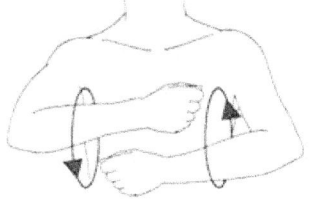 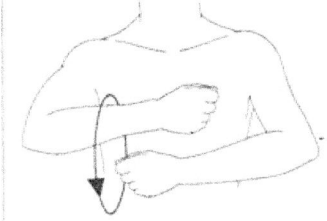

- Bend elbows, place forearms parallel to each other, and rotate the forearms about each other in a rapid rolling motion for 10 seconds in each direction
- Postitive test: the arm on the side opposite to the crerbellar lesion is stay still, while the other arm "orbits" around it

Rapid finger tapping

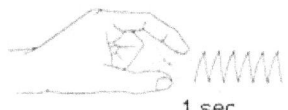 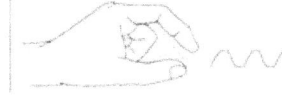

1 sec

➢ Special Tests for Unilateral Cerebral Lesions

- Tap the thumb and index finger together repeatedly at about two taps per second
- Positive test: the fingers on the side opposite to the cerebellar lesion tap more slowly, and may even look like the two fingers are sticking together

Adapted from: McGee SR. *Saunders/Elsevier* 2007, page 710.

- Perform a focused physical examination for **cavernous sinus thrombosis (CST), and for sagittal sinus thrombosis (SST).**

  o Cavernous sinus thrombosis (CST)
    - CN III, IV, VI, V – ophthalmic branch
    - Papilledema
    - Exophthalamus

  o Sagittal sinus thomsbosis (SST)
    - Crural dominance
      ▪ Paralysis and loss of sensation of the legs, from damage to the top of bottle cerebral cortices

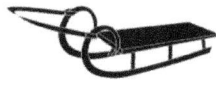

Dural Sinus Venus Thrombosis

➤ Causes/associations
  o Any cause of ↑ stasis
  o Inflammation
  o Cancer
  o Infection
  o Trauma
  o Pregnancy

➤ Clinical
• Give the usual presentation of central vein occlusion, or thrombosis of sinuses such as superior sagittal or cavernous sinus.
  o History severe headache - ↓ LOC (level of consciousness)
                              - Seizure
  o Physical
    - Papilledema (in about ½)
    - Ocula veins   ▪ Dilated
    - Periocular veins   ▪ Dilated
    - Central veins   ▪ Venous infarction
                           ▪ ICH (intracerebral hemorrhage)
    - CN (cranial nerve) changes ▪ III, IV, V (V1, V2), V1

• In the context of thrombosis of the cavernous sinus, give the **abnormalities in the cranial nerves (CN)**.
  o Eye – III, IV, VI
  o Face – V1, V2

➤ Diagnosis
  o CT head
    - Filling defects
    - Dural sinuses
    - Confluence of sinuses
      ▪ Empty delta sign
  o MRV (MR venography)

➤ Treatment
  o If no expanding hematoma needing surgical drainage
    - Heparin, flowed by warfarin for 6 mon (even if venous thrombosis causes venous infarction and ICH (intracerebral hemorrhage)
  o Treat associated causes of hypercoagulability e.g., infection, infiltration

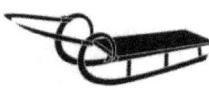

- Perform a focused physical examination for **obstruction at the base of the anterior spinal artery.**

  o Medial medullary syndrome

    - Corticospinal tracts
    - Medial lemniscus
    - Hypoglossal nerve (CN XII)

  o Which two areas of the spinal cord are especially prone to ischemic injury, and why?

    - Lower cervical region, just above the area where the segmental artery from the costo-cervical trunk enters; blood flow from this segmental artery flows downwards, thus not providing a second source of blood supply to the cord of the ASA is blocked.

    - Mid thoracic region, in the area between the additional supple from costo-cervical trunk, and the area where flow is supplemented by the artery of Adamkiewicz (usually on the left side); blood from this artery flows both upwards and downwards

    - The blood flow in the artery of Adamkiewicz may be damaged, and therefore ischemia of the mid thoracic spinal cord occur with

      - Dissection of the aorta
      - Nerve blocks to left lower nerve
      - Left lower thoracotomies

CLINICAL TIP

Temporal Arterial Insufficiency (TIA, transient ischemic attacks) may include symptoms and signs arising from ischemia of

  o Carotid artery
  o Basilar artery

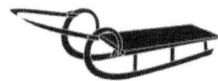

STROKE

➤ Definitions
- o Stroke – sudden, focal neurologic deficit caused by intracranial ischemia or hemorrhage with infarction on imaging
- o Transient ischemic attack (TIA)
  - Transcient, focal neurologic deficit lasting < 1 to 24h caused by intracranial ischemia with no infarction on imaging

➤ Types
- o Stroke
  - Ischemia (85%)
    - Large-artery atherosclerosis
    - Cardioembolic
    - Small-vessel disease
  - Hemorrhagic (15%)
    - Intracerebral (10%)
    - Subarachnoid (5%)

➤ Investigation
- o Heart
  - ECG
  - Echocardiogram
- o Head/neck
  - CTA (CT angiogram)
  - MRA (MR angiogram)
- o Neck
  - Caroti artery ultrasound

- Give the rationale for all patients with TIA/stroke require urgent CTA.

- o CTA (CT angiogram)
  - Determines if event was hemorrhagic, or ischemic, and there
  - Helps to direct optimal therapy
  - With physical examination, helps to implicate which artery was affected

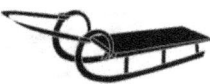

➢ Clinical

• Perform a focused physical examination to determine the likely blood vessel implicated in causing a stroke.

- o Anterior cerebral artery CL leg weakness

- o Middle cerebral artery
  - CL face, arm, leg weakness and sensory loss
  - Visual field defect
  - Aphasia, or neglect

- o Vertrbreal artery (lower cranial nerve defects)
  - Deviation
    ▪ Tongue, palate
  - Dysacthria
  - Dysphagia
  - Nystagmus
  - Vertigo

- o Posterior cerebral artery
  - CL visual defect

- o Deep/"lacunar"
  - CL motor/sensory defects
  - Clumsy hand-dysarthria syndrome
  - Ataxic hemiparesis

- o Basilar artery
  - Ocular defects, +/-
  - Ataxia plus
    ▪ Sensory/motor defection: side of face, plus sensory/motor defects on other side of body ("crossed" defects)

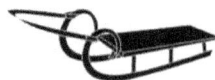

- Give the typical neurological deficiencies from areas of the cerebrovascular blood flow.

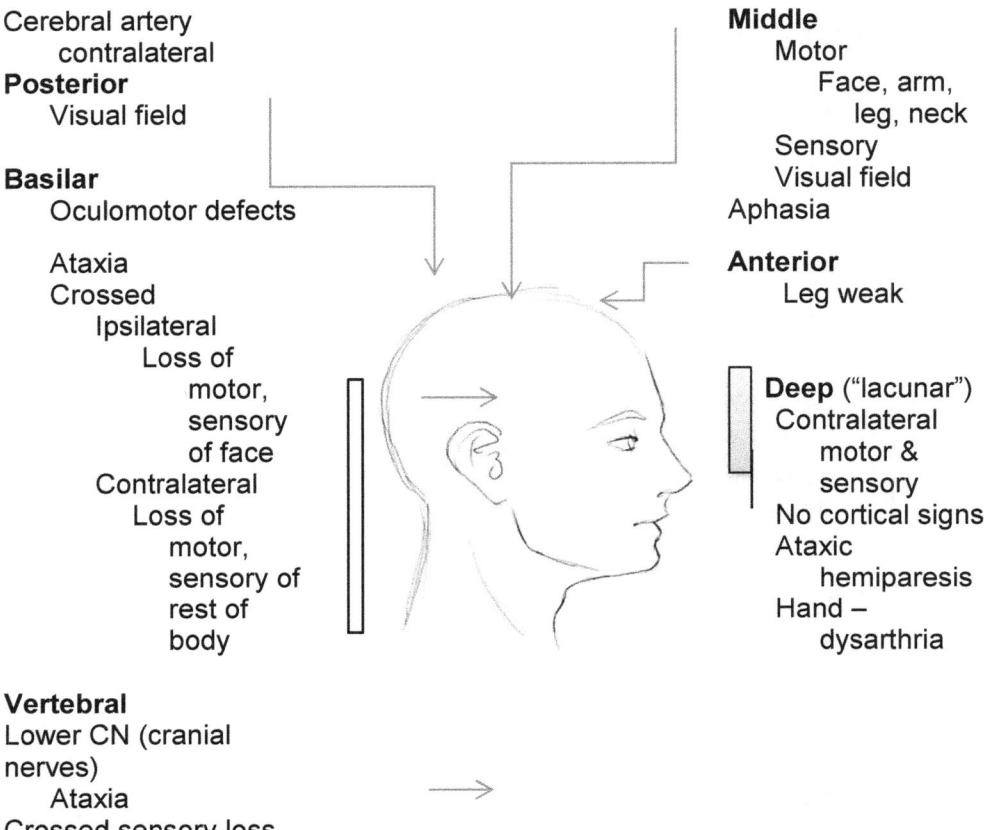

Cerebral artery
   contralateral
Posterior
   Visual field

Basilar
   Oculomotor defects

   Ataxia
   Crossed
      Ipsilateral
         Loss of
            motor,
            sensory
            of face
      Contralateral
         Loss of
            motor,
            sensory of
            rest of
            body

Middle
   Motor
      Face, arm,
         leg, neck
   Sensory
   Visual field
   Aphasia

Anterior
   Leg weak

Deep ("lacunar")
Contralateral
   motor &
   sensory
No cortical signs
Ataxic
   hemiparesis
Hand –
   dysarthria

Vertebral
Lower CN (cranial nerves)
   Ataxia
Crossed sensory loss

- Give the clinical findings in the **common stroke syndromes** (right-handed patient).

Affected artery	Clinical
o Left sided	– Aphasia
o Right sided	– Neglect of left space
	– Lack of awareness of deficit
	– Apathy
o Anterior cerebral artery (ACA)	– Contralateral weakness of the lower limb and shoulder shrug
o Middle cerebral artery (MCA)	– Contralateral motor, sensory and visual loss

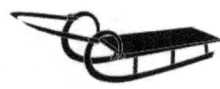

Affected artery	Clinical
o Posterior cerebral artery (PCA)	– Contralateral hemianopia and hemisensory loss
o Internal carotid artery (ICA)	– Contralateral MCA and ACA signs
	– Ipsilateral transient monocular blindness (amaurosis)
o Basilar artery	– Bilateral motor weakness, ophthalmoplegia and diplopia

Abbreviation: MCA, middle cerebral artery

Source: Filate W, et al. *The Medical Society, Faculty of Medicine, University of Toronto* 2005, page 171.

- Take a directed history and perform a focused physical examination for TIA-associated ischemia of carotid and MCA, as well as basilar artery and PCA.

    o Carotid and MCA
        - Eye
            ▪ Hemianopia
            ▪ Transient monocular blindness
            ▪ Horner syndrome
        - Speech
            ▪ Stuttering
        - Intellect
            ▪ Confusion
        - Motor
            ▪ Hemiplegia

    o Basilar artery and PCA
        - Hemianopia (optic radiation or occipital)
        - Dysarthria ⎤
        - Dysphagia |
        - Vertigo | -Pons and medulla
        - Facial pain |
        - Hemiplegia ⎦
        - "drop attacks" (reticular formation)
        - Temporal load signs & symptoms

Adapted from: Davies IJT. *Lloyd-Luke (medical books) LTD* 1972, page 258.

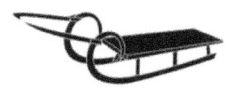

➤ Treatment

    o   IV normal saline for volume maintenance

    o   If > 38°C – acetaminphin

    o   If blood sugar- > 150 mg/dL insulin

    o   If LOC (level of consciousness) – intubation plus mechanical ventilation

    o   Hypertension
        – > 220/120 mm Hg, or (allow this level MAP > 140 mm Hg "permissive hypertension"

    o   Thrombolysis <u>not</u> planned
        – ASA 325 mg
        – DVT prophylaxis

    o   If seizure – anticonvulsion therapy
        – Target control at < 185/110 mm Hg
        – After recovery from acute event target < 140/90 mm Hg
            ▪ IV labetalol
            ▪ IV nicardipine

    o   Thrombolysis, yes
        – Ischemic (non-hemorrhagic stroke)
            ▪ Within 3h of brain onset, or
            ▪ Within 3h of last time patient known to be well, or
            ▪ Within 4.5 h in patient
               > 80 yr
               severe stroke
               diabetic, with previous stroke

No rtPA

    o   Intracerebral hemorrhage (now, or in the past)

    o   Seizure with stroke

    o   BP > 185/ > 110 mmHg

    o   Blood glucose < 50 or > 400 mg/dL

    o   INR > 1.7

    o   Platelets < 100,000/ µL

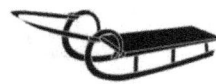

- o Time dependent, within
  2d- heparin Rx with ↑ PTT
  7d – arterial puncture at noncompressible site
  14d- major surgery/trauma
  21d- GI/GU bleeding

- o Videoflouroscopy swallowing study (VFSS)- before giving po food/fluids

- o Early stroke rehabilitation

- o Endarterctomy
  - – 24h after thrombolysis

- o ASA plus dipyridamole 48 hr after thrombolysis

- o Warfarin for associated
  - – Atrial fibrillation
  - – LA appendage thrombosis
  - – LV thrombus
  - – Cardiomyopathy, dilated with ↓ EF

Abbreviation: EF, ejection fraction; LA, left antrium; LV, left ventricle; MAP, mean arterial pressure; at PAs recombinant tissue plasminogen activator

- o Carotid endarterectomy for ipselateral carotid artery stenosis
  - – 50% t- 69% certain conditions may apply
  - – > 70%
    - ▪ If patient's life expectancy > 5yr
    - ▪ Non disabling stroke/TIN

- • A 60 year old presents in < 3 hr with symptoms suggestive of a stroke, with deficit detected on neurological examination. Her systolic blood pressure is 210/110 mmHg. Diagnostic imaging suggests a non-hemorrhagic stroke. Give the management.

  - o Immediate IV rtPA (recombinant tissue plasmogen activation, as long as there are no contraindications)

  - o After rtPA, administer labetalol to target systemic blood pressure < 180/105 mm Hg.

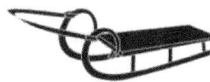

- In the patient for whom rtPA is indicated, the systemic blood pressure after IV rtPA must be < 180/105 mm Hg. Give the anti-hypertensive drug(s) of choice to maintain blood pressure < 180/105 after giving rtPA.

  - Nicardipine, or
  - Labetalol

Clinical Gem

- How to manage hypertension in the patient with an acute ischemic stroke, **not eligible for rtPA**, plus no end-organ damage.

  - Allow BP to be up to 220/120 mm Hg before treatment
  - End-organ damage: treat as appropriate
    - CNS
      - Encephalopathy
    - CVS.
      - Active CAD (coronary artery disease)
      - Aortic dissection
    - GU
      - AKI (acute kidney injury)
    - Pregnancy
      - Preeclampsia/eclampsia

- Perform urgent CT of head for CVQ / TIA to exclude intracranial/intracerebral hemorrhage.

  - Thrombolysis therapy with rtPA (recombinant tissue plasminogen activator)
    - Within
      - 3 hr of start of stroke
      - 3 hr of last time patient seen to be well
    - Unless excluded
      - Seizure with stroke
      - History
        - Intracerebral hemorrhage (ICH)
        - Ischemic stroke within 3 mon
        - Head trauma within 3 mon
        - Trauma within 3 wk
        - Bleeding (GI, GU) within 3 wk
        - Major surgery within 2 wk
        - Arterial puncture (non-compressible site within 1 wk)

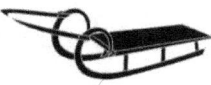

Mastering the Boards: Neurology   A.B.R. Thomson

- Heparin within 48 h, with ↑aPTT
- ↑ BP > 185/110 mm Hg
- Glucose < 50 or > 400 mg/dL
- INR > 1.7
- Platelets < 100,000 / μL

o Anti-platelet therapy within 24 hr (unless rtPA planned)
  - ASA plus dipyridamole
  - If > 220/ > 120 mm Hg, or MAP > 140 mm Hg

o Treat complications
  - Hypertension
    - IV labetalor plus IV nicardipine
    - Targets thrombolysis
      - Possible   < 185 / < 110 mm Hg
      - No possible 185 – 220 / 110-120 ("permissive hypertension") 140/90 after acute episode
  - Blood sugar
  - Fever
  - Maintain normal volume

o Anti-coagulation therapy (DVT prophylaxis) within 48 hr (use warfarin, do not use heparin)
  - AF (artrial fibrillation)
  - LA appendage thrombus

  - LV thrombus
  - Dilate cardiomyopathy with ↑ EF

o Ipsilateral end arterectomy
  - Within 2 wk for
    - Non-disabling strokes
    - Carotid stenosis > 70%
    - Life expectancy > 5 yr

o Statin
  - Regardless of lipid level

Abbreviations: EF, ejection fraction; LA, left atrium; LV, left ventricular

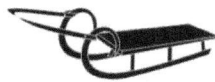

- Give what is best for **Secondary Stroke Prevention**

  o Clopidogrel is superior to ASA (aspirin) in
  - Prevention of
    - Stroke
    - Myocardial infarction (MI)
  - Death
  - In patient who has already had an
    - Ischemic stroke
    - MI
  - Who has PVD (peripheral vascular disease)

Ischemic Stroke

➤ Definition

  o Presence of cerebral infarction on imaging

  o Note: imprecise nature of definition – negative imaging does not exclude ischemic stroke

➤ Target artery atherosclerosis-associated Ischemic stroke

  o Mechanism of stroke
  - Emboli cerebral artery, or
  - ↓ local blood flow (stenosis)
  - Associated hypertension > 140 / 80 mm Hg

  o Vessels usually involved
  - Cerebral artery
    - Intracranial (ICA)
    - MCA (middle cerebral artery)
    - Vertebrobasilar arterial system

  o Risk of recurrent large artery atherosclerosis-associated stroke
  - 13% per year, especially when high degree of stenosis
  - Risk of recurrence highest in 2 wk following initial large artery atherosclerosis-associated ischemic stroke

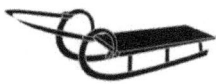

➢ Causes

Types	% of all ischemic strokes
o Cryptogenic	30%
o Subcortical infarcts, small	25%
o Cardioembolic	20%
o Large artery atherosclerosis	20%
o Others	5%

  – Cerebral artery
    ▪ Dissection
    ▪ Vasculitis

Cryptogenic stroke

  o Embolus from other than heart or large artery atherosclerosis about
    ~ ¼ have atrial fibrillation

Small subcortical infarcts (lacunae)

  o Definition: Small penetrating arteries from ACA (anterior cerebral
    artery), MCA (middle cerebral artery) or PCA (posterior cerebral
    artery) develop lipohyalinosis, usually in association with systemic
    hypertension, to cause lacunae, ischemic and small subcortical
    infarcts PCA.

  o Clinical: Depends upon which small penetrating arteries are blocked,
    and affect arterial blood flow to motor or sensory area, or areas
    affecting movement of eyes or gait.

Cardioembolic (ischemic) stroke

  o Cardiac source of emboli

- Arrhythmia	▪ Atrial fibrillation, flutter
- Intracardiac	▪ Thrombus
	▪ Tumour
- Function	▪ ↓ ejection
	▪ Fraction
- Valve	▪ Vegetation

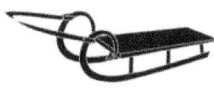

Hemorrhagic Stroke

- o Intracerebral hemorrhage (ICH; ~ 8% of all strokes)
- o Subarachnoid hemorrhage (SAH, ~ 8% of all strokes)

➢ Treatment

- o Non-contract CT head will establish major cerebral artery occlusion ischemic stroke
- o Evaluate for exclusion criteria to determine if thrombolysis is appropriate (non ICH stroke)
- o Mechanism of action of thrombolysis

$$\text{Plasminogen} \xrightarrow{\text{rtPA}} \underset{\text{fibrin}}{\text{plasmin}} \longrightarrow \text{Fibrinolysis} \longrightarrow \uparrow \begin{array}{l}\text{blood flow to ischemic/} \\ \text{non-infected brain tissue}\end{array}$$

- o Starting thrombolysis with rtPA (recombinant tissue plasminogen activator) within 3 hr recently (extended to 4.5 hr from onset of stroke) for ischemic (non-hemorrhagic) stroke improves functional outcome at 3 mon
- o Admission to ICU / stroke unit
- o Absolute IV rtPA exclusion criteria relate to high risk of bleeding from conversion of ischemic to hemorrhagic stroke:
    - Recent
        - Major surgery within 14 days
        - Systemic hemorrhage
    - Hemorrhagic stroke or possible SAH (subarachnoid hemorrhage) other stroke within 3 mon
    - Arterial puncture within 7 days at a site which cannot be compressed
    - Coagulopathy
        - ↑ PPT from heparin within 48 hr
        - INR > 1.7 platelets < 100 x 10^9 / L (< 100,000 / µL)
    - Hypertension
        - Sustained ≥ 185 / 110 mm Hg
        - Difficult to control

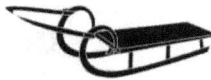

- When initially BP (blood pressure) > 185/110 mm Hg, treat with continuous IV labetalol or nicardipine infusion
  - If BP < 185 / 110 on treatment, give rtPA and continue IV labetalol or nicardipine infusion
  - If BP not controlled, or use of rtPA excluded, target control to < 220 / 120 mm Hg

---

SO YOU WANT TO BE A NEUROLOGIST!

- Give the reason why patients with an ischemic stroke who are eligible for rtPA do not have their hypertension treated to target < 185/110 mm Hg using nitroglycerin or nitroprusside, and why patient who are not eligible for rtPA have a target BP of < 220 / 120 mm Hg.
  - rtPA eligible
    - Nitroglycerin and nitroprusside may
      - ↓↓ systemic blood pressure
      - ↑ ICP (intracranial pressure)
  - rtPA ineligible
    - Target < 220 / 100 mm Hg in the hope of ↑ cerebral perfusion
  - Relative rtPA exclusion criteria relate to the stroke and the patient
    - Stroke symptoms
      - Minor
      - Rapidly improving
    - Seizure at onset
    - ↑ / ↓ blood pressure (< 2.8 or > 22.2 mmol/L; < 50 or 400 mg/dL)
    - Older age
  - Consider intra-arterial catheter thrombolysis for MCA ischemic stroke within 6 hr of onset
  - Consider endovascular treatment after IV rtPA

Intracerebral Hemorrhagic (ICH) Stroke

- Causes/associations
  - Hypertension
  - Angiopathy
  - AVM
  - Coagulopathy
  - Cocaine/alcohol use

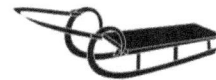

A Gem and a Pearl

- Give the commonest cause of bleeding into basal ganglia, cerebellium and thalamus

    o Hypertension

- Give the common cause of angiopathy in older people presenting with lobar hemorrhage.

    o Amyloidosis

- Perform a focused physical examination for the causes of **paraplegia**.

    o Congenital (cerebral palsy)
      - Hereditary ataxia

    o Infiltration
      - Abdominal
      - Anterior cerebral artery occlusions
      - Cord compression
      - Tumourous myelitis

    o Ischemia
      - Superior sagittal sinus thrombosis
      - Spinal artery occlusion (Erb's paraplegia)

    o Infection
      - Poliomyelitis

    o Degeneration
      - Motor neuron disease
      - Multiple sclerosis
      - Syringoyelia

    o Metabolic
      - Subacute combined degeneration

Adapted from: Burton JL. *Churchill Livingstone* 1971, page 84.

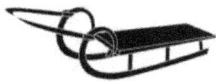

- Give the performance characteristics for **aspiration** after stroke.

Finding	PLR	NLR
o Neurologic examination		
– Drowsiness	3.4	0.5
– Absent pharyngeal sensation	2.4	0.03
o Other tests		
– Water swallow test	3.2	0.4
– Oxygen desaturation 0—2 min after swallowing	3.6	0.8

Note that several signs are not presented because their PLR was < 2: abnormal voluntary cough, dysphonia, dysarthria, abnormal sensation face and tongue, tongue weakness, bilateral cranial nerve signs, abnormal gag reflex.

Abbreviation: NS, not significant; likelihood ratio (LR) if finding present= positive LR (PLR); LR if finding absent=negative LR (NLR).

Adapted from: McGee SR. *Saunders/Elsevier* 2007, Box 56.1, page 699.

Probability

Decrease ← ⎯⎯⎯⎯⎯ Increase →

-45%	-30%	-15%		+15%	+30%	+45%	
NLR	0.1	0.2	0.5	1	2	5	10	PLR

Sen N out – <u>Sen</u>sitive test; when negative, rules <u>out</u> disease

Sp P in – <u>Sp</u>ecific test; when positive, rules <u>in</u> disease

Probability

Decrease ← ⎯⎯⎯⎯⎯ Increase →

-45%	-30%	-15%		+15%	+30%	+45%	
NLR	0.1	0.2	0.5	1	2	5	10	PLR

Sen N out – <u>Sen</u>sitive test; when negative, rules <u>out</u> disease

Sp P in – <u>Sp</u>ecific test; when positive, rules <u>in</u> disease

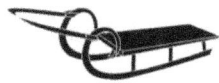

- Perform a focused physical examination to determine the site of pathology causing a person's motor defect.

Localizing Features of Motor Lesions

o Cerebral cortex	– Flaccid weakness – Flexors and extensors equally affected ("global weakness") – Cortical sensory loss may be present
o Internal capule	– Spastic weakness. – Hemianopia – Extensors more affected than flexors. – Distal limb muscles more affected than proximal muscles. Arm is greater than leg, if leg is greater than arm, suspect ant. Cerebral stem – Paralysis of head and eye movements so that patient looks away from the weak limbs
o Brain Stem	– Crossed hemiplegia, i.e., ipsilateral cranial nerve palsy with contralateral limb palsy. – Flaccid
o Cord lesion	– Flexors more affected than extensors – Lower motor neurone lesion
o Root & Peripheral Nerve	– Peripheral nerve lesions usually affect both motor and sensory function in muscles and skin supplied by the nerve. The following is a rough guide to the muscles supplied by clinically important motor nerve roots

C5 & 6	
C7 & 8	Biceps, deltoid
C7	Triceps

Localizing Features of Motor Lesions

C8	Finger extensors
T1	Finger flexors
L2 & 3	Small muscles of hand
L3 & 4	Adductors
L4 & 5	Quadriceps
L5 & S1	Dorsi flexors
S1 & 2	Hamstrings

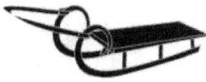

- Perform a focused physical examination to determine the location of lesions causing **sensory loss**.

Location of Lesion	Distribution of Sensory Loss	Examples of Causes
o Cortical (parietal)	– Able to recognize all primary modalities but localizes them poorly – Loss of secondary modalities	▪ Stroke, cerebral tumour, trauma
o Brainstem	– Pain and temperature: ipsilateral face, contralateral body	▪ Demyelination (young), brainstem stroke (older)
o Thalamic sensory loss	– All modalities; contralateral hemisensory loss (face, body) and pain –dysesthesia (e.g., burning feeling)	▪ Stroke, cerebral tumour, MS, trauma
o Spinal cord	– Depends on level of lesion and complete vs.. partial lesion	▪ Trauma, spinal cord compression by tumour, cervical spondylitis, MS
o Root or roots	– Confined to single root or roots in close proximity; commonly C5, 6,7 in arm and L4, 5, S1 in leg	▪ Compression by disc prolapse
o Peripheral nerve	– Distal glove and stocking deficit	▪ Diabetes mellitus, alcohol related B12 deficiency, drugs
o Single nerve	– Within distribution of single nerve; commonly median, ulnar, peroneal, lateral cutaneous nerve to the thigh	▪ Entrapment, most commonly in diabetes, mellitus, carpal tunnel syndrome, rheumatoid arthritis, and hypothyroidism; multiple (mononeuritis multiplex) = vasculitis
o Multiple nerves	– Mononeuritis – Multiplex, from involvement of multiple nerves	▪ Vasculitis

Abbreviations: MS, multiple sclerosis

Adapted from: Filate W, et al. *The Medical Society, Faculty of Medicine, University of Toronto* 2005, Table 16, page 168.

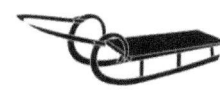

Mastering the Boards: Neurology   A.B.R. Thomson

XX

SO YOU WANT TO BE A NEUROLOGIST!

- From the physical examination, give how would you be able to differentiate between an obstruction of Heubner (medial striate) artery, and a more distal occlusion of the anterior cerebral artery?

    o Obstruction of Heubner artery (anterior damage to the limb of internal capsule and extrapyramidal nuclei)
        - Contralateral weakness and spasticity in the upper body
    o Obstruction of ACA
        - Contralateral flaccid weakness of the leg

XXXXXXXXXXXXXXXXXXXXXXXXXXXXXXXXXXXXXXXXXXXXXXXXXXXXXXXXXXXX

➤ Diagnosis
   o CT brain
   o Cerebral angiography for young (<45 yr) users of cocaine with ICH (↑ risk of associated vascular abnormalities)

➤ Diagnostic imaging

- Give the circumstances when computed tomography (CT) or magnetic resonance imaging (MRI) are preferred for neurologic Imaging

CT	MRI
o Suspected acute hemorrhage	– Subacute & chronic hemorrhage
o Skull fractures	– Ischemic stroke
o Meningiomas	– Posterior fossa & brainstem Tumour & lesion
o Hydrocephalus	– Diagnosis of multiple sclerosis
	– Evaluation of spinal cord

Abbreviation: SSRI, selective serotonin reuptake inhibitor

Adapted from: Ghosh AK. *Mayo Clinic Scientific Press* 2008, page 749.

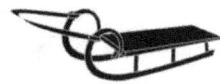

Mastering the Boards: Neurology   A.B.R. Thomson

```
╳╳╳╳╳╳╳╳╳╳╳╳╳╳╳╳╳╳╳╳╳╳╳╳╳╳╳╳╳╳╳╳╳╳╳╳╳╳╳╳╳╳╳╳╳╳╳╳╳
```

SO YOU WANT TO BE A NEUROLOGIST!

- Give the neurological conditions in which bladder disturbances are rare.
  - o Motor neuron disease
  - o Subacute combined degeneration
  - o Peripheral neuritis
  - o Extrapyramidal disease

```
╳╳╳╳╳╳╳╳╳╳╳╳╳╳╳╳╳╳╳╳╳╳╳╳╳╳╳╳╳╳╳╳╳╳╳╳╳╳╳╳╳╳╳╳╳╳╳╳╳
```

SO YOU WANT TO BE A NEUROLOGIST!

The signs of the foramen magnum pressure cone is caused by increased pressure in the foramen magnum.
- Give the bony conditions which may mimic
  - o Invagination of the base of the stull into the upper cervical spine, from
    - Congenital anomaly
    - Osteomalacia
    - Paget's disease
  - o Fusion of the cervical vertebrae
    - Congenital anomaly (aka Klippel-Feil deformity)

- Give what dysarthrias may be of psychological origin?

  - o Stuttering and stammering

```
╳╳╳╳╳╳╳╳╳╳╳╳╳╳╳╳╳╳╳╳╳╳╳╳╳╳╳╳╳╳╳╳╳╳╳╳╳╳╳╳╳╳╳╳╳╳╳╳╳
```

  - o Involvement of basal ganglia/cerebellum
    - High association with hypertension, especial in Asians
  - o Surface of the brain
    - Cerebral amyloid angiopathy, or
    - Hypertension

- ➤ Treatment
  - o Stop/reverse anticoagulation
  - o IV factor VII a
    - ↓ enlargement
    - No ↑ function/survival

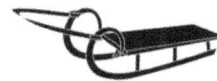

Mastering the Boards: Neurology   A.B.R. Thomson

- o ↓ ICP (intracranial pressure)
  - – IV manitol
  - – Hyperventilation
  - – Barbituarate coma
- o Central systemic blood pressure (SBP, 140-160 m Hg; MAP, 70-130 mm Hg)
  - – Labetalol
  - – Nicardipine
  - – Nitroprusside
- o Drainage
  - – Untraventricular
    - ventricles
  - – Cerebillar
    - posterior fossa

Intracranial Hemorrhage

➢ Treatment
- o Control of blood pressure (BP)
  - – > 180 / 130 > 200 / 150 mm Hg
    - IV labetalor or nicardipine → target
    - BP to 160/90
    - MAP to 110
- o If signs of ↑ ICP (intracranial pressure) develop when BP is controlled, consider possibility of
  - – Hematoma
  - – Edema
  - – Extension of blood into ventricles

Hydrocephalus

- o Stabilize intubate hyperventilate osmotherapy
  - – Ventricular surgery shunt
  - – Evacuation of hematoma > 30 mL
- o Repeat imaging 4 to 6 wk after ICH to exclude Tumour, infection, vascular malformation
  - – Mortality rate ICH > ischemic stroke

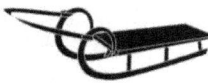

Subarachnoid Hemorrhagic (SAH) Stroke

Aneurysms > 7mm, particularly with posterior circulation where the risk of rupture is higher, requires surgical resection

➢ Causes of SAH

   o   Berry aneurysm, circle of Willis

   o   Arterovenous malformation (AVM)

   o   Dissection of cerebral artery

   o   Coagulopathy

   o   Use of cocaine

- Give 4 causes of sudden severe headache, in addition to SAH (subarachnoid hemorrhage)

   o   Intercerebral hemorrhage (ICN)

   o   Hypertensive crisis

   o   Arterial dissection

   o   Venous senses thrombosis

   o   Pituitary hemorrhafe (apoplexy)

CLINICAL PEARL

- Give the role of fundoscopy to diagnose suspected subarachnoid hemorrhage (SAH).

   o   The presence of subhyaloid hemorrhage (bleeding under the vitreous membrane is suggestive of SAH)

➢ Clinical suspicion

   o   Sudden, severe headache

   o   Focal neurological changes
       -   blood
       -   vacospasm

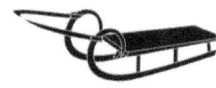

- o Pupil
  - – Unilateral dilated pupil
  - – Subhyaloid bleeding
- o Commonly associated with
  - – Severe headache
  - – Subhyaloid bleeding
  - – Focal neurological deficits
- o Performance characteristics of clinical features

Finding	PLR	NLR
– Neck stiffness	10.3	0.4
– Neurological findings not focal	5.9	0.4
– Seizures	2.2	NS

- o Mortality rate: SAH > ICH > ischemic stroke

Abbreviation: NS, not significant; NLR, negative likelihood ratio; PLR, positive likelihood ratio

Adapted from: McGee SR. *Saunders/Elsevier* 2007, Table 23.1, page 281.

- • Give the complication of SAH (subarachnoid hemorrhage) which becomes a risk factor on day 5 (day 2, rebleeding from aneurysm, and hydrocephalus), and give its diagnosis and treatment.

  - o Day 5 after SAH
    - – Cerebral arterial vasospasm
    - – May lead to cerebral infarction

  - o Diagnosis
    - – CT angiography

  - o Treatment
    - – Reduce hypertension
    - – Intra-arterial CCB (calcium channel blocker)
    - – Angioplasty to ↓ spasm of artery in question

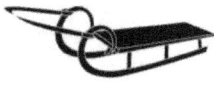

➤ Pathogenesis

  o Berry (saccular) aneurysm of the circle of Willis

  o Acute rupture of secular aneurysm of cerebral artery

  o If CT head negative, perform LP (lumbar puncture) for RBC, RBC-breakdown (xanthochromia)

➤ Diagnosis

  o Angiography, including CTA (CT angiogram)

  o CT (without contrast) is diagnostic in > 90%, and a
     – Positive CT is followed by
        ▪ Cerebral angiography
     – Negative CT is followed by
        ▪ Lumbar puncture
        ▪ RBCs
        ▪ Xanthochroma

  o Saccular aneurysm at major arterial bifurcation

  o Vasospams
     – Cerebral ischemia

                                    90% white density (blood)

  o CT or
  o Angiography (conventional)

                                    10% negative
                                    CSF to → RBC/xanthochromia

• Give the treatable risk factors for stroke, attention to which may ↓ risk of first stroke (primary prevention).

o Habit	– Use of	
		▪ Tobacco
		▪ Cocaine
	– Obesity	
o Heart	– Hypertension	
	– Atrial fibrillation	
o Endocrine	– Diabetes	
	– Dyslipidemia	
o Drugs	- Poorly controlled anti-coagulation	

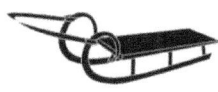

Mastering the Boards: Neurology   A.B.R. Thomson

➤ Treatment

o Early surgical clipping/coiling

o Complications
- Vasospasm nimodipine, 3 wks, to ↓ risk of vasospasm
- Rebleeding ⎫   urgent CT
- Hydrocephalus ⎭ → drain ventricles

Hemorrhagic Versus Ischemic Stroke

o Note – the specificity of the clinical examination for hemorrhagic stroke is sufficiently low, that the **diagnosis** of ischemic vs.. hemorrhagic stroke should be made by diagnostic imaging and not by clinical examination
- CT head, then
- MRI, brain
  ▪ Early images   - Infarction
  ▪ Later   - Vasogenic edema
            - Micro-hemorrhages

Just for olde-tyme clinical examinate forte, take a directed history and perform a focused physical examination for features which suggests that a stroke is hemorrhagic, rather than ischemic.

o History   - Seizure
       - Vomiting
       - Headache

o Physical - Coma
       - Meningism
       - DBP > 110 mm Hg

Abbreviation: DBP, diastolic blood pressure

➤ Treatment

o External shunting of CSF (cerebrospinal fluid)

o Control of
- Hypertension (systemic)
- ↑ intracranial pressure;
  ▪ Surgery ventricular drainage

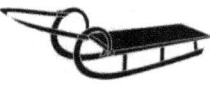

- Cerebral edema
- Vasospasm nimodipine to ↓ vasospasm and ↑ blood flow
- Nimodipine
  - 21 days
  - For post-SAH vasospasm, stroke
- Ischemia systemic vasopressor

- Surgery (cliporcoil) within 48-72 hr

- Small, unruptured aneurysm
  - Follow up

Abbreviation: ICP, intracerebral pressure

XXXXXXXXXXXXXXXXXXXXXXXXXXXXXXXXXXXXXXXXXXXXXXXXXXXXXXXXXXXXXXXXXXX

SO YOU WANT TO BE A NEUROLOGIST!

- Many conditions may increase intracranial pressure (e.g. hemorrhagic stroke, brain abscess or tumour with cerebral), and cause "coning" (nastral-candal herniation of the uncus of the temporal lobe, followed by compression of the brainstem). Your question: give the signs which display the layer-by-layer loss of function which occur with the progression of coning.

  o Ipsilateral cerebral posturing
    - Decortication, then
    - Decerebration

  o Loss of painful stimuli

  o Ipsilateral dilated pupil

  o Ipsilateral loss of oculo cephalic reflex ("doll's head")

  o Corneal reflex tests become positive

  o Contralateral paratonic muscle resistance, and positive contralateral plantar extensor ("Babinski") reflex.

Source: Mangione S. *Hanley & Belfus* 2000, page 429.

XXXXXXXXXXXXXXXXXXXXXXXXXXXXXXXXXXXXXXXXXXXXXXXXXXXXXXXXXXXXXXXXXXX

XXXXXXXXXXXXXXXXXXXXXXXXXXXXXXXXXXXXXXXXXXXXXXXXXXXXXXXXXXXXXXXXXXX

A TRICK QUESTION FOR THE "WANTABE" NEUROLOGIST!

- Give the only non-surgical intervention which decreases the mortality at 1 yr to yr 10 from stroke.

  o Admission to multi-disciplinary stroke centre

XXXXXXXXXXXXXXXXXXXXXXXXXXXXXXXXXXXXXXXXXXXXXXXXXXXXXXXXXXXXXXXXXXX

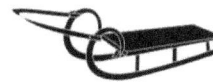

Secondary Prevention of Stroke

o   Physical and occupational therapy may contribute to benefit of stroke units, and general patient well-being.

o   Smoking cessation

o   Hypertension-controlled to < 140/80 mm Hg

o   Dyslipidemia
-   Statin therapy if LDL-C > 2.59 mmol/L (> 100 mg/dL)

o   Warfarin/anti-thrombotic (ASA, clopidogrel)

    –   Stroke from intracranial atherosclerosis (large vessel stroke)
        ▪   ASA, 325 mg/d
    -   Give ASA within 48 hr of onset of stroke
    -   For TIA or stroke in association with AF (atrial fibrillation)
    -   Possibly also for intracardiac thrombus
    -   Use heparin in setting of acute ischemic stroke only
    -   For stroke from AF (atrial fibrillation) after cardiac surgery
    -   For stroke associated with mechanical heart valve
    -   Cervicocephalic arterial dissections

    –   Aortic arch atheroma

    –   Warfarin, or anti-platelet agents

    –   Atrial fibrillation (AF) plus
        ▪   Recurrent falls
        ▪   Previous ICH

o   Small vessel stroke, or cryptogenic stroke
-   ASA, or warfarin

o   Recurrent ischemic stroke
-   Clopidogrel, or
-   ASA plus dipyridamole

o   Stroke prevention without AF
-   ASA 81 mg/d

o   Stroke prevention plus PVD (peripheral arterial disease)
-   Clopidogrel

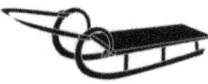

SURGERY

Carotid Revascularization for Intracranial Carotid Artery (ICA) **Atherosclerosis**

- o Risk of recurrence of stroke
  - Symptomatic
    - \> 70% stenosis of ICA is associated with 2.6% risk of recurrent stroke
  - Asymptomatic
    No carotid revascularization unless Doppler ultrasound shows
    - No vasodilation with CO_2
    - Signs of microemboli
- o Similar beneficial outcome with
  - Angioplasty and stenting
  - Carotid end arterectomy
- o Perioperative complications different for these two procedures
  - Angioplasty and stenting
    - ↑ risk of stroke
  - Carotid end arterectomy
    - ↑ risk of MI (myocardial infarction)

Hemicraniectomy

- o MCA (middle cerebral artery) ischemic infarctions (> 50% of MCA perfusion area) cause marked brain damage and herniation
- o Hemicraniectomy performed within 48 hr of stroke causes ↓ mortality and severe morbidity (76% → 25%)

Closure of patient foramen ovale (PFO)

- o Closure of PFO is equivalent to ASA plus warfarin to ↓ risk of recurrent ischemic stroke
  - Treat conditions associated with worsening of stroke
- o Mechanisms
  - Extension of territory of ischemia
  - Additional stroke
  - Conversion of ischemic to hemorrhagic stroke
    - Do not treat hypertension while using rtPTA

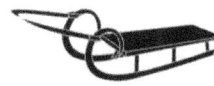

Mastering the Boards: Neurology   A.B.R. Thomson

- o Associated conditions
  - Seizure
  - Sedation excess
  - Infection
    - UTI (urinary tract infection)
    - Pneumonia (aspiration)
  - Hypoglycemia/diabetes
  - Cardiac
    - HF (heart failure)
    - Myocardial infarction
    - Arrhythmia
    - Hypertension
    - Cardiomyopathy
  - DVT 9deep vein thrombosis)
  - PE (pulmonary embolus)
  - MSK
    - Falls
  - CNS
    - Depression
    - ↓ cognition

- Give the conditions associated with the increased risk of **perioperative stroke** after types of surgery.

Type of surgery	Cause of ↑ risk	Type of stroke
o Cardiothoracic surgery	- Post-operative • Atrial fibrillation • Hypotension	Ischemic
o Valve replace	- Pre-existing symptomatic carotid artery disease - CABG (coronary artery bypass graft)	Ischemic
o Aortic grafting	- Aortic dissection	Spinal cord

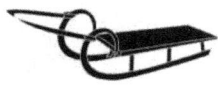

➢ Long-term prognosis

• Give the patient's clinical picture 6 months after CVA.

Clinical picture	~ % of survivors
o Functional independence	50
o Hemeparesis	50
o Require assistance to walk	40
o Incontinence (bladder)	30
o Aphasia	20
o Institutional care	20

• Give the main factor which predicts best the long-term disability of the stroke survivor.

    o The severity of the initial neurological deficit

➢ Treatment (intracerebral hemorrhage)
    o IV factor VIIa to reduce early enlargement of hemorrhage
    o Manage associated
      – Hypertension
      – Anticoagulation
      – Abuse of alcohol, cocaine
    o Maintain SBP (systolic blood pressure) 140 to 160 mm Hg (MAP 70 to 130 mm Hg)
      – IV
        ▪ Labetalol
        ▪ Nicardipine
        ▪ Nitropusside
    o Correct ↑ ICP (intracranial pressure) bleeding
      – Intraventricular
        ▪ Drain
      – Cerebellar
        ▪ Drain posterior fossa
      – Do not use corticosteroids to ↓ ICP

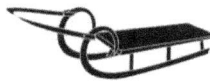

Carotid Bruit and Stenosis

➤ The presence of a carotid bruit increases the likelihood of a 70-99% carotid stenosis:

Patient	Ipsilateral Bruit		
o Asymptomatic	Yes	4.0-10.0	PPV 22%
	No	Uncertain	
o Symptomatic*	Yes	3.0 (1.3-7.1)	PPV 50%
	No	0.49 (0.36-0.67)	

*Carotid-territory cerebrovascular symptoms.
- The presence of a carotid bruit cannot be used to rule it stenosis, nor can its absence be used to rule it out (JAMA, Chapter 9, page 109).

Abbreviations: CB, carotid bruit; PPV, positive predictive value; TIA, transient ischemic attack

Source: Simel DL, et al. *JAMA* 2009, Table 9-5 and 9-6, page 110.

Transient Ischemic Attack (TIA)

➤ Definition: "……. a transient deficit resulting from focal brain spinal cord or retinal ischemia without acute infarction" (defined now on basis of diagnostic imaging , i.e., brain MRI or CT head diffusion-weighted imaging)

  o A TIA is a stroke syndrome with neurological symptoms lasting from a few minutes to as long as 24 hours followed by complete functional recovery. A RIND (reversible ischemic neurological deficit) is a condition in which a person has neurological abnormalities similar to acute completed stroke, but the deficit disappears after 14 to 36 hours, leaving few or no detectable neurological sequelae.

➤ Clinical
  o The symptoms include:
    - Intention tremor (29%)
    - Hypotonia
    - Dysdiadochokinesia (47-69%)
    - Arm drift (44-69%)
    - Rebound
    - Balance
      ▪ Rhomberg test, Pull test
      ▪ Gait- Normal gait, Toe walking, Heel walking, Tandem gait, Ataxia
      ▪ Reflexes reduced

Values in brackets represent mean or range of common findings.

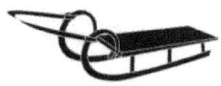

Adapted from: Jugovic PJ, et al. *Saunders/ Elsevier* 2004, page 165; Talley NJ, et al. *Maclennan & Petty Pty Limited* 2003, page 431; McGee SR. *Saunders/Elsevier* 2007,Table 61.1, page 198.

- o The importance of recognizing and treating TIA is to **prevent progression** to a stroke or a new vascular event
- o Useful statistics for the person with TIA
  - 25% risk of a new vascular event
    - Another TIA
    - Stroke (in about 40% of ischemic strokes, there is a preceeding TIA)
    - Death
  - 10% risk of stroke at 3 mon

- o **Risk stratification** of TIAs-ABCD^2 Scoring System

Risk of stroke by day 2	Score
0-1	0%
2-3	1.3%
4-5	4.1%
6-7	8.1%

- o Admission to hospital
  - ABCD^2 score ≥ 3, or
  - Transient monocular blindness, regardless of score

- Take a directed history of differentiated between a carotid or vertebrobasilar transient ischemic attack (TIA).

➢ Carotid TIA
  - o Hemiparesis
  - o Aphasia or transient loss of vision in only one eye (amaurosis fugax)

➢ Vertebrobasilar TIA
  - o Vertigo, dysphagia, ataxia, drop attacks (at least two of these should occur together)
  - o Bilateral or alternating weakness or sensory symptoms
  - o Sudden bilateral blindness in patients aged over 40 years

Source: Baliga RR. *Saunders/Elsevier* 2007, page 122.

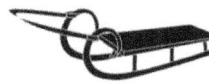

Internal Carotid and Vertebral Artery Dissection

- Pathology
  - Vessels
    - Extracranial
      - Internal carotid artery
    - Intracranial
      - Vertebral artery
  - Hematoma develops in tunica media layers of arteries
  - Dissection → thrombus → artery-to-artery embolism → ischemia, mass effect
- Clinical
  - Unilateral pain in eye, head, neck
  - Ipsilateral
    - Monocular Δ vision
    - Horner syndrome
  - Contralateral
    Muscle weakness and numbness
- Diagnosis
  - MRA
    Irregularity of artery
    Crescent-shaped hematoma
- Treatment
  - Heparin, followed by ASA for 6 mon

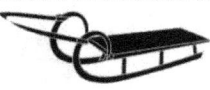

BODY TEMPERATURE DISORDERS

- Give the characterisitcs of disorders of body temperature.

Diagnosis	Characteristics
o Heat Cramps	– Core body temperature is normal; skin is moist and cool – Occurs in muscles following vigorous exercise in the heat – Caused by salt depletion from excess sweating combined with hypotonic fluid replacement, resulting in dilutional hyponatremia

o Heat Exhaustion	– Core body temperature is minimally increased and is between 37°C and 40°C
	– Consequence of salt and water losses
	– Symptoms:
	  ▪ Muscle cramps
	  ▪ Diaphoresis
	  ▪ Headache
	  ▪ Nausea / Vomiting
	  ▪ Orthostatic syncope

o Heat Stoke	– Core body temperature ≥40.6°C
	– *Classic*: develops over several days during heat waves and affects primarily the elderly or those suffering from chronic illness
	– *Exertional*: occurs acutely with workers, endurance athletes or soldiers submitted to conditions of high heat and humidity without appropriate access to salt and water
	– Signs and symptoms:
	  ▪ Dehydration
	  ▪ No smoking
	  ▪ Central nervous system dysfunction (delirium, seizure, coma)
	  ▪ Hot, dry skin
	– Complications:
	  ▪ Disseminated intravascular coagulation (DIC)
	  ▪ Rhabdomyolysis
	  ▪ Renal failure (acute)
	  ▪ Seizures
	  ▪ Permanent neurologic damage
	– Treatment (supportive care, as needed)
	  ▪ Cooling
	  ▪ IV fluids
	  ▪ O_2
	  ▪ Benzodiazepines for shivering

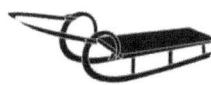

Mastering the Boards: Neurology   A.B.R. Thomson

Diagnosis	Characteristics

o Malignant Hyperthermia

- Drug-induced reaction characterized by genetic susceptibility (family history) to generalized and sustained skeletal muscle contraction after exposure to depolarizing muscle relaxants such as succinylcholine or volatile anesthetic agents, such as halothane or isoflurane
- Sustained muscle contraction and increased metabolism result in
  - Hyperthermia
  - Metabolic acidosis
  - Increased serum creatine kinase (CK)
- Duchenne disease and myotonic muscular dystrophy have been associated with an increased incidence of malignant hyperthermia
- Family history
- History of exposure to anesthetics
- Treatment: Dantrolene (plus supportive measures)

o Neuroleptic Malignant Syndrome (NMS)

- Drug-induced idiosyncratic reaction (dopamine D2 receptor antagonist) characterized by
  - Hyperthermia
  - Altered mentation
  - Muscle rigidity
  - Autonomic instability (e.g.,cardiac arrhythmias)
- Drugs implicated are most often
  - Haloperidol
  - Fluphenazine
  - L-dopa cessation (sudden)
  - Phenothiazines (e.g.,chlorpromazine) and butyrophenones (e.g.,haloperidol)
  - Withdrawal of a dopaminergic agent (e.g.,levodopa) resulting in reduced central dopamine neurotransmission
  - Treatment
    - Dantrolene (plus supportive measures)

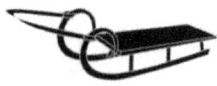

Diagnosis	Characteristics

o Serotonin syndrome	– SSRI (serotonin reuptake inhibitor) plus MAO (monoamine oxidase) inhibitor
	– Serotoninergic medication
	– History of use of SSRIs
	  ▪ ↑ dose
	  ▪ Adding second medication which causes ↑ dose effect
	
	– Unique signs in a hyperthermic patient
	  ▪ Shivering
	  ▪ Myoclonus
	  ▪ Confusion
	  ▪ ↑ reflexes
	  ▪ Myoclonus
	  ▪ Ataxia
	– Treatment
	  ▪ Supportive measures, as per heat stroke

Reproduced with permission: Therapeutics Choices. Sixth Edition. Ottawa, Canada: *Canadian Pharmacist Association* 2012, Table 1, page 187.

Neuroleptic Malignant Syndrome (NMS)

➤ Definition: Neuroleptic malignant syndrome (NMS) is a drug-induced, idiosyncratic serious medical emergency which can occur at any dose of antipsychotics, and is characterized by

- o Autonomic dysfunction
  - Fever (hyperthermia)
  - Labile blood pressure
  - Sweating
  - Tachycardia (> 100 bpm)
  - Extrapyramidal signs
    - Rigidity
    - Dystonia, and
    - Elevated muscle enzyme levels
- o Varying level of consciousness
- o Dehydration
- o Leucocytosis
- o ↑ CK (creatine kinase)
- o Delirium

Source: MKSAP 16 2012, Neurology, page 56)

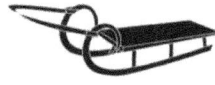

- ➤ Cause/association
  - ○ Therapeutic doses of D2 receptor blockers
- ➤ Clinical
  - ○ In the context of psychosis, perform a focused physical examination for NMS (neuroleptic malignant syndrome).
- ➤ Treatment
  - ○ ABC's of supportive care
  - ○ Bromocriptine (D2 [dopamine] agonist)
  - ○ Dantrolene (torelax muscle contractions)
  - ○ Note: receiving the D2 receptor blocker which caused the NMS may or may not precipitate the disorder

"The future will bring personalized medicine based on genetics."

Grandad

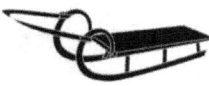

ALTERED LEVEL OF CONCIOUSNESS (LOC)

To be covered here

- o Coma
- o Delirium
- o Syncope
- o Confusion
- o Dizziness
- o Fainting

- Give the common causes of syncope

  - o Volume depletion and drugs
    - – Volume depletion
      - Diarrhea
      - Diminished oral intake
      - Polyuria
    - – Drugs
      - ACE inhibitors
      - Alcohol
      - Alpha- and beta-adrenergic blockers
      - Antiparkinsonian drugs
      - Diuretics
      - Nitrates
      - Phosphodiesterase type 5 inhibitors (sildenafil, tadalafil, vardenafil)
      - Vasodilators

  - o Orthostatic intolerance disorders
    - – Reflex syncope syndromes
      - Carotid sinus hypersensitivity
      - Vasovagal syncope syndromes
    - – Autonomic neuropathies
      - Pure autonomic failure syndromes
      - Multiple system atrophy syndromes

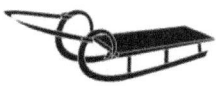

- o Arrhythmias
  - – Bradycardias
    - Complete (third degree) and bifasicular heart block
    - Sinus node disease
  - – Tachycardias
    - Supraventricular arrhythmias (uncommon)
    - Torsades de pointes polymorphic ventricular tachycardia
    - Ventricular tachycardia

- o Obstruction
  - – Aortic stenosis
  - – Pulmonary emboli
  - – Many other rare causes

Reproduced with permission: Therapeutics Choices. Sixth Edition. Ottawa, Canada: *Canadian Pharmacist Association* 2012, Table 1, page 597.

"Mediocrity is metric modulation-bringing people back (regression) to the mean."

Anonymous

 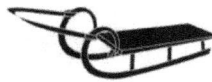

TRAUMA / HEAD INJURY

Traumatic Brain Injury (TBI)

➢ Approach
  o Diagnostic imaging
    – Acute injury
      ▪ CT head, using bone windows 9skull fracture, hematoma
    – Chronic
      ▪ MRI of head (parenchymal changes)
  o Access severity
    – Using Glasgon Coma Scale (GCS)
  o Post-concussion syndrome
  o Epidural and subdural hematoma

Concussion

➢ Definition
  o Closed head trauma-induced alteration in mental status +/- LOC (loss of consciousness)

Grade	Confusion	Amnesia	LOC*	Duration, min	Abnormalities > 1 wk need for CT head / MRI brain
1	+	-	-	< 15	-
2	+	+	-	> 15	+
3	+	+	+	Brief – seconds	+
				Prolonged - minutes	

*LOC, level of consciousness

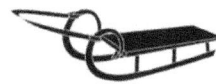

Mastering the Boards: Neurology   A.B.R. Thomson

✕✕✕

CLINICAL CHALLENGE

- Perform a focused neurological examination of a 12 year old hockey enthusiast who is hit in the head and demonstrates confusion.

  - Cognition (MOL) – Memory
  - – Orientation
  - – Language

  - Vision (AVE) – Acuity
  - – Visual fields
  - – Eye movements

  - Gait – Atagia
  - – Extremities

✕✕✕

➢ Treatment

- Give the management of the above hockey player if s/he has a neurological examination suggestive a concussion.

Action	1	2	Stage 3-Brief (seconds)	Stage 3-Prolonged Minutes	Stage 3-Second Occurrence
○ Remove from game	+	+	+	+	+
○ Examine					
– Immediately	+	+	Neuro' exam' normal-home observation	ER for CT / MRI	ER for CT / MRI
– 5 min intervals	+	+			
○ Remove from game if symptoms clear in < 15 min	-	+	+	+	+
○ Second concussion of similar grade on same day, remove from game	+	+	+	+	+
○ No competition until asymptomatic					
– For weeks					
▪ 1 concussion	1	1	1	2	4
▪ 2 concussion	1	2			
– Return to baseline ImPACT			+	+	+

Abbreviation: ImPACT, Immediate post-concussion assessment and cognitive testing (neurocognitive assessment)

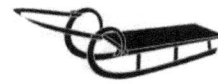

Mastering the Boards: Neurology   A.B.R. Thomson

Post-Concussion Syndrome (PCS)

➢ Causes/associations

    o Concussion

        – Closed head injury

    o "Whiplash"

        – Extension-flexion injury to cervical spine

Within 2 weeks of the head injury, the hockey player develops symptoms of headache.

➢ Clinical

• Take a directed history for PCS (post-concussion syndrome)

o Pain	– Headache	
	– Neck pain	
o Neurological symptoms	– Eyes	▪ Blurring vision
		▪ Diplopa
		▪ Light sensitivity
	– Ears	▪ Dizziness
		▪ Vertigo
		▪ Ringing (tinnitus)
		▪ Noise sensitivity
	– Taste/smell loss	
	– Memory/concentration loss	
o Psychological	– Anxiety	
	– Depression	
	– Irritability	
o Somatic	– ↓ appetite	
	– ↓ energy	
	– Sleep disorder	▪ Insomnia
		▪ Hypersomnia
	– ↓ libido	

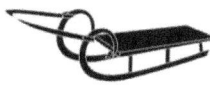

Coma

- ➢ Definition
  - ○ Coma is a leading to a state of unarousable unresponsiveness (BB 2013, page 240)
  - ○ Condition in which there is diffuse, bilateral dysfunction of the cortex due to disease in either the cortex or in the reticularis activating system (RAS) in the brainstem.
  - ○ Loss of response to external stimulation, which may progress to irreversible brain damage

- ➢ Terms
  - ○ Coma "a state of unrousable unresponsiveness" Board Basics, 2012, page 240
    - – Multiple causes, some potentially reversible
  - ○ Common plus meningism
    - – Meningitis, memengecephalitis
    - – Subarachnoid hemorrhage (SAH)
  - ○ Coma plus focal signs
    - – Stroke- ICH- Tumour-abscess
  - ○ Coma plus
    - – Brain stem function, and sleep-wake cycles
    - – Vegetative state
    - – Quadriplegic, mute, vertical eye movement intact
    - – "locked-in" state pontine infarction hemorrhage
  - ○ Coma plus **no** brain stem function, plus apnea
    - – "brain dead"

A Matter of "Life or Death"

Presense of respiratory drive (no apnea) plus "motor posturing signs" (brain stem function) excludes brain death.

Board Basics, 2012, 241

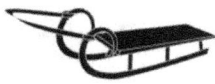

- ➢ Causes
  - o Inherited (inborn errors of metabolism)
  - o Infection
  - o Ischemia
  - o Introgenic drugs and toxins
  - o Metabolic

  - o Damage to both cerebral hemispheres
  - o Damage to one cerebral hemisphere plus damage to reticular activating system (RAS) in brain stem
  - o Damage to RAS
  - o Thalamus (first and upper most)
    - Response to painful stimulus to supraorbital ridge, nail bed, or to the sterna
    - Decorticate posture
      - Mild dysfunction of thalamus
      - Ipsilateral arms
        - Flexon ipsilateral
      - Legs
        - Extension
        - Internal rotation (de-cor-tication hand points to heart [cor])
    - Decerebratic posture
      - Moderately severe dysfunction of thalamus
      - Arms
        - Ipsilatteral extension
      - Legs
        - Ipsilateral extension
        - Internal rotation
    - Severe thalamic damage
      - No response to painful stimulation, or
      - Bending of knees from a spinal reflex

Source: Mangione S. *Hanley & Belfus* 2000, page 422.

- ➢ Definition of brain death
  - o Coma
  - o Apnea
  - o No brainstem reflexes

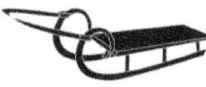

- Perform a focused physical examination for coma (determine Glasgow coma scale [GCS]).

Response	Score
o Eye opening	
– Spontaneous	4
– On your verbal command ('open your eyes')	3
– In response to painful stimulus	2
– No response	1
o Motor response	
– Correct response to 'show me two fingers'	6
– Localises painful stimulus and tries to stop it	5
– Withdraws from painful stimulus to fingernail	4
– Abnormal flexor response of forearms, wrists and fingers	3
– Abnormal extensor response of arms and legs	2
– No response	1
o Verbal response to the question: What year is this?	
– Correct year	5
– Wrong year	4
– Words but no year	3
– Incomprehensible sounds	2
– No response	1

o Total Points

Glasgow Coma Scale points	
14-15 =	5
11-13 =	4
8 - 10 =	3
5 - 7 =	2
3- 4 =	1

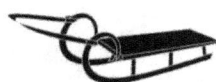

Mastering the Boards: Neurology   A.B.R. Thomson

SO YOU WANT TO BE A NEUROLOGIST!

- Give the differential diagnosis of coma (Note: NOT the differential diagnosis of the causes of coma).

  o Locked-in-state
    - Damage to junction between upper one third and lower two thirds of pons
    - No function below the pons, but there may be enough RAS function for person to be awake
    - Control of only CN III/VI (blinking eyes)

  o Hysteric coma
    - Hand dropping test, falling gently to side

  o Catatonic coma
    - Preexisting depression, in which an intercurrent major illness then leds to catatonia

Source: Mangione S. *Hanley & Belfus* 2000, page 428.

- Give the reason it is important to examine the comatous patient for brain stem reflexes.
  o The presence of brain stem reflexes suggests a vegetative state rather than brain death

- Give the methods of eliciting deep pain.

  o Abadie sign – the loss of pain sense in the Achilles tendon.

  o Biernacki sign – the absence of pain on pressure on the ulnar nerve.

  o Haenel sign – analgesia to pressure on the eyeballs.

  o Pitres sign – loss of pain on pressure on the testes.

Source: Baliga RR. *Saunders/Elsevier* 2007, page 201.

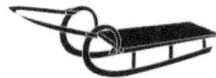

- Perform a focused physical examination to determine the cause of a patient's coma as arising from the cerebral cortex or brainstem.

  - Cortical coma
    - All layers of the brainstem are normal on examination

  - Brainstem coma (cortex is dysfunctional because of defect in reticular activating system [RAS] of brainstem)
    - Midbrain (second layer)
      - Pupillary reflex
        Midposition (neither pin-point or dilated
        Fixed (nonresponsive light, ipsilateral and contralateral)
    - Pons
      - Pupillary light reflex
        - Bilateral small pupils
        - React very slightly to light
      - Oculocephalic reflex (aka "doll's eye reflex)
        - Loss of the function of the medial longitudinal fasciculus (MLF), which connects CN III in the midbrain to CN VI in the upper pons
        - Loss of oculocephalic reflex on the ipselateral side
        - MLF is surrounded by RAS, so dysfunction of MLF is a surrogate marker to damage to the RAS. Both eyes move to the opposite side eyes fixed in midline
        - Awake
          - Rotating head
          - Loss of MLF/RAS
        - Comatose, preserved MLF /RAS
          - Rotating head
      - Corneal reflex
      - Abnormal breathing
        - Cheyne-Strokes respiration
        - Progressive increase in depth $\pm$ frequency of breathing, followed by a short interval of apnea
        - Apneustic breathing deep inspiration – breath holding – rapid expiration

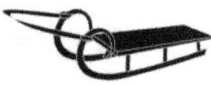

Mastering the Boards: Neurology   A.B.R. Thomson

- Medulla (fouth and lower most layer)
  - Ataxic vantillation
    - Irregular irregularity of breathing, with fluctuation and hypoventilation/apnea
  - Apnea test
    - Loss of integrity of cardiopulmonary function
    - Loss of ability to take a spontaneous breath
    - Death is associated with a loss of all brainstem function

- In the patient with no doll's eye conjugate movement on turning the head back and forth, and no eye movement towards the side irrigated with ice water, give causes other than bilateral pontive disease.

  o Prior CNS disease
    - Progressive external opthalmoplegia
  o Drugs
    - Barbiturates
    - Paralytics
    - Phenytoin

In the patient with delirium or coma, examination of the eyes for conjugate movement on turning the head from side-to-side (doll's eyes movement, oculocephalic test) is performed.
- Give the alternate test which is performed of the same patient is suspected as having traumatic injury to the cervical spine.

  o Cold calorie sculovestibular test
    - Normal
      - Eyes move to side in which ice water was placed
    - No movement
      - Suggests possible bilateral pontive lesion
    - Gaze at rest ("gaze preference")

Side relative to lesion	crossing midline	site of lesion
o Ipselateral	No	
o Contralateral	yes	Frontal lobe

  o Dysconjugate- brainstem lesion

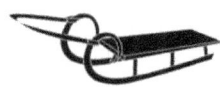

- ➢ Laboratory
  - ○ Indication
    - – Suspected infection e.g.,meningitis ⎤ ensure no signs of
    - – New symptom of headache ⎦ ↑intracranial pressure

- ➢ Diagnostic imaging
  - ○ CT of head
  - ○ MRI of head
    - – CT nondiagnostic
    - – Lesion
      - ▪ Posterior fussa
      - ▪ Ischemic
      - ▪ Parenchymal

- ➢ Functional testing EEG (electroencephalography)
  - ○ Seizure
    - – Diagnosis
    - – Typing
  - ○ PLEDs (periodic lateralized epileptiform discharges)
    - – HSV encephalitis
  - ○ Triphasic
    - – Liver
    - – Kidney
      - ▪ Hepatic ⎤ encephalopathy
      - ▪ uremia ⎦
  - ○ B activity/low voltage
    - – Drug/toxin poisoning

- ➢ Treatment
  - ○ ABCs
    - – Airway
    - – Breathing
    - – circulation

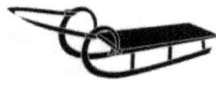

Mastering the Boards: Neurology   A.B.R. Thomson

- o Empiric management for suspected
  - – Hypoglycaemia
    - ▪ Finger prick → IV glucose plus thiamine
  - – Opiod overdose
    - ▪ IV naloxone
  - – Benzodiazepine overdose
    - ▪ flamazenil
- o CT lead
  - – Routine or for suspected
    - ▪ Abscess,communicating hydrocephalus, enhalytic temporal love edema, ICH, SAH, Tumour,
- o Urgent ECG
  - – If suspected nonconvulsive status epilepticus

Abbreviations: ICN, intracerebral hemorrhage; SAH, subarachnoid hemorrhage

Confusion

➢ Definition: Assessment of Confusion
  - o Acute onset with fluctuating course
  - o Inattention
  - o Disorganized thinking
  - o Altered level of consciousness

Function	Normal	Diencephalon	Midbrain	Pons
o Respiration	Normal	Cheyne-Stokes	Regular, hyperventilation	Irregular, erratic
o Pupil size and response to light	Normal	Small, Reactive	Mid Position, fixed	Pinpoint Reactive
o Oculo-vestibular reflex	Suppressed	Constant (tonic) deviation	Dysconjugate gaze	No response
o Motor response to pain	Appropriate	Decorticate (arms flexor response)	Decerebrate (all extensor response)	No response

Reproduced with the permission of Dr. B. Fisher, U of A

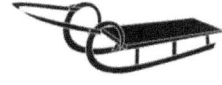

Mastering the Boards: Neurology   A.B.R. Thomson

- Give the use of the mini mental test for confusion.

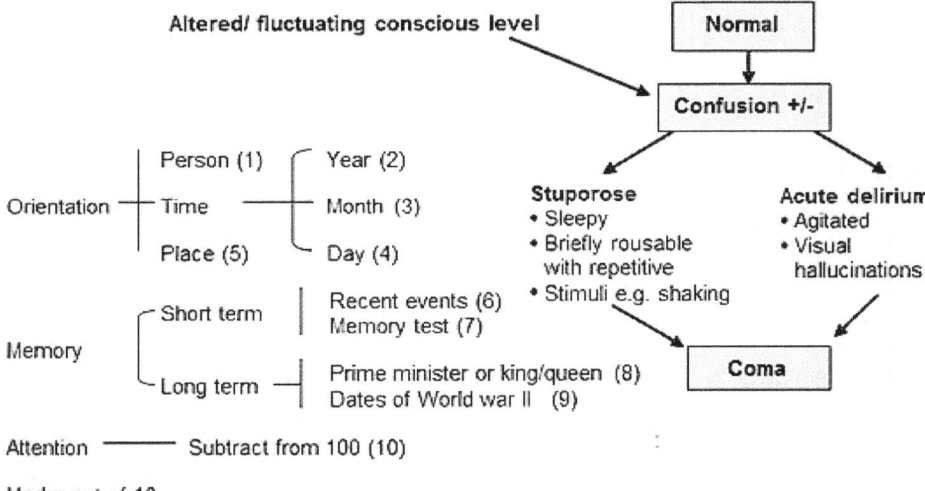

Marks out of 10

Adapted from: Davey P. *Wiley-Blackwell* 2006, page 138.

Delerium

➢ Definition

- o Acute onset and fluctuating cause of inattention, altered level of consciousness, and disorganized thinking

- o Sudden onset of
  - – Confusion
  - – Disorientation
  - – Restlessness

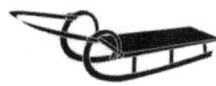

- o Rapid and often fluctuating ↓ cerebral function, associated with
  - − ↓ attention
  - − ↓ cognition
  - − ↓ level of consciousness
  - − ↑ confusion
  - − Hallucinations
- o Due to ↓ cerebral function from disease which is
  - − Multifocal
  - − Diffuse

➢ Causes
  - o Infection
    - − In or outside of CNS (asymptomatic or symptomatic urinary tract infection is a common output in the elderly)
  - o Ischemia (CVA)
  - o Trauma
  - o Toxins/drugs e.g., alcohol
    - − Sedative – hypnotics
    - − Anticholinergic agents
    - − NSAIDs (nonsteroidal anti inflammatory drug)
    - − Adrenergic blockers
    - − Antipsychotic agents
  - o Metabolic
    - − Hypoglycemia
    - − Hypocalcemia
    - − Hypernatremia
    - − Hypotension
    - − Hypoxia
    - − Hepatic/renal failure
  - o Others
    - − Korsakow psychosis
    - − Puerperal psychosis
    - − Post-seizure confusion

➢ Clinical
- Take a directed history for delirium.
  - o Initial screen
    - − Assesses hearing/vision
    - − Assesses orientation (person, place, time)
    - − Elicits chief complaint

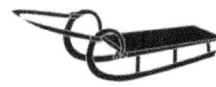

- o Description of symptoms
  - – Onset, duration, and course of current complaint(s)
  - – Palliating/provoking factors
  - – Limitations in functioning (ADLs, IADLs)

- o Depression symptoms
  - – Assesses depression symptoms (low mood, anhedonia, sleep disturbance, etc.)
  - – Assesses suicidality and homicidality
- o Anxiety symptoms
  - – Anxiety symptoms (phobias, obsessions, compulsions, etc.)

- o Perception disturbances
  - – Psychotic symptoms (hallucinations, delusions, ideas of reference etc.)

- o Personality and behavioural disturbances
  - – Changes in personality
  - – Behavioural abnormalities (apathy, agitation, odd behaviours, etc.)

- o Past and family medical history
  - – Hx of alcohol/drug abuse
  - – Medications and Hx of adverse drug reactions
  - – Hx of psychiatric illness
  - – Hx of other metabolic or systemic illness(es)

- o Collateral history from family member
  - – Elicits concerns
  - – Confirms history
  - – Inquiries about safety, home fire risks, driving, wandering

- Perform a focused examination to determine the site of disease causing a person's delirium or coma.

- ↑ ICP (intracranial pressure)

  - o CNS
    - – Eyes
      - Papillerdema
    - – CN VI
    - – Visual changes
    - – LOC (changes in level of consciousness)

  - o CVS.
    - – Hypertension (↑ BP)
    - – Bradycardia (↓ PR)

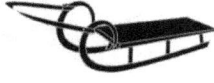

Mastering the Boards: Neurology   A.B.R. Thomson

- o GI
  - – Vomiting

- Herniation
  - o Supratentorial
    - – Uncus
      - ▪ Unilateral
    - – CNS
      - ▪ ↓ LOC
    - – Eyes
      - ▪ Pupil
        - –Dilated
        - –Ipsilateral
    - – MSK
      - ▪ Hemiparesis
        - –Contra → unilateral
    - – Central
      - ▪ Bilateral/medial
    - – CNS
      - ▪ Δ LOC (altered level of consciousness)
    - – Eyes
      - ▪ Pupils
        - –Midposition
        - –Unreactive
        - –Upward gauge
    - – Breathing
      - ▪ Cheyne-Stokes
    - – MSK
      - ▪ Posturing of extremities
  - o Posterior fossa
    - – Cerebellar tonsils
      - ▪ Medullary compression
        - –CNS
          - ▪ Δ LOC
        - –Breathing
          - ▪ Irregular
          - ▪ Apneic

Abbreviation: Δ, altered (as in Δ LOC); LOC, level of consciousness

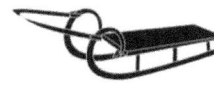

- Level of Consciousness
  - o **Glasgow coma scale** (GCS)
- Breathing
  - o Hyperventilation
    - – Brainstem disease/injury
    - – Lung disease
      - ▪ Acidosis, metabolic
      - ▪ Hypoxemia
      - ▪ Pulmonary disease
  - o Cheyne-Stokes
    - – "rhythmic crescends- decrescends hyperpnea alternating with periods of apnea"
    - – Causes
      - ▪ Supratentorial lesions
      - ▪ Metabolic
      - ▪ Lung disease
      - ▪ Heart failure (HF)
  - o Apnec
    - – Brainstorm disease/injury
  - o Clusters (short bursts "clusters" of breathing)
  - o Ataxic (no pattern)

- Pupils
  - o Isocordia (symmetrical changes)
    - – Reactive, small
      - ▪ Pons
      - ▪ Metabolic endephalopathy
      - ▪ Drugs – narcotics
    - – Fixed, midposition
      - ▪ Transtentorial
      - ▪ Midbrain
    - – Fixed, dilated
      - ▪ Amoxicencephalopathy
      - ▪ Drugs/toxins
        - –Anticholinergics
        - –Methanol

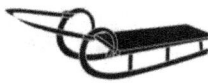

- Eye movements
  - Conjugate
    - Head turning
      - Conjugate eye movement to opposite side → normal (oculocephalic doll's eye test)

    - No movement
      - Perform cold cabric (oculovestibular test) → normal if eyes move to side in which ear was irrigated with ice water → no eye movements → bilateral pontive lesion.

SO YOU WANT TO BE A NEUROLOGIST!

In a person with delirium or coma, you note their reduced level of consciousness, dilated pupils, and hemiparesis. You suspect a supratentorial lesion with hermiation of the uncus.

- Give the meaning of the **Kernohan notch syndrome**.

  - With uncal hermiation, the hemiparesis is initially contralateral to the lesion, and then progresses to be ipselateral to the mass.

  - This phenomenon of contra → ipselateral hemiparesis is known as the Kernohan notah syndrome.

- ➢ Diagnosis
  - Acute onset, with fluctuating course
  - Inattention
  - Disorganised thinking
  - Altered level of consciousness
  - Diagnosis of delirium requires the presence of 1 and 2 and either 3 or 4
  - Clinical diagnosis (confusion assessment method) presence of
    - Acute onset
    - Fluctuating course
    - Inattention
    - Consciousness level altered
      +/-
    - Thinking disorganized

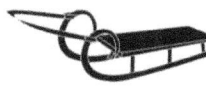

- Give the indication for a CT head or MRI in a person with delirium.

  o Possible subdural hematoma from a fall

  o Focal neurological changes suggesting a space-occupying lesion

➤ Differential

  o Slow loss of
    - Short-term memory
    - Intellect (reasoning and making correct judgements)
    - Understanding new ideas
    - Social awareness

  o Inattention
    - Loss of hygiene and aspects of personal care

  o Confusion

  o Delusions

  o Affect
    - Depression
    - Anxiety
    - Mania

➤ Treatment

  o Treat any precipitating factors e.g.,
    - Drugs
    - Infection
    - Disorientation
    - Electrolyte abnormalities
    - Pain
    - Disturbances
      ▪ Sleep
      ▪ Vision
      ▪ Hearing
    - Immobility

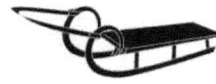

- o Correct precipitants
  - – Drugs
  - – Infection
  - – Fluid/electrolyte disorder
  - – Hypoxemia
  - – Pain (poorly controlled)
  - – ↓ vision/hearing
  - – Immobility
  - – Restraints
  - – Catheters/lines
- o If persistent or agulated
  - – Haloperidol
  - – Rasperidone

SO YOU WANT TO BE A NEUROLOGIST!

- In delirium, there is abnormal perception and motor activity. Give the difference between hallucination and illusion?

  - o Hallucination – sensory impression, without sensory stimulus

  - o Illusion – sensory impression which is incorrectly interpreted

---

THERAPEUTIC ALERT

- Give the reason why antipsychotics are **used with great caution** in dementia

  - o Dererium
  - o Psychosis   ↑ mortality rate
  - o Behaviour outbreaks

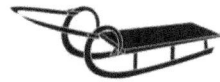

DEMENTIA

➢ Definition
   o "Dementia is a ......progressive, deteriorating......syndrome of acquired global impairment of cognitive function sufficient to interfere with normal activities" (Rockwood K, et al. Chapter 4. In: Therapeutic Choices. Grey J, Ed. 6th Edition, *Canadian Pharmacists Association*: Otttawa, ON, 2011, page 45).
   o Dementia is a progressive deterioration of cognitive function severe enough to impair occupational or social functioning ...., and which is measurable by standardized tests"
   o Dementia is a syndrome of acquired global impairment of cognitive function sufficient to interfere with normal activities.
   o The most common causes are
      – Alzheimer disease
      – Vascular dementia
      – Mixture of the two
         ▪ Lewy body dementia
         ▪ Frontotemporal dementia.
   o Dementia is also recognized as a complication of Parkinson disease.
   o Dementias are almost always progressive, deteriorating illnesses in which treatment opinions are different at different stages of the illness.

	Onset	Course	Dysfunction	Activities of Daily Living
o Delirium	Acute	Fluctuating	Attention	↓/N
o Consciousness			Thinking	
o Mild Cognitive Impairment (MCI)	chronic	progressive	memory	N Impairment (MCI)
o Alzeimer	chronic	progressive	memory	↓↓ disease thinking (delusional) agnosia aphasia apraxia attention executive function "L-R confusion"

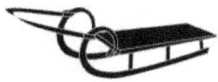

➤ Differential diagnosis

- ○ Structural
  lesions
  - Normal-pressure hydrocephalus
  - Subdural hematoma
  - Neoplasm
  - Vascular dementia

- ○ Infections
  - Chronic meningitis
  - Neurosyphilis
  - HIV dementia
  - Encephalitis
  - Meningitis
  - Abscess
  - Creutzfeldt-Jakob disease
  - Cryptococcal meningitis

- ○ Inflammatory/immune disorders
- ○ Vasculitis
  - SLE vasculitis
  - Sarcoidosis
  - Granulomatosis with polyangiitis

- ○ Hashimoto/autoimmune encephalopathy
- ○ Tumour
  - Intracranial (especially frontal)

- ○ Degenerative
  dementia
  - Alzheimer disease
  - Diffuse Lewy bosy disease
  - Frontotemporal dementia (including Pick disease)
  - Huntington disease
  - Progressive supranuclear palsy
  - Multiple sclerosis

- ○ Associated with Parkinson disease

- ○ Drugs (e.g.,anti-cholinergics)

Abbreviation: HIV, human immunodeficiency virus

Adapted from: Hauser SC, et al. *Mayo Clinic Gastroenterology and Hepatology Board Review*. 3rd Review, page 753; Burton JL. *Churchill Livingstone* 1971, page 71.

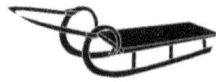

Buzz Words suggestive of cause of dementia

- o Alzeimer
  - ↓ executive function
  - Delusional thinking
  - L-R confusion
  - The "A's": agnosia, aphagiam apraxia, inattention
- o Crentzfeld-Jacob (CJ) disease – early age, rapidly progressing, myoclonus
- o Frontotemporal – behaviour and personality changes (e.g., disinhibition)
- o Huntington disease- choreonthetosis, family history (AD)
- o Lewg body- delusions, hallucinations (visual), Parkinsonism (mild)
- o Normal-pressure hydrocephalus – dementia, gait shuffling, incontinence (urine)
- o Progressive supranuclear palsy – vertical gaze palsy, axial rigidity, bradykinesia, retropulsion

Abbreviations: AD, autosomal dominant

➢ Clinical

- Take a directed history for the differential diagnosis.
  - o **D**rugs (alcohol, barbiturates, bromides)
  - o **E**motion (depression, schizophrenia)
  - o **M**etabolic (Wernicke-Korsakoff syndrome, B12/folate deficiency, hyper/hypothyroid)
  - o **E**ye and ear (severe visual and auditory impairment)
  - o **N**eurodegenerative (Huntington's, Parkinson's, Alzheimers disease)
  - o **T**rauma (head injury, dementia pugilistica), tumour (subfrontal meningioma)
  - o **I**nfection (HIV, syphilis, viral encephalitis, Creutzfeld-Jacob disease)
  - o **A**rteriosclerotic and vascular (multi infarct dementia, vasculitis, cerebral hemorrhage)

Adapted from: Ghosh A.K. *Mayo Clinic Scientific Press* 2008, Table 10-4, page 390; FOS, page 131. Data from Inouye SK, et al. *Ann Intern Med.* 1991;114 (11):991-992; Jugovic PJ, et al. *Saunders/ Elsevier* 2004, Box 4-1, page 131 M, page 51.

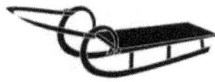

- Perform a focused physical examination for dementia.

  - Signs of fluctuating delirium
    ↓ in [ACCD] ACCD plus AC
    - Attention
    - Concentration
    - Coherence
    - Disorientation, plus
    - Agitated Confusion

  - Signs of cortical dementia: ↓
    - Memory
    - Language fluency
    - Calculation
    - Executive function

  - Signs of subcortical dementia
    - Parkinsonism
    - Apathy
    - Depression
    - Tremor
    - Bradykinesia
    - Ataxia

- Perform a focused physical examination for the causes of dementia
  - Alzheimer disease
  - Vascular dementia
  - Combination of Alzheimer and vascular dementia
  - Lewy body dementia
  - Frontotemporal dementia
  - Nutrient deficiencies
    - Intake
      - B12 deficiency
      - Thiamine deficiency
    - Infection
      - Abscess
      - Meningitis
      - HIV
      - Syphilis
      - Encephalitis, viral
      - Whipple disease
    - Infiltration
      - Tumour
      - Subdural hematoma
      - Paraneoplastic disease

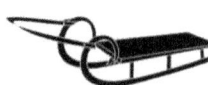

- – Iatrogenic
  - Drugs withdrawal, alcohol, heavy metal
- – Trauma
  - Post-concussion
- – Psychiatric
  - Depression
  - Schizophrenia
  - Catatonia
- – Endocrine
  - Hypo/hyperthyroidism
  - Hypoparathyroidism

o Primitive neurological reflexes
  - – Grasp
  - – Root
  - – Snout
  - – Glabella
  - – Palmomental
  - – Retropulse

o Later signs
  - – Aggression
  - – Agitated
  - – Anxious
  - – Belligerent
  - – Delusion (reidentity)
  - – Demanding
  - – Disinhibition
  - – Incontinence
  - – Paranoid
  - – Posture, flexion
  - – Psychosis
  - – Self-centred ($\downarrow$ empathy)
  - – Sleep disturbance

MCQ Trick

- Give the physical findings found in a person with Pick presenile dementia.
  - o Same findings as disturbed function of the frontal lobe of the cerebral cortex

---

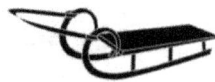

- Take a directed history and perform a focused physical examination for dementia.
- History
  - Initial screen
    - Assesses hearing/vision
    - Assesses orientation (person, place, time)
    - Elicits chief complaint
  - Description of symptoms
    - Onset, duration, and course of current complaint(s)
    - Palliating/provoking factors
    - Limitations in functioning (ADLs, IADLs)
  - Depression symptoms
    - Assesses depression symptoms (low mood, anhedonia, sleep disturbance, etc.)
    - Assesses suicidality and homicidality
  - Anxiety symptoms
    - Anxiety symptoms (phobias, obsessions, compulsions, etc.)
  - Perception disturbances
    - Psychotic symptoms (hallucinations, delusions, ideas of reference etc.)
  - Personality and behavioural disturbances
    - Changes in personality
    - Behavioural abnormalities (apathy, agitation, odd behaviours, etc.)
  - Past and family medical history
    - Hx of alcohol/drug abuse
    - Medications and Hx of adverse drug reactions
    - Hx of psychiatric illness
    - Hx of other metabolic or systemic illness(es)
  - Collateral history from family member
    - Elicits concerns
    - Confirms history
    - Inquiries about safety, home fire risks, driving, wandering
- Physical examination
  - Inspection
    - Dress and grooming
    - Speech
    - Attitude and behaviour in office

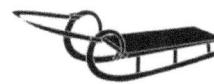

- o **Folstein mini mental status exam**
  - Orientation (place, time: 5pt for each)
  - Registration (name 3 objects: 1 pt for each)
  - Attention and concentration (serial 7's, world, months: 5 pt total)
  - Recall (recall 3 objects: 1 pt for each)
  - Language:
    - identify 2 objects pointed to:2 pt total
    - ask no ifs ands or buts: 1 pt total
    - perform 3 stage command: 3 pt total
    - read and obey written command: 1 pt total
    - write a sentence: 1 pt total
    - draw intersecting pentagons: 1 pt total

- o Additional cognitive tests
  - Perseveration (ask patient to copy a series of loops)
  - Construction ability (draw hands of clock for diff. times)
  - Concrete thinking (compare word similarities)
  - Abstract thinking (describe meaning of proverb)

Adapted from: Ghosh AK. *Mayo Clinic Scientific Press* 2008,Table 19-3; Jugovic PJ, et al. *Saunders/ Elsevier* 2004, pages 129-131.

SO YOU WANT TO BE A DEMENTIA EXPERT!

- Give indications for performing a **lumbar puncture** (LP) and analysis of the cerebrospinal fluid (CSF) in the patient with possible dementia.

  - o Patient
    - – < 60 yr
    - – Rapidly progressing dementia

  - o Associated conditions
    - – Infection
      - Positive VDRL (serology for syphilis)
    - – Inflammation/inflammatory autoimmune
    - – Infiltration
      - Systemic cancer
    - – Immunosuppression

  - o Note: CSF tau proteins and B-amyloid protein are not yet considered to be diagnostic for Alzheimer Diease (AD)

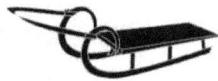

➢ Stages of dementia

• Give the stages of dementia.

Stage	Characteristics	Corresponding FAST Rating[a]
○ Preclinical	– Subjective complaints accompanied by very mild objective cognitive decline; functioning is unimpaired – This stage has considerable overlap with normal aging and may or may not progress to dementia.	3

○ Mild	– Impaired instrumental activities of daily living (IADL), e.g.,
	  ▪ Driving
	  ▪ Medication use
	  ▪ Finances
	  ▪ Use of telephone and housekeeping
		4

○ Moderate	– In addition to IADL impairment, personal activities of daily living (PADL) such as
	  ▪ Bathing
	  ▪ Feeding
	  ▪ Dressing
	  ▪ Toileting can be done only with prompting
		5

○ Severe	– PADL cannot be done even with prompting	6
○ Terminal	– Patients must be fed and become immobile and mute	7

[a] Included because many jurisdictions use the Functional Assessment Staging Tool (FAST) in adjudicating reimbursement for dementia medications.

Reproduced with permission: Therapeutics Choices. Sixth Edition. Ottawa, Canada: *Canadian Pharmacist Association* 2012, Table 1, page 45.

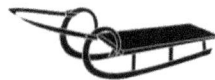

➢ Causes

- • Take a directed history and perform a focused physical examination for the causes of dementia.

  - o Infection
    - – Meningitis
    - – Encephalitis
    - – Abscess
    - – Malaria
    - – Septicemia

  - o Ischemia
    - – Thrombosis, embolism, hemorrhage
    - – Hypertensive encephalopathy
    - – Causes of syncope

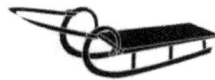

- o Metabolic
  - – Alcoholism
  - – Drugs
  - – Uremia
  - – Hepatic failure
  - – Myxedema
  - – B 12 deficiency
  - – Pellagra

- o Trauma

- o Pressure effects
  - – Space-occupying lesions
  - – Hydrocephalus

- o Hyper- or hypo-thermia

- o Hysteria or hypnosis

Adapted from: Burton JL. *Churchill Livingstone* 1971, page 72.

- ➢ Diagnosis
  - o "Mini Mental" (Folstein Mini-Mental State Examination) test score
    - – < 24 – dementia
  - o Screen for
    - – Depression
    - – Infection   } sudden worsening of dementia
    - – Rx errors

  - o ECG
    - – Triphasic sharp waves in Crentzfeld-Jakob disease
  - o CSF
    - – With delirium or rapidly progressing dementia
    - – Suspected infection (syphilis serology positive), carcinomatous meningitis
    - – Protein 14-3-3 (CJ disease)

  - o Clinical   – Suggested by a score < 24 on Folstein Mini-Mental State Examination (FMMSE)

             – Screen for associated
               ▪ Depression
               ▪ Infection
               ▪ Medication errors

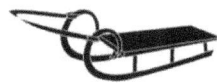

- o Diagnostic imaging
  - – Obtain CT or MRI
  - – Consider performing lumbar puncture for
    - Associated delirium
    - Rapid progression
    - Risk for
      - - Carcinomatous meningitis
      - - CNS infection
      - - Positive serology for syphilis

- Give the indications for performing a CT of the head.

  - o Patient
    - – < 60 years
    - – Recent head injury
    - – History and cancer
    - – Use of anticoagulants

  - o Dementia
    - – Rapidly progressive
    - – Unusually cognitive symptoms (e.g., early delusions or hallucinations)

  - o Neurological
    - – Focal or lateralizing signs
    - – Gait disorder
    - – Early urinary incontinence

Grey J, Therapeutic Choices. 6th Edition, *Canadian Pharmacists Association*: Otttawa, ON, 2011, page 46.

- For an excellent consideration of how to take a focused history to evaluate competency in medical decision-making, please see: Jugovic PJ, et al. *Saunders/ Elsevier* 2004, page 206.

➢ Determine site of cause
  - o Cortical coma (brainstem functions are present)

    - – Brainstem coma
      - Response to pain
      - Decerebrate – mild
        - – Upper extremity flexion (hands point towards heart)
        - – Lower extremity extension and internal rotation
      - Moderate
        - – Upper and lower extremities – extension and internal rotation
      - Severity

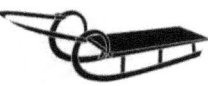

- Midbrain
  - Fixed pupils
- Pons
  - Doll's eye reflex eyes – remain fixed in the midline when head is turned (CNI; normally, touching cornea on one side causes a wink response on both sides with a unilateral disturbance of V, wink response does not occur on either side when affected side is stimulated)
  - Loss of corneal reflex
  - Loss of jaw reflex (CN) jaw will deviate towards the side of the lesion
- Medulla
  - Dysfunction of cardiopulmonary centres
- Corticol pontine
  - Impaired conjugate eye movement (cerebral or basilar artery thrombosis)
    - Death
  - Global absence of brainstem function on two neurological examinations 12 hours apart, and exclusion of toxic-metabolic cause

Adapted from: Burton JL. *Churchill Livingstone* 1971, page 72; Talley NJ, et al. *Maclennan & Petty Pty Limited* 2003, Table 10.38, page 439.

- Take a directed history to **differentiate** between delirium and dementia.

	Delirium	Dementia
o Onset	– Rapid	▪ Progressive
o Course	– Fluctuates over time	▪ Constant or may slowly worsen
o Orientation	– Disoriented to time and place	▪ Disoriented to time and place usually only in late stages
o Psychosis	– More likely present	▪ Less likely present
o Other	– Perceptual disturbances, sleep wake cycles disturbed, ↑ or ↓ psychomotor activity	▪ Loss of judgment, changes in personality present
o Reversible	– Often	▪ Very rarely

Adapted from: Filate W, et al. *The Medical Society, Faculty of Medicine, University of Toronto* 2005, page 277 and Jugovic PJ, et al *Saunders/ Elsevier* 2004, page 131.

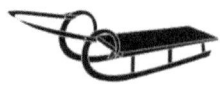

- Give the performance characteristics for test for dementia and delirium.

Finding	PLR	NLR
o Dementia		
– Abnormal clock drawing test	5.3	0.5
o Mini mental status examination: 3 levels		
≤ 20	14.5	…
21 to 25	2.2	…
≤ 23	8.1	0.2
o Delirium		
– Positive test using "Confusion Assessment Method"	10.3	0.2

Abbreviation: PLR, positive likelihood ratio; NLR, negative likelihood ratio

Source: McGee SR. *Saunders/Elsevier* 2007, Box 4-1, page 51.

In a MCQ if a "buzzword" is used, a particular cause of memory dysfunction may be implied.

- Give the likely cause of **memory impairment** associated with 6 of the following buzzwords.

Buzzwords	Suggested diagnosis
o ↓ executive function	– Alzheimer disease
o Left-right confusion	
o Myoclonus, abnormal EEG	– CJ (Creutzfeldt-Jakob disease)
o Personality changes	– Frontotemporal dementia
o Disinhibition	
o Impulsive behaviour	
o Choreoathetosis	– Huntington disease
o Family history	
o Parkinsonism	– Lewy body dementia
o Delusions	
o Visual hallucinations	
o No cognitive deficit	– Mild cognitive impairment
o Dementia	– Normal-pressure hydrocephalus
o Shuffling gait	
o Urinary incontinence	

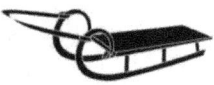

Buzzwords	Suggested diagnosis
o Vertical gaze palsy	– Progressive supranuclear palsy
o Stepwise confusion	– Vascular dementia
o Multiple infarction CT / MRI	

➢ Treatment
- o Cholinesterase inhibitor (anti-cholinesterase)
- o If "Mini-Mental" 3 to 14, add memantine
- o For depression do not use amitriptyline or imipramine
- o Avoid antipsychotics (↑ mortality rate)
- o Avoid anticholinergics

- o Associated conditions
  - – Depression
    - ▪ SSRIs
  - – Infection
    - ▪ Psychosis
    - ▪ Antipsychotics
  - – Parkinsonism
    - ▪ Quetapine
- o Mini-mental 3-14
  - – Memantine (slows decline in Alzheimer disease), +/ cholinesterase inhibitor
- o Alzheimer disease
  - – Cholinesterase inhibitor
    - ▪ Donepezil
    - ▪ Galantamine
    - ▪ Rivastigmine
- o Vascular dementia
  - – ASA

- o CSF drainage
  - – Normal-pressure hydrocephalus

In dementia with Lewis bodies, in addition to the dementia, delusions and visual hallucinations, there may be mild Parkinsonism.
- Give the reason for the use of atypical psychotic agents, such as quetiapine, in this setting.

  - o Quetiapine is less likely to ↑ extrapyramidal syndromes

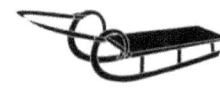

THERAPEUTIC ALERT

In demented patients with depression, use SSRIs rather than TCAs, because the latter may ↑ confusion.

Abbreviations: SSRI, selective serotonin reuptake inhibitor; TCA, tricyclic antidepressants

Common Types of Dementia

- To be considered here
    - Alzheimer disease
    - Frontotemporal dementia
    - Lewy body dementia
    - Mild cognitive impairments
    - Normal pressure hydrocephalis
    - Vascular dementia

Alzheimer Disease (AD)

➤ Pathogenesis
- Give the pathogenesis of non-familial Alzheimer disease (AD).

APP (amyloid precursor protein) in neuronal membranes

↓

Normal: proteolysis by secretases

AD: abnormal proteolysis

Non-toxic products

B-amyloid and hyperphosphorylated tau microtubular protein

↓

Neuronal damage and AD

↓

Brain cholinergic deficit

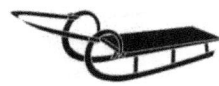

Mastering the Boards: Neurology　　　　　　　　A.B.R. Thomson

SO YOU WANT TO BE A GOLD MEDALIST!

- Give the comparison of the histology features of the brain in the octagenerian without (NA, normal aging) and with Alzheimer disease (AD).

Histological findings	NA	AD
o Cerebral atrophy	+	+
o Loss of cortex	Especially in medial temporal lobes	Diffuse loss, especially - Hypocampus - Temporal lobe - Basal nucleus of Meynert
o Neurons		
- Shrinkage amyloid-containing plaques	+	+
- Neurofibrillary tanges	-	+
- Granulovascular degeneration	-	+

- Give the characteristics of the neurofibrillary tangles in Alzheimer disease).

    o Knotted loops of neurons
    o Silver-stained strands in neuronal bodies
    o Helices of hyperphosphorylated tau microtubular protein

➢ Treatment
    o Alzheimer disease (AD) is associated with a brain cholinergic deficit, so it is not surprising that cholinesterase inhibitors (such as donepezile, rivastigmine, tacrine) are used to slow the progression of the disease.

- Give the classes of pharmaceuticals used to treat Alzheimer disease besides anti-cholinesterase inhibitors.

    o Agonists   - Nicotinic receptor
    o Inhibitors   - N-methyl-D-aspartate
                       - To the ↑ production of tau protein

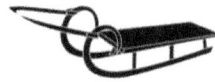

SO YOU WANT TO BE A NEUROLOGIST!

- In the context of Alzheimer dementia, give the meaning of **Capgras syndrome.**

    o Capgras syndrome is a "misidentification delusion"

    o In this misidentification delusion, persons with Capgras syndrome "...... believe their family members or caretakers are imposters" (Source: MKSAP 16 2012, Neurology, page 43), i.e.,

    o Loss of recognition and emotional familiarity

    o Treatment is that of the underlying condition, such as AD

- Give the classes of drugs to which persons with dementia are very susceptible, such that these drugs must be **prescribed with precaution.**

    o **Anti-cholinergics**

    o **Benzodiazepines**

Frontotemporal Dementia

➤ Definition: "....a heterogeneous clinical syndrome of behavioural and cognitive deterioration combined with Parkinsonism and motor neuron disease" (MKSAP 16 2012, Neurology, page 46).

➤ Pathophysiology

    o Accumulation of hyperphosphorylated tau protein in neurons and glia in frontotemporal lobes

    o One form is inherited with chromosome 17-associated genetic changes in tau protein

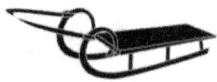

➤ Clinical

- o Cognitive decline in
  - Memory
  - Verbal fluency
  - Executive function
- o Behaviour changes
  - Apathy
  - Depression
  - Obsessive
  - Impulsive
  - Perseveration
  - ↓ judgement

Lewy Body Dementia

➤ Demographics

- o Affects ~ 20% of persons with dementia, especially in persons with Parkinson disease (and especially with axial distribution)
- o ~ 80% of persons with Parkinson-associated dementia have Lewy body dementia

➤ Pathophysiology

- o Unknown
  - α-synuclein aggregates in neurons

➤ Clinical

- o Cognitive decline, plus
  - Common psychiatric changes
    - Apathy
    - Depression
    - Personality changes
    - Psychiasis
    - Hallucination (↑ by levodopa, or dopamine agonists)
  - Abnormal dreams (dreams enactment)
  - Motor signs of Parkinsonism
- o May be overlap of Lewy body and Alzheimer dementia

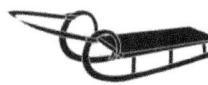

Mild Cognitive Impairments (MCI)

➢ Definition:
- o ↓ memory, learning, problem solving
- o > than expected for age and level of education
- o Does not interfere with occupational function

MCI (mild cognitive impairment) progresses to probable Alzheimer disease at the rate of 10% to 15% per year

- • Give the features which ↑ risk of MCI (mild cognitive impairment) progressing to AD (Alzheimer disease).
    - o History/testing
        - – Memory deficit
            - ▪ > 1.5 SD (standard deviations) below normal tests of cognitive function
        - – Tests of cognitive function
            - ▪ Montreal cognitive assessment: www.mocatest.org
            - ▪ Folstein Mini-mental state examination
            - ▪ Using either tests, a score < 22 indicates dementia
    - o Family history
        - – Positive for AD
    - o Laboratory
        - – Positive for allele for apolipoproteins E4
    - o Neuroimaging
        - – Atrophy of brain, diffuse
        - – ↓ volume of hippocampus
        - – ↑ sulci
        - – ↑ ventricles

Clinical Pearl

- o In the patient with idiopathic intracranial hypertension, the patient may have a "false-localizing sign related to ↑ ICP (intracranial pressure) and not to focal pathology.

- o Note: current research explores an even milder stage of cognitive impairment (CI) where the patient/family are concerned that there may be CI.

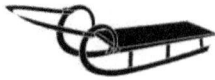

Mastering the Boards: Neurology   A.B.R. Thomson

Vascular Dementia

- ➢ Definition
  - o Dementia due to progressive brain ischemia resulting from
    - Multiple strokes
    - Spread (confluence) of cerebral ischemia

- ➢ Causes
  - o Frequent and recurrent ischemic strokes, e.g.,
    - Endocarditis
    - Vasculitis
  - o Progressive leucoencephalopathy
    - MS (multiple sclerosis, advanced)
    - PML (progressive multifocal leukoencephalopathy)

- ➢ Diagnosis
  - o Diagnostic imaging
    - Evidence of cerebral ischemia

"Action is the foundational key to all success."
Pablo Picasso

 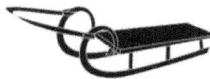

SYNCOPE AND DIZZINESS

➢ Definition: a transient loss of consciousness with spontaneous recovery.

➢ Causes

- o Cardiogenic syncope
  - Structural heart disease
  - Coronary artery disease
  - Rhythm disturbance
  - Vasovagal
  - Carotid sinus hypersensitivity
  - Dysrhythmia e.g., AF, BBB
  - Orthostatic hypotension
  - After exercise
  - Coronary artery disease, previous myocardial infarction
  - Structural heart disease
  - Left ventricular dysfunction
  - Congestive heart failure

- o Neurologic
  - In patients who present with a prodrome (e.g., nausea, diaphoresis), a neurocardiogenic mechanism is likely.
  - Patients who experience rapid recovery (less than 5-10 minutes) rarely have neurologic cause for syncope and are most unlikely to have syncope due to seizure or 'brain hypoperfusion' because recovery in such circumstances takes hours.
  - For cases in which recovery from syncope is rapid and no residual neurologic signs or symptoms are present, detailed (and expensive) neurologic evaluation should be avoided.

- o Metabolic

- o Psychiatric

- o Situational

- o Lung
  - Tussive
  - Valsalva maneuver
  - Sneeze

 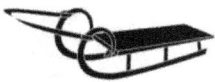

- o GI
    - – Deglutition
    - – Defecation
    - – Glosspharyngeal neuralgia
    - – Postprandial

- o GU
    - – Micurition

- o Miscellenous
    - – Oculovagal
    - – Instrumentation
    - – Diving

Adapted from: Hauser SC, et al. *Mayo Clinic Gastroenterology and Hepatology Board Review.* 3rd Review, page 90; Shen W-K, et al. Syncope: mechanisms, approach, and management. In: Low PA, ed. Little, *Brown and Company* 1993, pages 605-640.

➢ Clinical associations

- o Prodrome
    - – Warm
    - – Sweating
    - – Nausea

- o Position
    - – Prolonged standing
    - – Orthogenic

- o Provocation
    - – Pain
    - – Emotion
    - – Swallowing (or postprandial)
    - – Defecation
    - – Urination
    - – Coughing

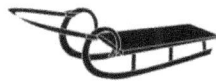

Mastering the Boards: Neurology   A.B.R. Thomson

➢ More associations

- ○ Angina   – ↓ LV outflow   ▪ AS (aortic stenosis)

- ○ Exercise   ▪ HCM (hypertrophic cardiomyopathy)
  - ▪ PE (pulmonary embolus)
  - ▪ PHT (pulmonary hypertension)

- ○ Upper extremity exercise   – Subclavian steal syndrome

- ○ Pressure on neck   – Hypersensitivity of carotid sinus

- ○ Sudden loss of consciousness without prodome or changes in position   – Arrhythmia, heart block

---

Clinical Gem

Assessment of orthostatic hypotension may be simple, but also access for hypovolemia, drug effects, and disorders of the autonomic nervous system such as diabetes, Parkinsonism.

➢ Clinical

- Take a directed history to determine the cause of a patient's dizziness.

  - ○ Physiological
    - – Motion sickness
    - – Space sickness
    - – Height vertigo

  - ○ Psychological
    - – Acute anxiety
    - – Agoraphobia (fear & avoidance of being in public places)
    - – Chronic anxiety

  - ○ Eyes
    - – High magnification & lens implant
    - – Imbalance in extraocular muscles
    - – Oscillopsia

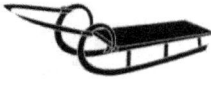

- o Balance
  - – Brain stem, cerebellar or temporal cortical lesions
    - Pontine infraction or haemorrhage
    - Vertebro-basilar insufficiency
    - Basilar artery migraine
    - Temporal lobe epilepsy
    - Disseminated sclerosis
    - Tumours
    - 'Benign post traumatic positional vertigo', etc.
  - – Vestibular lesions
    - Physiological
    - Labyrinthitis
    - Meniere disease
    - Drugs e.g., quinine, salicylates, alcohol
    - Otitis media
    - Motion sickness
  - – Vestibular nerve lesions
    - Acoustic neuroma
    - Drugs e.g., streptomycin
    - Vestibular neuronitis
  - – Disequilibrium
    - Lesions of basal ganglia, fromtal lobes, & white matter
    - Hydrocephalus
    - Cerebellar dysfunction
  - – Ear
    - Vertigo
      - – Peripheral
      - – Central

- o CVS.
  - – Orthostatic hypotension
  - – Vasovagal attacks
  - – Impaired cardiac output
  - – Hyperventilation

- o Multisensory dizziness

Adapted from: Hauser SC, et al. *Mayo Clinic Gastroenterology and Hepatology Board Review.* 3rd Review, Table 19.13, page 763; Burton JL. *Churchill Livingstone* 1971, page 76.

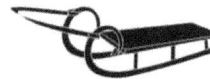

VERTIGO

➢ Definition

  o A sensation of rotation on movement

➢ Causes

  o Peripheral
    – Benign positional vertigo
      ▪ Short multiple attacks from rapidly changing position
    – Vestibular neuritis (labyrinthitis)
      ▪ Acute, severe symptoms lasting for hours-days
    – Maniere disease
      ▪ Multiple attacks
      ▪ Severe vertigo
      ▪ ↓ hearing (fluctuating)
      ▪ Tinnitus
      ▪ Multiple brain stem findings

  o Central
    – Vascular
      ▪ Vertebrobasilar insufficiency
      ▪ Intracerebral hemorrhage
      ▪ Symptoms of TIA/stroke
    – Infiltration
      ▪ Tumour (acoustic neuroma)
      ▪ Multiple sclerosis optic neuritis, symptoms/signs of neurological defects in different areas of brain, brainstorm and spinal cord, and at different times

---

CLINICAL CHALLENGE

  o When vertigo is associated with
    – ↑ sensory loss/tingling when neck is flexed
    – An affected eye cannot be adducted ("Buzzword"- internuclear opthalneoplegia), or
    – Optic neuritis
- Give the relapsing/remitting cause that do you think?
  o Multiple sclerosis

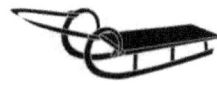

➢ Clinical

➢ Treatment (peripheral causes)

Type	Cortico-steroids	Meclizine	Rehabilitation Program	Surgery Epley Canal Repositioning	Na Intake Diuretic
o Benign positional	-	-	+	-	-
o Vestibular neuritis	+	+	+	-	-
o Meniere disease	-	+	-	+	+

The Plague:
"When originality may not be genuine, check it on 'Turn it in.com.' Even Deans deviate."
Grandad

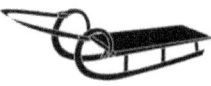

Mastering the Boards: Neurology   A.B.R. Thomson

THE EYE: CN II

➤ The eyes, and cranial nerve II (Optic)-vision (sensory)

    ○ Visual acuity (Snellen visual chart)

    ○ Visual fields by confrontation

    ○ Colour test

    ○ Reflex
       - Papillary light reflex (perform at time of fundoscopy: tests CN III)

    ○ Accommodation to light

    ○ Red reflex

    ○ Fundoscopy
       - Retinal vessels
       - Optic disc
       - Macula
       - Lesions

➤ Translational Neuroanatomy

    ○ Ganglion cells of retina
       ↓

    ○ Optic nerve
       ↓

    ○ Chiasma tract
       ↓

    ○ Lateral geniculate body
       ↓

    ○ Visual radiation through posterior limb of internal capsule

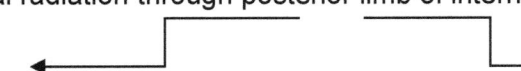

Medial aspect of occipital lobe   - descending horn of lateral ventricle
(fibres from upper retinal quadrants)   (fibres from lower retinal quadrants)
                                   ↓
                       Parietal and temporal lobe

➤ Fibres from

    ○ Upper retinal quadrant cuneate gyri above calcoume fissure

    ○ Lower retinal quadrant lingular gyri below

    ○ Macula
       – Posterior aspect of occipital ple
       – Bilateral cortical representation

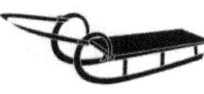

Lesions of the Visual Fields

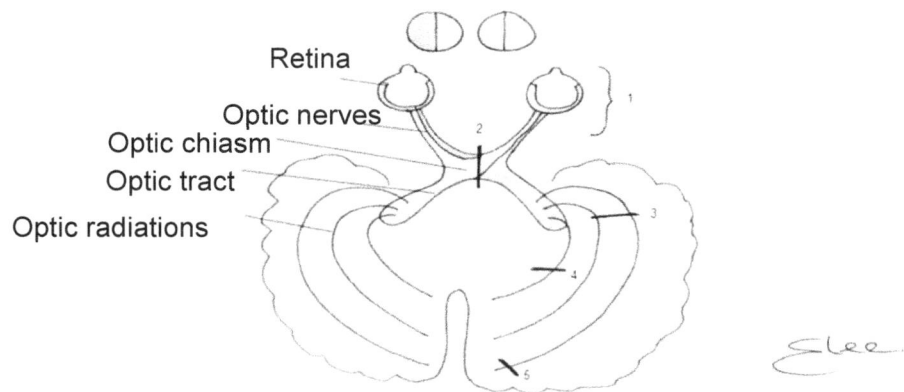

ANTERIOR LESIONS	**CHIASMAL**

1. Constricted visual field

2. Bitemporal hemianopia

1. Arcuate scotoma

3. **POSTCHIASMAL LESIONS**
Left homonymous superior quadrantanopia

1. Altitudinal defect

4. Left homonymous inferior quadrantanopia

1. Central scotoma

5. Left homonymous hemianopia (macular sparing)

Adapted from: Talley NJ, et al. *Maclennan & Petty Pty Limited* 2003, page 363; McGee S. R. *Saunders/Elsevier* 2007, pages 664-5; and Davey P. *Wiley-Blackwell* 2006, page 99.

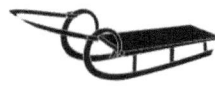

The Visual Pathways

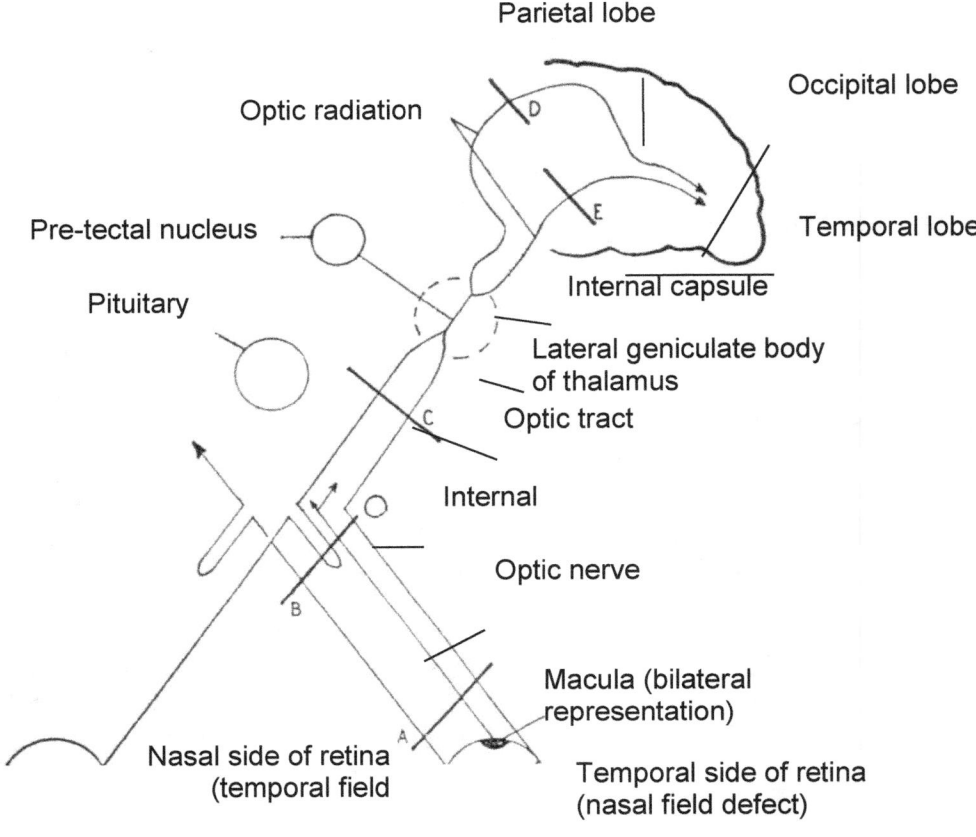

Parietal lobe

Optic radiation

Occipital lobe

Pre-tectal nucleus

Temporal lobe

Pituitary

Internal capsule

Lateral geniculate body
of thalamus

Optic tract

Internal

Optic nerve

Macula (bilateral
representation)

Nasal side of retina
(temporal field

Temporal side of retina
(nasal field defect)

- o Note the pituitary in relation to nasal fibres from both ratinae.
- o The optic radiation.
- o The internal carotid artery.
- o The macular fibres passing to both optic tracts.

➢ Visual Field Defects

- o Monocular defects are usually due to a problem in the affected eye, whereas binocular visual field defects are usually intracranial in origin

- o III Nerve palsy: affected side dilated (mydriasis), ptosis, weak extraocular muscle except lateral rectus and superior oblique

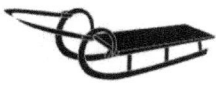

Lesion Location	Anatomy	Signs and Symptoms
o One eye	– Anterior to optic chiasm	▪ Glaucoma ▪ Retinal hemorhage ▪ Optic neuropathy ▪ Central retinal artery occlusion (leads to potential monocular blindness [amaurosis fugax])
o Both eyes (bitemporal hemianopia)	– At optic chiasm	▪ Upper > lower – inferior chiasmal compression (pituitary adenoma) ▪ Lower > upper – superior chiasmal compression
o Both eyes (homonymous hemianopia)	– Behind optic chiasm	▪ Cerebral infarcts ▪ Hemorrhage ▪ Tumours

Source: Filate W, et al. *The Medical Society, Faculty of Medicine, University of Toronto* 2005, page 158.

Blindness

- Give the causes of **sudden blindness.**
  - o Brain
    - – Trauma- ocular or post head injury
    - – CVA
    - – Migraine
    - – Hysteria Vitreous haemorrhage, especially in diabetics
  - o CN II
    - – Cranial arteritis
    - – Toxins e.g., methanol
    - – Retrobulbar neuritis
  - o Retinal vessels
    - – Embolism of retinal artery
    - – Thrombosis of retinal vein
  - o Retina
    - – Retinal detachment
  - o Intraocular
    - – Acute glaucoma

Adapted from: Burton JL. *Churchill Livingstone* 1971, page 82.

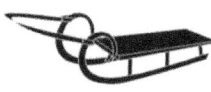

> Clinical

- Perform a focused physical examination for the causes of sudden blindness.
  - o Artery
    - – Embolus
    - – Arteritis
  - o Vein
    - – Thrombus
  - o Retinal detachment
    - – Trauma
    - – Tumour
    - – Toxemia
    - – Myopia
  - o Retinal hemorrhage
    - – Diabetes
    - – Edwards
  - o Glaucoma
  - o CVA
  - o Migraine
  - o Hysteria
  - o Drugs/toxins

- Take a directed history and perform a focused physical examination for AION (**anterior ischemic optic neuropathy**).

- History
  - o Sudden, total loss of vision in one eye (infarction of optic disc or nerve head)

- Physical
  - o Afferent pupillary defect in affected eye (Marcus Gunn pupil)
  - o Pale optic nerve head
  - o Dyschromatopsia
  - o May be associated signs of temporal (giant cell) arteritis

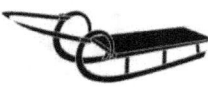

- Perform a focused physical examination to distinguish between the retinal vein and artery.

  - Retinal vein
    - Larger than artery (3:2 diameter)
    - Darker
    - Spontaneous pulsations
    - No light reflex

Adapted from: Mangione S. *Hanley & Belfus* 2000.

- Give the causes of **gradual blindness.**

  - CNS – Migraine

  - CN III
    - Optic neuritis
    - Atrophy
    - Papilloedema

  - Retina – Retinal degeneration

  - Intraocular – Glaucoma

  - Lens – Cataracts

"Walk tall. Walk steady. Walk together."

Catherine Zahn

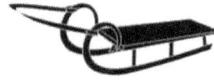

SO YOU WANT TO BE A NEUROLOGIST!

- In the context of blindness, give the meaning of **amaurosis fugax**?
    - A transient monocular blindness due to episodic retinal ischemia, usually associated with ipsilateral carotid artery stenosis or embolism of the retinal arteries resulting in a sudden, and frequently complete, loss of vision in one eye.

Source: Jugovic PJ, et al. *Saunders/ Elsevier* 2004, page 150.

- Give the reason why obstruction of the PCA distal to the thalamic branch not affect the macula.
    - Because the macula is supplied by both the MCA and the PCA

- From the physical examination, give the way in which you determine if the patient had cortical blindness (CB) from occlusion of the PCAs, versus damage to the optic tracts (OT), optic nerve (ON) or the retina (R)?

	Finding	OT/ON/R	CD
o	Pupillary reflexes	+	normal
o	Fundus	+	normal
o	Awareness when light shone in eyes	+	no

- In the context of an abnormal examination of the eyes, give the meaning of Eale Disease.
    - Periodic vitreous hemorrhage and pre-retinal (subhyaloid) hemorrhages.
    - Disease of young man attributed to tuberculosis periphlebitis.

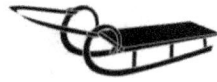

- Give the causes of concentric diminution (**tunnel vision**).

  o Brain
    - Anterior calcarine cortex
    - Migraine
    - Hysteria
    - Occipital cortex

  o CN II
    - Papilloedema
    - Retroneuritis

  o Retinal vessels

  o Retinal disease

  o Glaucoma

  o Causes of bitemporal hemianopia (Central chiasmal lesions)
    - Pituitary or peri-sellar tumour
    - Inflammatory, vascular or traumatic lesions

  o Binasal hemianopia
    - Bilateral lesions confined to the uncrossed optic fibres.

  o Causes of homonymous hemianopia (HN)
    - Optic tract lesions – usually due to tumours, which produce a
      progressive hemianopia, which bisects the macula, commonly due
      to thombosis of the posterior cerebral vessels.

  o Causes of homonymous quadrantanopia
    - Anteriorly placed lesions of the optic radiation, especially temporal lobe
      tumours. More posterior lesions of the optic radiation become more hemianopic.

Source: Burton JL. *Churchill Livingstone* 1971, page 79.

- Give the causes of **central scotoma***.

  o Brain   – Demyelinating disorders (multiple sclerosis)

  o CN II   – Optical nerve compression by Tumour, aneurysm
                   – Toxins – methanol, tobacco, lead, arsenical poisoning
                   – Hereditary disorders – Friedreich's ataxia, Leber's optic atrophy

  o Retinal   – Ischemia
    vessels   ▪ Central retinal artery occlusion(thromboembolism)
                     ▪ Temporal arteritis
                     ▪ Syphilis
                     ▪ Idiopathic acute ischemic neuropathy

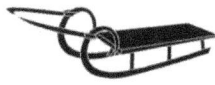

o Retina   – Secondary to retinitis pigmentosa

o Intraocular   – Glaucoma

o Metabolic   – Vitamin B_{12} deficiency

*Scotoma is a small patch of visual loss within the visual field.
Adapted from: Baliga RR. *Saunders/Elsevier* 2007, page 135.

Retina

➢ Causes

• Give the causes of **retinal hemorrhage**.

- o CNS
  - – Subarachnoid hemorrhage
  - – Raised IC pressure
- o Retinal vessels
  - – Arteritis (PN, cranial arteritis, etc.)
  - – Retinal vein thrombosis
- o Retina
  - – Trauma
  - – Retinal detachment
- o Hypertension
- o Diabetes
- o Hematology
  - – Severe anemia, especially PA
  - – Bleeding diathesis-defect in platelets, vessels or coagulation factors

Affected pupil size may be dilated, depending on the cause of the CN III palsy, (e.g., intracranial aneurysm).

Abbreviation: PA, pernicious anemia; IC, intracranial nerve; PN, polyarteritis nodosum

Adapted from: Burton JL. *Churchill Livingstone*, 1971, page 82.

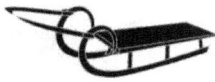

➢ Clinical

- Perform a focused physical examination for the causes of retinal hemorrhage.

  - o Brain — ↑ ICP, including subarachnoid hemorrhage

  - o Eye — Eye – trauma

  - o Retinal vessels — Artery
    - HBP
    - Arteritis
    — Vein
    - Thrombosis
  - o Retina — Retinal detachment, including tumour

  - o Hematology — Anemia (severe)
    — Bleeding diathesis (severe)
  - o Diabetes

Abbreviations: CNS, central nervous system; ICP, intracranial pressure; HBP, hypertension

Adapted from: Burton JL. *Churchill Livingstone* 1971, page 22.

- Perform a focused physical examination of the fundus for **hypertensive retinopathy**.
  - o Vasoconstrictive phase
    - Constriction of 2nd or 3rd branching point of the
      - Retinal arteries usually not visible with direct
      - Examination with ophthalmoscope
  - o Sclerotic phase
    - Narrowing of arteries
    - AV nicking (narrowing of retinal vein where crossed by the artery)
    - light reflex (from thickening of anterior wall of retinal artery)
  - o Exudative phase
    - Flame-like hemorrhages
    - Exudates, hard
    - Cotton-wool spots

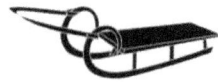

- Perform a focused physical examination of the fundus for **diabetic retinopathy**.

    o Microaneurysms

    o Dot and blot hemorrhages

    o Cotton-wool spots, and hard exudates

    o Neovascularization PDR (proliferative diabetic retinopathy)
        - Cotton-wool spot followed by development of tiny, irregular vessels
        - Preretinal or vitreous hemorrhages
        - Traction retinal detachment
            ▪ Whitish area of retina
            ▪ Fine surface folds
            ▪ Loss of light reflex
    o Almost always followed by diabetic nephropathy (Kimmel stiel-wilson glomerular disease)

- Perform a focused physical examination of the eye for **macular degeneration.**

    o "Dry" type
        - Drusen yellow, round, distinct deposits
        - Loss of pigmentation
        - Prominent choroidal vessels (because of the loss of the retinal pigment epithelium)

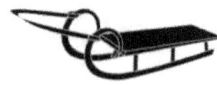

Mastering the Boards: Neurology   A.B.R. Thomson

- o "Wet" type
  - – Grey/ green area
  - – Hemorrhage and exudates
  - – Scaring of the macula

- o Complications
  - – Central retinal artery occlusion (CRAO)
    - ▪ Fundus – pale
    - ▪ Retina – swelling
    - ▪ Macula – cherry – red
    - ▪ Afferent papillary defect
  - – Branch retinal artery occlusion (BRAO)
  - – Central retinal vein occlusion (CRVO)**
    - ▪ Veins
      - - Engorgement
      - - Dilation – microaneurysm
    - ▪ Retina
      - - Multiple dot or flame hemorrhages in all parts of retina
      - - Cotton-wool spots
    - ▪ Optic disc – edema
  - – Branch retinal vein occlusion (BRVO)***
    - ▪ Occlusion of branch vein produces changes only in that quadrant
    - ▪ Flame hemorrhages
    - ▪ Cotton-wool spots
    - ▪ Vein distal to occlusion
      - - Dilated
      - - Tortuous

Source: Mangione S. *Hanley & Belfus* 2000, page 96.

Retinal Lesions

- Give the physical findings which suggest a lesion of the retina

  - o Cotton-wool spots ("soft" exudates); small retinal infarcts due to occlusion of the end-arteriole.
    - – White
    - – Opaque
    - – Indistinct
    - – Can obscure adjacent vessels

  - o Hard exudates (leaky vessels)
    - – Whitish yellow
    - – Distinct

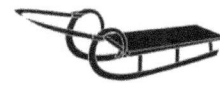

- o Drusen deposit
  - – Yellow
  - – Located in the macula or in the peripheral retina
  - – Distinct
  - – Round

- o Myelinated nerve fibre
  - – White
  - – Obscure blood vessels
  - – Bright
  - – No clinical significance

Source: Mangione S. *Hanley & Belfus* 2000, page 97.

- • Give the causes of **cotton-wool spots** and **hard exudates** in the retina.

  - o Metabolic
    - – Hypertension
    - – Diabetes

  - o Infiltration
    - – Leukemia
    - – Lymphoma

  - o Infection
    - – Bacterial endocarditis
    - – HIV-associated CMV

  - o Vascular
    - – Microemboli
    - – Anemia
    - – Increased intracranial pressure (papilledema)

- • Give the causes of **red spots** in the retina.

  - o Microaneurysms

  - o Blot and dot hemorrhages –
    - – arise from bleeding in the middle retinal layer in the retina
    - – Common in diabetes

  - o Flame and splinter hemorrhages
    - – Arise from bleeding in the superficial nerve fibre layer in the retina
    - – Parallel to orientation of nerve fibres running out from the optic disc
    - – Common in hypertension

  - o Preretinal hemorrhages (including dubhyaloid hemorrhages)

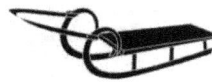

- o Roth spots
  - – Red (hemorrhage) with white (fibrinous) centre
  - – SBE, diabetes, intracranial bleed

Source: Mangione S. *Hanley & Belfus* 2000, page 99.

- • Give the causes of **dark-coloured spots** in the retina.

  - o Retinitis pigmentosa
    - – Pigment arranged in a spicule formation

  - o Retinal pigment epithelial hypertrophy
    - – Pigmented lesions
      - ▪ Numerous (>4)
      - ▪ Bilateral
      - ▪ Varying sizes and shapes
      - ▪ The grouping together of the pigmented spots suggest "bear tracks"
      - ▪ Normal vision
      - ▪ 78% sensitive, and 95% specific for Gardner's syndrome

  - o Choroid pigmentation
    - – Benign nevi
      - ▪ Flat
      - ▪ Grey/green
      - ▪ Indistinct borders
    - – Melanoma raised

  - o Healed chorioretinitis

  - o Laser scars, treated diabetic retinopathy

Source: Mangione S. *Hanley & Belfus* 2000, page 18.

- • Give the causes of **retinitis pigmentosa**.

  - o Congenital (associated with cataract and deaf mutism)

  - o Laurence Moon Biedl syndrome

  - o Hereditary ataxia

  - o Familial neuropathy i.e., Refsum disease

Abbreviation: CSF, cerebrospinal fluid
Source: Talley NJ, et al. *Maclennan & Petty Pty Limited* 2003, Table 10.5, page 363.

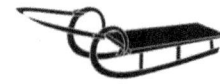

Eye Pain

➤ Causes

- Give the causes of eye pain.

    o Cornea, conjunctiva (by blinking)
    - Corneal abrasions
    - Foreign bodies
    - Keratitis

    o Iris (photophobkia)
    - Inflammation of the iris
    - Middle layer of the eye corneal irritation

    o CN II (by moving eye)
    - Optic neuritis

    o Artery (forehead)
    - With brow or temporal pain (e.g., may indicate temporal arteritis)

    o Intraocular (headache, nausea)
    - Acute angle-closure glaucoma

Adapted from: Filate W, et al. *The Medical Society, Faculty of Medicine, University of Toronto* 2005, page 201.

Pupils

➤ Definition

    o Anisocoria is a difference ≥ 0.4 mm in diameter of the pupils

    o Represents either a problem with the papillary constrictor muscle (parasympathetic denervation, iris disorder, pharmacologic pupil) or the papillary dilator muscle (sympathetic denervation, simple anisocoria)

➤ Clinical

- Unequal size of the pupil (anisocoria) may occur congenitally. In the comatose patient, how do you determine by physical examination if the anisocorm is due to a pathological process?

    o Pathological anisocoria is asymmetry of the pupils plus loss of reaction of the pupils to light.

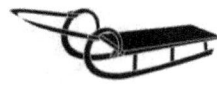

- Give in what eye disease it is not possible to properly assess anisocoria.
  - With iritis, the patient may have so much photophobia that it is not possible to determine if the size of the pupils is not equal.
  - Horner syndrome
  - Pharmacological
  - Blindness or amblyopia in one eye (pupil larger in the affected eye)
  - Cerebrovascular accidents
  - Severe head trauma
  - Hemianopia due to optic tract involvement

Adapted from: McGee SR. *Saunders/Elsevier* 2007, page 217-219; Baliga RR. *Saunders/Elsevier* 2007, page 129.

- Perform a focused physical examination of the eye to distinguish the unequal size of the pupils (anisocoria) due to a defect in the hippus or an afferent pupillary defect.
  - Hippus
    - Normal (physiological) constant changing in the size of the pupil, in which the pupil, initially constricts to light
  - Afferent pupillary defect (aka Marcus Gunn pupil)
    - The pupil from the affected eye initially dilates, in response to light
    - Due to optic nerve lesion (optic neuritis, optic neuropathy), or massive retinal lesion (retinal artery occlusion)

- Isolated palsies may occur in CN III (oculomotor), IV (trochlear) or VI (abducens). Give the commonest cause of a isolated CN palsy of each of these 3 nerves.
  - III ischemia
  - IV head trauma, idiopathic, ischemia
  - VI neoplasm, ischemia

Source: McGee SR. *Saunders/Elsevier*, 2007, Table 55-1, page 680.

Useful background: Pupils

Finding	Sensitivity (%)	Specificity (%)	PLR	NLR
➢ Detecting intracranial structural lesion in patients with coma				
o Anisocoria > 1mm	39	96	9.0	0.6
o Absent light reflex in at least one eye	83	77	3.6	0.2

Source: McGee SR. *Saunders/Elsevier* 2007, Box 19-1, page 222.

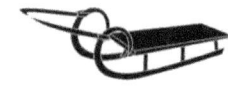

Mastering the Boards: Neurology   A.B.R. Thomson

- Perform a focused physical examination for the causes of the Argyll Robertson pupil.

  o Infection
    - Neurosyphillis – tabes dorsalis
    - Brainstem encephalitis
    - Sarcoidosis
  o Infiltration
    - Pinealoma
    - Tumours of the posterior portion of the third ventricle
  o Metabolic
    - Diabetes mellitus and other conditions with autonomic neuropathy
    - Lyme disease
  o Degenerative
    - Multiple sclerosis
    - Syringobulbia

Adapted from: Baliga RR. *Saunders/Elsevier* 2007, page 128.

- Give the causes of **abnormal reaction to light or to accommodation**.

  o Pupil fails to constrict to light, but does constrict with accommodation (Argyll Robertson pupils)
    - Syphilis, tertiary
    - Diabetes
    - Alcohol (Wernicke encephalopathy)
  o Pupil fails to constrict to light and to accommodation (Adie pupil)
  o Pupil fails to constrict to light, and actually dilates
    - Marcus Gunn pupil (aka afferent pupillary defect) seen in optic neuritis or severe retinal damage such as central retinal artery occlusion)

Source: McGee SR. *Saunders/Elsevier* 2007, pages 213 and 223.

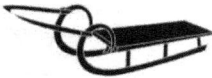

SO YOU WANT TO BE A NEUROLOGIST!

- Give the meaning of **Argyll Robertson pupil**; give its clinical features, its the underlying neuroanatomy and give a systemic approach to its causes.

  ➢ Definition: The Argyll Robertson pupil is a pupil which reacts to accommodation, but not to light.

  ➢ Neuroanatomy
    o Unlike the pupillary light reflex, the efferent fibres of the accommodation reflex do not pass through the ciliary ganglion
    o Thus, a lesion of the oculomotor (CN III) nerve fibres damages the area of the ciliary ganglion will prevent the light reflex but not the accommodation reflex
    o Sympathetic innervation may also be impaired

  ➢ Clinical features
    o Pupils react to accommodation but not to light
    o Pupils are not always small
    o Pupils may react a little to light (constriction), but with constriction not being maintained
    o Small irregular pupil
    o Patchy atrophy of iris
    o Depigmentation of iris

SO YOU WANT TO BE A NEUROLOGIST!
- Give how to distinguish between Argyll Robertson pupils (ARP), and the pupils of the patients with aberrant regeneration of CN III (AR III).

Clinical	AR III	ARP
o Constriction of pupil during convergence, but not to light	Unilateral	Bilateral
o Associated anisocoria, ptosis, diplopia	Yes	No

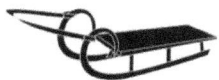

Tonic pupil (Holmes-Adie pupil)

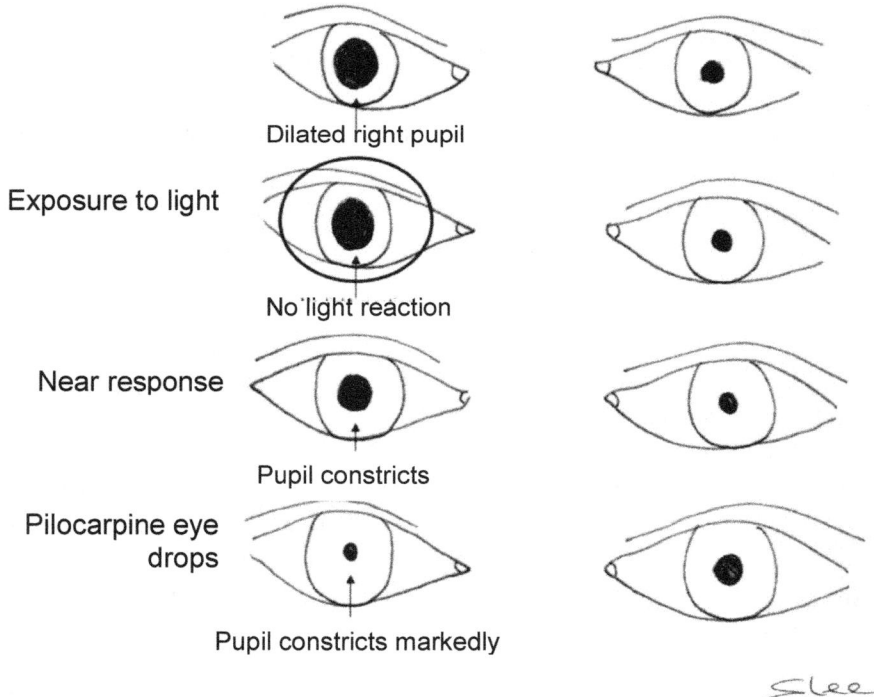

Dilated right pupil

Exposure to light

No light reaction

Near response

Pupil constricts

Pilocarpine eye drops

Pupil constricts markedly

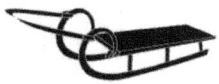

➢ The patient in this figure has a right tonic pupil.

  o At baseline, there is anisocoria with the right pupil larger than the left (first row).

  o The dilated pupil fails to react to light (second row) but constricts slowly (i.e., 'tonic' contraction) when the patient focuses on a near object (third row).

  o After instillation of dilute pilocarpine eye drops (fourth row), the pupil constricts markedly.

Adapted from: McGee S. R. *Saunders/Elsevier* 2007, page 223.

SO YOU WANT TO BE A NEUROLOGIST!

- Give the meaning of the Holmes-Adie pupil.
  o Large pupil
  o Reacts slowly to accommodation, but not to light
  o Unilateral
  o Usually occurs in women
  o Associated with slow deep tendon reflexes

- Be prepared to differentiate between the pupils in Argyll Robertson versus Holmes-Adie syndrome.
  o Please see answers below.

SO YOU WANT TO BE A NEUROLOGIST!

- Give the causes of miosis.
    o Old age
    o Pilocarpine (treatment for glaucoma)
- Give the non-neurological conditions which cause an eccentric pupil.
    o Trauma
    o Iritis

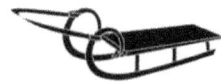

- Perform a focused physical examination of the patient with a large pupil (regular or irregular, oval or circular) which reacts slowly to light and accommodation (Holmes-Adie Syndrome).

➢ Eye
  o Near vision
    - ↓ constriction in response to near vision.
    - ↓ re-dilation after near vision.
  o If a strong and persistent stimulus is used
    - The pupil contracts excessively to a very small size
    - When the stimulus is removed, the pupil slowly returns to its former size (known as the "myotonic" pupil).
  o Segmental palsy and segmental spontaneous movement of iris

➢ Ankle reflexes – absent

Adapted from: Baliga RR. 250 *Saunders/Elsevier* 2007, page 130.

SO YOU WANT TO BE A NEUROLOGIST!

- A "fixed pupil" is a pupil which does not react to light or to accommodation. A fixed pupil which is dilated may be due to iritis or to oculomotor (CN III) lesion. How can you distinguish between the two by examining the eyes?

  o Iritis
    - Fixed, dilated, irregular pupil
    - Does not react to light or accommodation
  o Retrobulbar neuritis
    - Fixed dilated pupil
    - Reacts slowly to direct light

- In the context of the Argyll Robertson pupil (ARP), what is the Adie pupil (AP)?

	Light	Accommodation
- ARP	No	Yes
- AP	No	No

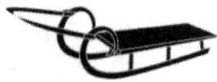

➢ Causes

• Give the causes of **dilated pupils** and **contracted pupils.**

  o Normal variant

  o CN III palsy

  o Unilateral blindness (affected eye is dilated)/ eye disease)
    – Iritis
    – Acute angle closure glaucoma
    – Trauma
    – Previous surgery
    – Congenital

  o Dilated
    – CN III
      ▪ Third nerve lesion
      ▪ Holmes-Adie syndrome (degeneration of nerve to the ciliary ganglion)
    – Iris
      ▪ Blunt trauma to the iris (pupil may be irregularly dilated and reacts sluggishly to light – post-traumatic iridoplegia)
    – Lens
      ▪ Lens implant
      ▪ Iridectomy
    – Drugs
      ▪ Mydriatic eye drops
        - Drug overdose, e.g., cocaine, amphetamine
        - Poisoning, e.g., Belladonna
    – Coma, death
      ▪ Deep coma
      ▪ Death

  o Contracted
    – Old age
    – CN III
    – Pons
      ▪ Argyll Robertson pupil (distinguish)
      ▪ Pontine lesion
      ▪ Narcotics
    – Sympathetic nerve disorders
      ▪ Horner syndrome
    – Drugs
      ▪ Pilocarpine eye drops

Adapted from: Baliga RR. *Saunders/Elsevier* 2007, page 131.

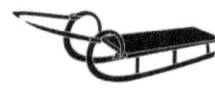

- Give causes of **pin-point pupils**.
  - o Pin-point pupils are caused by
    - – Opiates
    - – Pontine hemorrhage

Papilledema

- ➤ Causes
- Give the causes of papilledema.

  - o Increased intracranial pressure
    - – Space occupying lesion (causing raised intracranial pressure), or a retroorbital mass
    - – Benign intracranial hypertension (pseudotumour cerebri) (small or normal sized ventricles)
      - ▪ Idiopathic
      - ▪ Oral contraceptive pill
      - ▪ Addison's disease
      - ▪ Drugs- e.g., nitrofurantoin, tetracycline, vitamin A, steroids
      - ▪ Head trauma
  - o Increased formation of CSF- e.g., choroids plexus papilloma (rare)
  - o Decreased absorption of CSF
    - – Tumour causing venous compression
    - – Subarachnoid space obstruction from meningitis
  - o Decreased outflow
    - – Hydrocephalus (large cerebral ventricles)
    - – Obstruction (a block in the ventricle, aqueduct or outlet to the fourth ventricle) e.g., tumour
  - o Communicating hydrocephalus
  - o Systemic hypertension (grade 4)
  - o Central retinal vein thrombosis

Adapted form: Baliga RR. *Saunders/Elsevier* 2007, page 81.

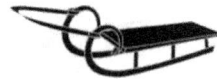

➢ Clinical

- Perform a funduscopic examination for papilledema (edema of optic nerve disc, papilla).
  - o Bilateral changes
  - o Disc
    - – Blurred margins
    - – Swelling
    - – No loss of cupping (cup-to-disc ratio, < 50%)
  - o Retinal veins
    - – Loss of spontaneous pulsations

Source: Mangione S. *Hanley & Belfus* 2000, page 93.

- Give causes of **optic neuritis**.
  - o Infective
    - – Local: retinitis, periostitis
    - – Systemic: syphilis, toxoplasmosis, typhoid fever, mumps
  - o Toxins
    - – Lead
    - – Methyl alcohol/benzene
    - – Tobacco
  - o Metabolic
    - – Diabetes mellitus
    - – B12 deficiency
    - – Intestinal or uterine haemorrhage
  - o Demyelinating disease eg.
    - – Multiple sclerosis (MS)
    - – Devic disease
    - – Schilder disease
  - o Hereditary degenerations
    - – Leber disease
    - – Marie disease
    - – Freidreich ataxia
  - o Giant cell arteritis
  - o Trauma

Source: Burton JL. *Churchill Livingstone* 1971, page 81.

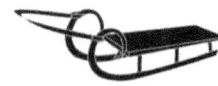

- Perform an examination for **acute angle closure glaucoma**.

  - Cornea
    - Haziness (edema)
    - Halos, with rainbow-cloured fringes around points of light
    - Ciliary flush (circumcorneal erythema)
  - Conjunctiva
    - Redness
    - Tearing
  - Pupils
    - Partially dilated
    - Non responsive
  - Optic disc
    - ↑ optic cup-todisc ratio, > 50%
    - ↓ visual acuity

Adapted from: Mangione S. *Hanley & Belfus* 2000, page 92.

- Take a directed history and perform a focused ocular examination for **papillitis/optic neuritis** (a form of papillitis is optic neuritis).

  - History
    - Eye pain
    - Acute, unilateral loss of vision

  - Physical
    - Loss of vision in one eye
    - Defect in colour vision
    - Swelling of the optic disc, without ↑ ICP
    - Afferent pipillary defect (Marcus Gunn pupil) on the affected side

---

CLINICAL CHALLENGE

- From fundoscopic examination of the ocular vessels, how can you distinguish between choriodosis and retinitis?

  - Choriodosis – exudate is under the vessel (superficial to the exudate)
  - Retinitis – exudate interrupts the vessel

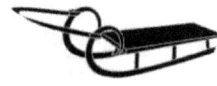

- Perform a focused physical examination to distinguish between papilledema vs. papillitis.

Papilledema	Papillitis
o Optic disc - Swollen without venous pulsation	- Optic disc swollen
o Visual acuity - Normal (early)	- Poor
o Blind spot - Large	- Large central scotoma
o Visual fields of peripheral constriction - Usually slow onset and bilateral	- Onset usually sudden and unilateral
- Colour vision normal	
- Eye movement- no pain	- Painful

Adapted from: Baliga RR. *Saunders/Elsevier* 2007, page 128.

"Old age makes you redundant

but

It's OK to be redundant – but only if you're a gene!"

Grandad

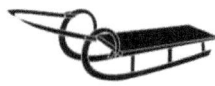

Mastering the Boards: Neurology A.B.R. Thomson

CRANIAL NERVES

Remember: You need to establish **where** is the lesion, and **what** is the likely lesion.

> Terminology

- o Olfactory (I)
  - – Smell

- o Optic (II)
  - – Vision

- o Oculomotor (III)
  - – All ocular muscles, except superior oblique and lateral rectus
  - – Ciliary muscle
  - – Sphincter papillae
  - – Levator palpebrae superioris

- o Trochlear superior oblique muscle (IV)
  - – Oculomotor tested by asking patient to look down and inwards

- o Trigeminal (V)
  - – Sensory for face, cornea, sinuses, nasal mucosal, teeth, tympanic membrane and anterior two thirds of tongue
  - – Motor to muscles of mastication

- o Abducens (External rectus muscle) (VI)
  - – Oculomotor

- o Facial (VII)
  - – Motor to scalp and facial muscles of expression
  - – Taste in anterior two thirds of tongue (via chorda tympani)
  - – Nerve to stapedius muscle

- o Auditory and vestibular components (VIII)

- o Glossopharyngeal (IX)
  - – Sensory for posterior one third of tongue, pharynx and middle ear
  - – Taste fibres for posterior one third of tongue
  - – Motor to middle constrictor of pharynx and stylopharyngeus

- o Vagal (X)
  - – Motor to soft palate, larynx and pharynx (from nucleus ambigus)
  - – Sensory and motor for heart, respiratory passengers and abdominal viscera (from dorsal nucleus)

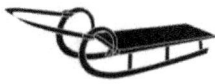

- o Spinal accessory (XI)
  - – Motor to sternomastoid and trapezius
  - – Accessory fibres to vagus (XII)
- o Hypoglossal Motor to tongue and hyoid bone depressors

Source: Burton JL. *Churchill Livingstone* 1971, page 73.

➢ Neuroanatomy

- o Medial longitudinal bundle
  - – Interconnects the cranial nerve nuclei
  - – Co-ordinates movements of face and eye

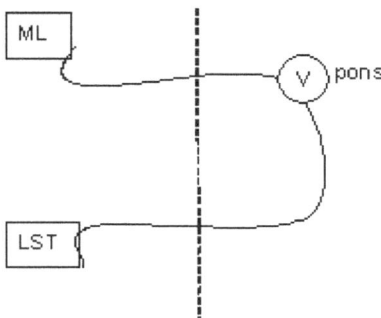

- o CN V (trigeminal nerve)
  - – Ascending tract
    - ▪ Fibres/or proprioception and left touch (just like the posterior colums)
    - ▪ Ascending tract (AT) fibres cross the midline and join the medial lemniscus (ML)
  - – Descending tract (of CN V)
    - ▪ Fibres for pain and temperature (just like the lateral spinothalamic tracts
    - ▪ Descending tract (DT) fibres descend to C2 on the same side
    - ▪ From C2, DT fibres cross the midline to join the lateral spinothalamic tract (LST)
- o Tractus solitarium
  - – Fibres for taste
- o Corticospinal tracts

The medial lemniscus terminates in the thalamus.

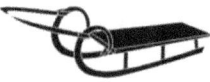

SO YOU WANT TO BE A NEUROLOGIST!

Crossed hemiplegia may be caused for example by a CVA, causing hemiplegia on one side of the body, but weakness on the other side of muscles suppied by cranial nerves IX to XII.

- Give other causes of crossed hemiplegia.

    o Weber syndrome   -   Ipselateral cranial nerve III LMN lesion, with contralateral hemiplegia

    o Miller-Gubler syndrome   -   Ipselateral cranial nerve VI lesion (supplies the lateral rectus muscle), with contralateral hemiplegia

    o Foville syndrome   -   The eyes are fixed towards the side of the hemiplegia (paralysis of conjugate deviation towards the side of the lesion

- Give, by looking at the eyes whether a patient's hemiplegia is due to a lesion in the internal capsule or brainstem (Foville syndrome).

    o Conjugate deviation towards side of lesion - Foville syndrome

    o Conjugate deviation away side of lesion   - Internal capsule

➢ Nuclei of the cranial nerves

  o Midbrain

  o Oculomotor
    – Trochlear

  o Pons
    – Abducens
    – Trigeminal
    – Facial
    – Auditory

  o Medulla
    – Glossopharyngeal
    – Vagus
    – Accessory
    – Hypoglossal

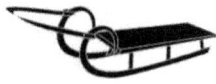

Sensory pathway

Cerebral cortex (conscious discrimatory functions)
↑
Thalamus
↑
Sensory input
←⌐

Cord   Decussation, except for spinocerebellar tracts

- Perform a focused physical examination of the cranial nerves (CN).
    - I (Olfactory) smell (sensory) (detecting non irritating odours)
        - Coffee, mint, vinegar

Translational Neuroanatomy

CN I
    - Nerve endings in ciliated receptors in mucous membrane of upper part of nasal cavity
        ↓
    - Cribriform plate of ethnoid bone
        ↓
    - Olfactory bulb and tract
        ↓
    - Mammillary bodies of hypothalamus
        ↓
    - Uncinate and hippocampal gyri of both temporal lobes

- Give the causes of **multiple cranial nerve palsies**.

    - Inherited   – Arnold Chiari malformation

    - Infection   – Guillain Barre syndrome (spares sensory nerves)
                       – Tuberculosis
                       – Sarcoidosis

    - Infiltration   – Nasopharyngeal carcinoma
                       – Hematological malignancy,
                       – Brainstem Tumour (eg in the cerebellopontine angle) have similar signs

    - Vascular   – Brainstem vascular disease causing crossed sensory or motor paralysis (i.e., cranial nerve signs on one side and contralateral long tract signs).

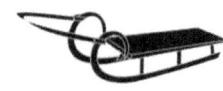

o Trauma

o Metabolic   – Paget disease
                   – Mononeuritis multiplex (rarely, e.g., diabetes mellitus)

Abbreviations: LMN, lower motor neurons; MS, Multiple sclerosis; UMN, upper motor neurons

Adapted from: Talley NJ, et al. *Maclennan & Petty Pty Limited* 2003, Table 10.7, page 384.

Ptosis

- Perform a focused physical examination for the causes of unilateral ptosis.

    o Third cranial nerve (III) palsy
    o Horner syndrome
    o Myasthenia gravis
    o Congenital or idiopathic

Horner Syndrome

➢ Definition

     o Miosis

     o Ptosis (at rest, but not on looking upwards)

     o Anhydrosis

     o Lack of tears

     o Interruption of the sympathetic innervation of the eye

➢ Causes

     o Neck
         – Malignancy- e.g., Thyroid
         – Trauma, surgery lymphadenopathy

     o Lower trunk brachial plexus lesions
         – Trauma
         – Tumour

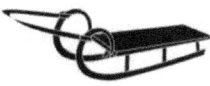

- o Carotid arterial lesion
    - – Carotid aneurysm or dissection (vascular lesions)
    - – Pericarotid tumours (Raeder's syndrome- sweating not affected since Tumour involves internal carotid artery)
    - – Cluster headache
- o Brainstem lesions
    - – Vascular disease (especially the lateral medullary syndrome)
    - – Tumour
    - – Syringobulbia
- o Syringomyelia (rare)
- o Lung
    - – Carcinoma (usually squamous cell carcinoma) of the apex of the lung

Adapted from: Talley NJ, et al. *Maclennan & Petty Pty Limited* 2003, Table 10.10, page 389; Baliga RR. *Saunders/Elsevier* 2007, page 126.

- ➢ Clinical

- • Perform a focused physical examination for the causes of Horner Syndrome.
    - o *Partial ptosis* (as sympathetic fibres supply the smooth muscle of both eyelids)
    - o *Constricted* pupil (unbalanced parasympathetic action) which reacts normally to light
    - o Decrease in the *sweating* over each eyebrow
    - o As part of the lateral medullay syndrome
    - o Syringomyelia
        - – Dissociated sensory loss
        - – Bilateral Horner syndrome)
    - o Nystagmus to the side of the lesion
    - o Ipsilateral fifth (pain and temperature)
    - o Ninth and tenth cranial nerve lesions
    - o Ipsilateral cerebellar signs
    - o Contralateral pain and temperature loss over the trunk and limbs

Adapted from: Talley NJ, et al. *Maclennan & Petty Pty Limited* 2003, page 389.

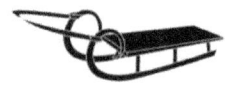

╔══╗

SO YOU WANT TO BE A NEUROLOGIST!

- Give how you would distinguish congenital from non-congenital Horner syndrome.
  - In congenital Horner syndrome, there are all the usual features of miosis, ptosis, enopthalmos, and elevation of the lower lip, plus there would be heterochromia of the iris (i.e., the iris remains grey-blue).

- In the patient with ipsilateral Horner syndrome and contralateral loss of pain and temperature sensation, give the Wollenberg syndrome.
  - Wollenberg syndrome is also known as the lateral medullary syndrome, which usually presents with the above features in the person who has suffered a stroke.

- Give one cause of intermittent Horner syndrome.

  - Easy- Migraine.

╚══╝

╔══╗

- In Horner syndrome, give how would you differentiate clinically whether the lesion is above (peripheral) or below (central) the superior cervical ganglion.

Position of Lesion Related to Superior Ganglion

Test	Above	Below
○ Sweating	– May not affect sweating – The main outflow to the facial blood vessels is below the superior cervical ganglion	▪ Affect sweating over the entire head, neck, arm, and upper trunk ▪ Lesions in the lower neck affect sweating over the entire face

Source: Baliga RR. *Saunders/Elsevier* 2007, page 127.

╚══╝

➢ Pupillary Light Reflex

  - CN III → ciliary ganglion → parasympathetic → constrictor pupillary muscle

  - CN V (ophthalmic division)→ ciliary ganglion → cervical sympathetic nerves → dilator pupillary muscle

  - Pupillary light reflex → optic nerve afferents → lateral geniculate body → biliary nuclei in midbrain

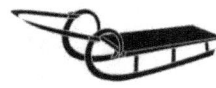

Mastering the Boards: Neurology A.B.R. Thomson

➤ Accommodation

- ○ Afferent component: Frontal cortex-efferent component: CN III (note: unlike the pupillary light reflex, the efferent fibres do not pass through the ciliary ganglion)
  - – Output
    - ▪ Convergence of eyes (medial recti)
    - ▪ Contraction of ciliary muscle
    - ▪ Constriction of pupil

➤ Oculosympathetic pathway involved in Horner syndrome

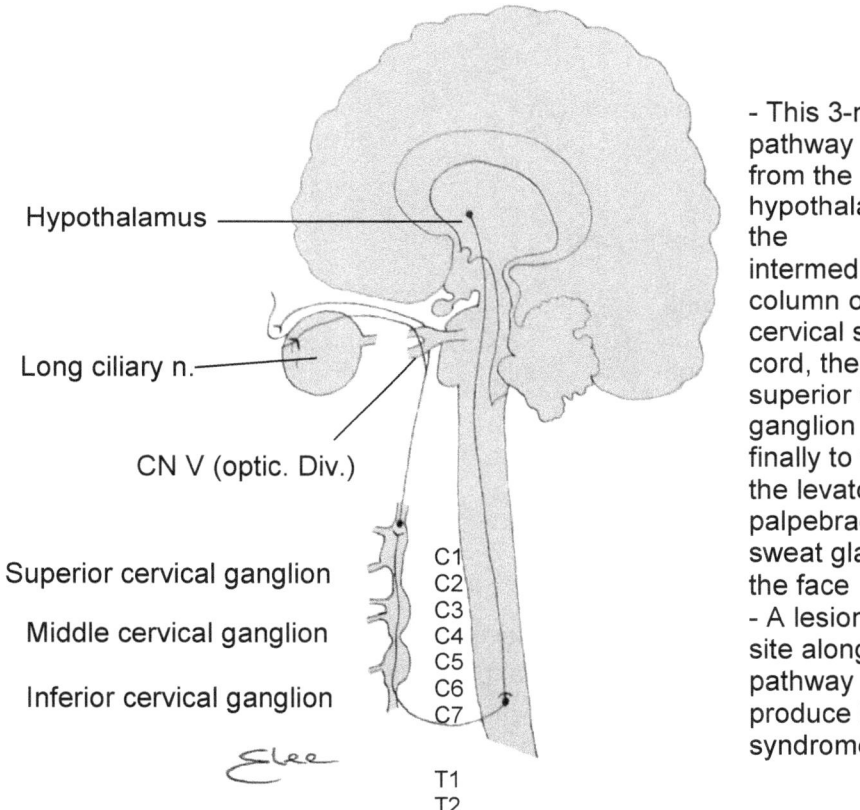

Hypothalamus

Long ciliary n.

CN V (optic. Div.)

Superior cervical ganglion

Middle cervical ganglion

Inferior cervical ganglion

C1
C2
C3
C4
C5
C6
C7

T1
T2

- This 3-neuron pathway projects from the hypothalamus to the intermediolateral column of the cervical spinal cord, then to the superior cervical ganglion and finally to the pupil, the levator palpebrae and the sweat glands of the face
- A lesion at any site along the pathway can produce Horner syndrome

Adapted from: Talley NJ, et al. *Maclennan & Petty Pty Limited* 2003, Figure 10.23, page 388.

- o Miosis
  - No sympathetic activity to balance parasympathetic action: paralysis of the dilator of the pupil
- o Ptosis
  - Damage to sympathetic nerves of eyelids, with paralysis of upper tarsal muscle.
  - Often, slight elevation of brow lid, due to paralysis of lower tarsal muscle
  - Rarely, enophthalmos due to paralysis of the muscle of muller.
- o Anhydridosis (not always present)

- ➤ **Translational Neuroanatomy**: Sympathetic Fibres to Eye and Face
  - o Hypothalamic ganglia
    ↓
  - o Superior colliculus of midbrain
    ↓
  - o Tectospinal tract
    ↓
  - o Lateral horns of spinal cord
    ↓
  - o Preganglionic rami
    ↓
  - o Anterior nerve roots
    ↓
  - o Cervical sympathetic chain
    ↓
  - o Superior cervical ganglion
    ↓
  - o Postganglionic fibres
    ↓
  - o Internal carotid and cavernous sinus plexus -→ Ciliary nerve of eye (from V1)
    - o Levator pulpebrae superioris
      ↓
    - o Dilator pupillae
  - o Same side of face ←--------vasomotor and sweat fibres
  - o Associated neurological signs
    - Ipsilateral
    - Nystagmus
    - V (pain/ temperature)
    - IX, X
    - Lower cranial nerves, recurrent laryngeal nerve palsy (hoarseness)
    - Loss of cerebellar function
    - Contralateral – loss of pain/ temperature over trunk and limbs

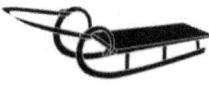

- o Associated non-neurological signs (see causes below)
  - – Clubbing, weak finger abduction, abnormal respiratory examination of lung apices, lymphadenopathy, thyroid mass, (carcinoma), carotid aneurysm or bruit
  - – Test for syringomyelia, with central cord, lesions (look for disassociated sensory loss, and possible bilateral Horner syndrome)

Marcus Gunn Pupil

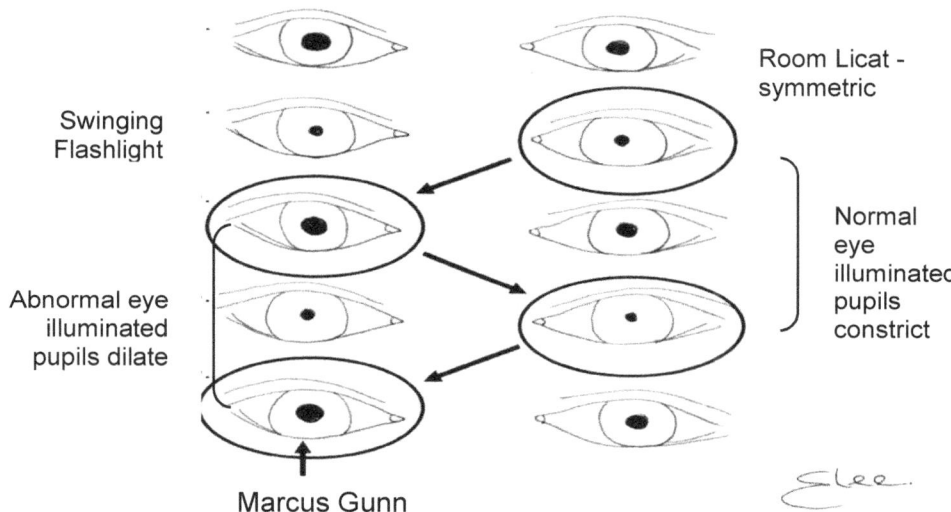

Marcus Gunn

- o A relative afferent papillary defect (Marcus Gunn Pupil)
- o This figure shows a patient with an abnormal right optic nerve.
- o The pupil that dilates during the swinging flashlight test has the 'relative afferent papillary defect, and is labelled the 'Marcus Gunn pupil'.

Adapted from: McGee SR. *Saunders/Elsevier* 2007, page 213.

➢ Clinical

- • Perform a focused pupil examination to distinguish between Argyll Robertson and Marcus Gunn.
  - o Argyll Robertson pupils: normal pupillary constriction with accommodation, but not to light (light-near dissociation, usually bilateral; seen mostly in diabetics, alcoholics (Wernick encephalopathy) and tertiary syphilis
  - o Marcus Gunn Pupil (afferent pupillary defect): swinging a light back and forth from one eye to another, the eyes affected by an optic nerve lesion (e.g., optic neuritis) or massive retinal lesion (e.g.,central retinal artery occlusion)

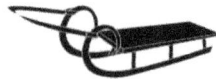

SO YOU WANT TO BE A NEUROLOGIST!

- Give the translational neuroanatomical basis for the Marcus Gunn pupil (afferent pupillary defect).

  o Afferent stimulus from
    - Disease eye weak
    - Contralateral healthy eye strong
  o Efferent system
    - Normal in diseased and healthy eye
  o With the swinging flashlight test
    - Light in normal eye
      - Normal pupil constricts
    - Light taken away from normal eye to diseased eye
      - Loss of constriction signal from to normal eye
      - No afferent pathway from diseased eye to cause constriction of pupil on that side
      - The pupil in the affected eye initially dilates in response to light, rather than constricting as would be normal

SO YOU WANT TO BE A NEUROLOGIST!

- What is the neurological changes associated with **hyperparathyroidism**.
  o Cataracts
  o Papilloedema
  o Basal ganglia defects
  o Benign intracranial hypertension

Source: Burton JL. *Churchill Livingstone* 1971, page 81.

We all know that **blue slerae** are seen in new borns, and are associated with ostegenesis imperfecta.

- Give the name of 3 other associations.
  o Anemia (especially severe iron deficiency)
  o Marfan syndrome
  o Pseudo-pseudo hypoparathyroidism
  o Newborns, small children, some "normal" adults

Source: Mangione S. *Hanley & Belfus* 2000, page 83.

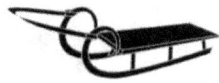

Mastering the Boards: Neurology   A.B.R. Thomson

> Other common visual eye symptoms and disease states

Visual Symptoms	Possible Causes
o Coloured haloes around light	– Acute angle closure glaucoma, – Opacities in lens or cornea
o Difficult seeing in dim light	– Myopia – Vitamin A deficiency – Retinal degeneration – Cataract – Diabetic retinopathy
o Distortion of vision	– Retinal detachment – Macular edema – Wet age-related macular degeneration – Macular pucker – Central serous retinopathy
o Flashes (photopsias)	– Migraine, retinal tear – Detachment – Posterior vitreous detachment – Chorroiditis – Retinitis
o Glare, photophobia	– Iritis – Meningitis – Encephalitis – Syphilis – Migraines – Foreign bodies – Corneal deposits
o Loss of visual field or presence of shadow or curtain	– Retinal detachment or hemorrhage – Branch retinal vein or arterial occlusion – Chronic glaucoma
o Spots/floaters (usually of no significance)	– Retinal tear/detachment – Vitreous hemorrhage

Printed with permission: Filate W, et al. *The Medical Society, Faculty of Medicine, University of Toronto* 2005, page 202.

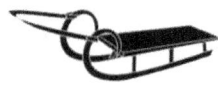

Mastering the Boards: Neurology   A.B.R. Thomson

Cataracts

➢ Causes
- o Inherited
  - – Rubella syndrome
  - – Down's syndrome
  - – Hepatolenticular degeneration
  - – Galactosemia
  - – Dystrophia myotonica

- o Senility

- o Heat, radiation

- o Secondary to ocular disease
  - – Glaucoma
  - – Opthalmitis
  - – Trauma (contusion cataract)
- o Metabolic
  - – Diabetes mellitus
  - – Hypoparathyroidism (lamellar cataract)
  - – Corticosteroid therapy
- o Trauma
- o Miscellaneous causes
  - – Atopic eczema

Adapted from: Burton JL. *Churchill Livingstone* 1971, pages 80 and 186.

Optic Atrophy

➢ Causes
- o Glaucoma

- o Chronic papilledema

- o Retinal lesions
  - – Chorio-retinits, meningitis
  - – Intra-ocular hemorrhage, etc.
- o Optic neuritis (retrobulbar neuritis)

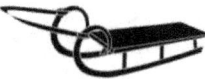

- o Pressure on an optic nerve
  - – Tumour
    - ▪ Pituitary
    - ▪ Optic Nerve
  - – Aneurysm
    - ▪ Intracavernous aneurysm of internal carotid artery
  - – Paget's disease

- o Division of optic nerve
  - – Surgery
  - – Trauma

- o Lesions of optic tract

Adapted from: Burton JL. *Churchill Livingstone* 1971, page 79.

- Give the name of 3 examples of physical findings of the optic disc, and their interpretation.
  - o Normally the disc is pales, sharply defined but with slight blurring of nasal margin, and slightly paler on temporal than on the nasal side
    - – Increased temporal palor
      - ▪ Multiple sclerosis
    - – Increased nasal blurring
      - ▪ Papilledema
    - – Pink disc
      - ▪ Papilledema
      - ▪ Papillitis
    - – Pale disk
      - ▪ Optic atrophy

Red Eye

- Give the clinical findings of causes of red eye for which the patient should be referred urgently to an ophthalmologist.

Site	Key Findings
o Conjunctivitis	–Herpes zoster rash
	–Purulent discharge
o Iridocyclitis and keratitis	–Photophobia
	–Corneal irregularity
o Acute angle-closure glaucoma	–Unilateral severe eye pain
	–Fixed non-reactive pupil
o Scleritis	–↑ pain in eye with movement or light
	–Raised red lesion

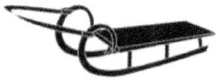

- Give causes of red eye.

  - Conjunctiva
    - Conjunctivitis
      - No blurred or lost vision
      - Improved vision with blinking
      - Scratchy discomfort, but no pain
      - No photophobia dischart
        - Yellow – bacterial infection
        - Clear – viral infection
      - Prepuricular lymphadenopathy

  - Cornea
    - Keratitis (inflammation of the cornea)

  - Episclera
    - Episcleritis (inflammation of the connective tissue between the sclera and the conjunctiva

  - Sclera
    - Scleritis

  - Iris and ciliary body
    - Iridocyclitis
      - Anisocoria

  - Adnexal structures
    - Rainbow-like ring around a point of like, looking like a halo
      - Pupil, mid-dilated non reactive to light

  - Intraocular acute glaucoma

"We are inherently critical as scientists, and inherently kind as physicians."

Grandad

Mastering the Boards: Neurology   A.B.R. Thomson

- Perform a focused physical examination to differentiate between the causes of a red and painful eye

Disease		Distribution of redness	Corneal surface		Pupil		Vision		Iris		Discharge
➢ Bacterial conjunct-tivitis	o o	Peripheral conjunctiva Bilateral	- Normal	o o	Normal Reactive	o	Normal	o	Normal	o	Muco-puralent
➢ Acute iritis	o o	Around cornea Unilateral	- Dull	o o o	Irregular shape Miotic Slowly reactive	o o	↓/ blurred Photo-phobia	o	Normal	o	Watery
➢ Acute closure glaucoma	o o	Around cornea Unilateral	- Dull	o	Oval partially dilated	o	↓/ blurred	o	Corneal edema	o	Watery
➢ Corneal ulcer/ abrasion	o o	Around cornea Unilateral	- Dull - Fluo-rescein dye stains ulcer -Irregular light reflex	o o	Normal Reactive			o	Defect shadow	o	Watery/ muco-purulent
➢ Sub-conjunctival hemorrhage	o o	Localised hemorrhage No posterior limit	- Normal								
➢ Conjunctival hemorrhage	o o	Localised hemorrhage Posterior limit present	- Normal								

Adapted from: Talley NJ, et al. *Maclennan & Petty Pty Limited* 2003, page 385; Davey P., *Wiley-Blackwell* 2006, page 112.

- Perform a focused physical examination of the eye to differentiate between a red eye caused by conjunctivitis (conj) versus/ keratitis (kera).

	Conjunctivitis	Keratitis
o Vision Blurred	No	Yes
- Improvement with blinking	yes	No
o Sensation	Scatchy	Pain
o Photophobia	No	Yes
o Discharge	Yes	No
o Anisocoria	No	Yes
o Preauricular lymphadenopathy	Yes	No

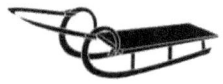

- Perform a focused physical examination for a CN IV lesion (of the right side in this example).
  o Looking down and *left*

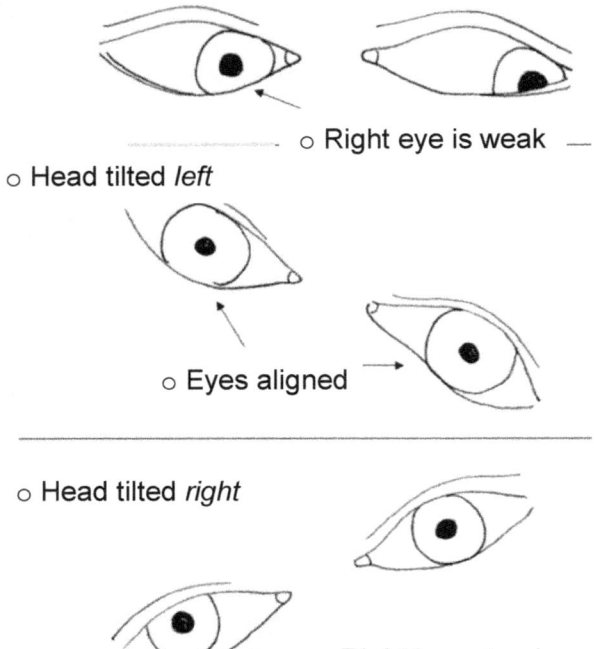

o Right eye is weak

o Head tilted *left*

o Eyes aligned

o Head tilted *right*

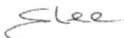

o Right hypertropia

- – Simple inspection (first row) reveals that the right eye lags behind left eye, indicating that the weak muscle is indeed on the right side (e.g., right superior oblique).

- – Tilting the head away from the affected side (e.g., to the left side, away from the weak right superior oblique, aligns the eyes normally).

- – Tilting the head toward the affected side (e.g., to the right side, third row) brings out a prominent right hypertropia (e.g., the right eye is higher than the left eye).

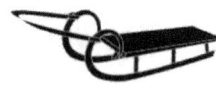

- Give the causes of **uveitis** (Uveal tract= iris, ciliary body and choroid)

  o MGI
    - Ulcerative colitis
    - Crohn disease

  o MSK
    - Ankylosing spondylitis
    - Rheumatoid arthritis
    - Reiter disease
    - Behcet disease

  o Lung
    - Sarcoidosis
    - TB

- o Infections
    - – Spirochaetal
    - – Syphilis
    - – Relapsing fever
    - – Weil disease
    - – Protozoal: Malaria, toxoplasmosis
    - – Nematode larvae: Toxocara of dog or cat

- o Ocular disease
    - – Ophthalmitis
    - – Trauma

- o Idiopathic

Adapted from: Burton JL. *Churchill Livingstone* 1971, page 81.

SO YOU WANT TO BE A NEUROLOGIST!

- Give how to distinguish clinically from the red eye caused by conjunctivitis versus uveitis.

    - o Conjunctivitis
        - – Diffuse red edemators, sclera and palpebral conjunctivae
        - – Discharge (bacterial-purulent/mucopurulent; viral and chemical – watery discharge

      Discomfort, with scratchy feeling of sand in eye

    - o Uveitis
        - – Circumcorneal injected vessels (at the limbus) (aka ciliary flush)
        - – Photophobia
        - – Deep, aching pain, not relieved with a topical anesthetic

Source: Mangione S. *Hanley & Belfus* 2000, page 83.

- Is the cornea reflex lost if a patient has weakness of the face as a result of damage to the facial nerve and LMV lesion?

    - o No, since there is bilateral innervation of the orbicularis oculi.

- Give causes of retinal artery **microaneurysms**.

    - o Diabetes

    - o Systemic hypertension

    - o Thrombosis of retinal vein

    - o Sickle cell anemia

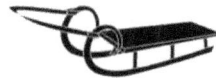

Eye Movement: CN III, IV, VI

Cranial nerve (CN)	EOM	Movement of globe of eye
III	Medial rectus	Medial
III	Inferior rectus	Down and out
III	Superior rectus	Up and out
III	Inferior oblique	Up and in
IV	Superior oblique	Down and in
VI	Lateral rectus	Lateral

Abbreviation: EOM; Extra ocular movement

Useful background: Cardinal positions of gaze

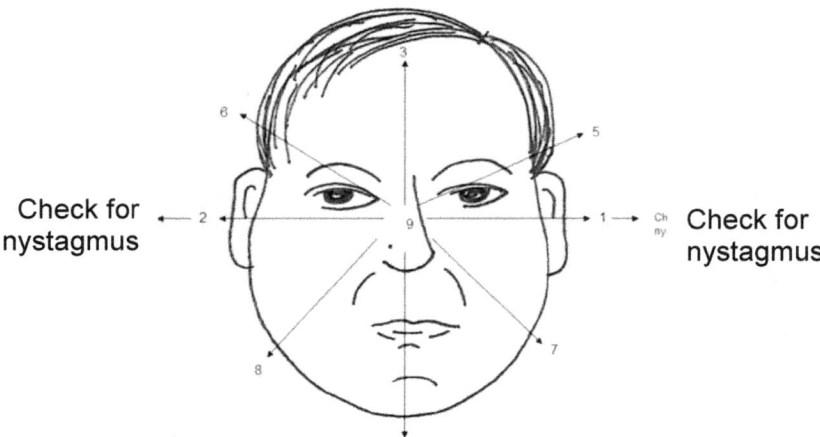

Check for nystagmus   Check for nystagmus

Adapted from: Filate W., et al. *The Medical Society, Faculty of Medicine, University of Toronto* 2005, page 159

➤ III (Oculomotor), [IV (trochlear), VI (abducens)] (motor)
  o Eye alignment
  o Gaze (6 position movements)
  o Endpoint nystagmus
  o III only – lid elevation, pupillary constriction to light (direct and consensual) or on a near object (accommodation)
  o Papillary light reflex
  o Ciliary muscle
  o Sphincter papillae
  o Levator palpebrae superioris

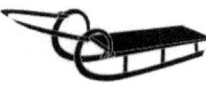

Translational Neuroanatomy

The cranial nerve (CN) III, IV, VI have a long and common intracranial pathway

- o   Within the brainstem
- o   On the meninges
- o   Pierce the dura
- o   In the cavernous sinus
- o   Through the superior orbital fissure

Midbrain

- o   Nuclei at level of superior corpora quadrigemina

    ↓

- o   Connected by the posterior longitudinal bundle near aqueduct of Sylvius in grey matter

    ↓

- o   4 nuclei close together

    - -   2 nuclei for each muscle
    - -   1 nucleus for light reflex
    - -   1 nucleus for accommodation

    ↓

- o   Interpeduncular space

    ↓

- o   Nerves emerge between cerebral peduncles
(close to circles of Willis and hypothalamus)

    ↓

- o   Nerves pass between posterior cerebral artery and superior cerebellar artery

    ↓

- o   Middle fossa CN III, with IV, V, VI

    ↓

- o   Cavernous sinus

    ↓

- o   Through dura

    ↓

- o   Superior orbital fissure

    ↓

- o   Orbit, supplying extraocular muscles, as well as levator palpebrae superioris and sphincter papillae

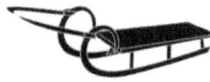

Afferent Pathway	Efferent Pathway

> Light reflex
- o Optic nerve
  ↓
- o Chiasma
  ↓
- o Optic tract
  ↓
- o Superior corpora quadrigemina (same side)

- o CN III
  ↓
- o Ciliary ganglia
  ↓
- o Short ciliary nerve
  ↓
- o Sphincter pupillae
  ↓
- o Constriction of pupil

> Accommodation convergence reflex
- o Same afferent and efferent pathways as for light reflex
- o Constriction of pupils, ptosis, convergence

Cranial Nerve III (Oculomotor)

- Perform a focused physical examination for CN III palsy.

  - o Paralytic squint
  - o Diplopia
  - o Defective ocular movement
  - o Dilated pupil
  - o Loss of light and accommodation reflexes
  - o Ptosis

"A journey of a thousand miles begins with a single step."

Lao Tzu

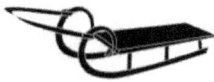

- Perform a focused physical examination for a CN III lesion (of the left side in this example).

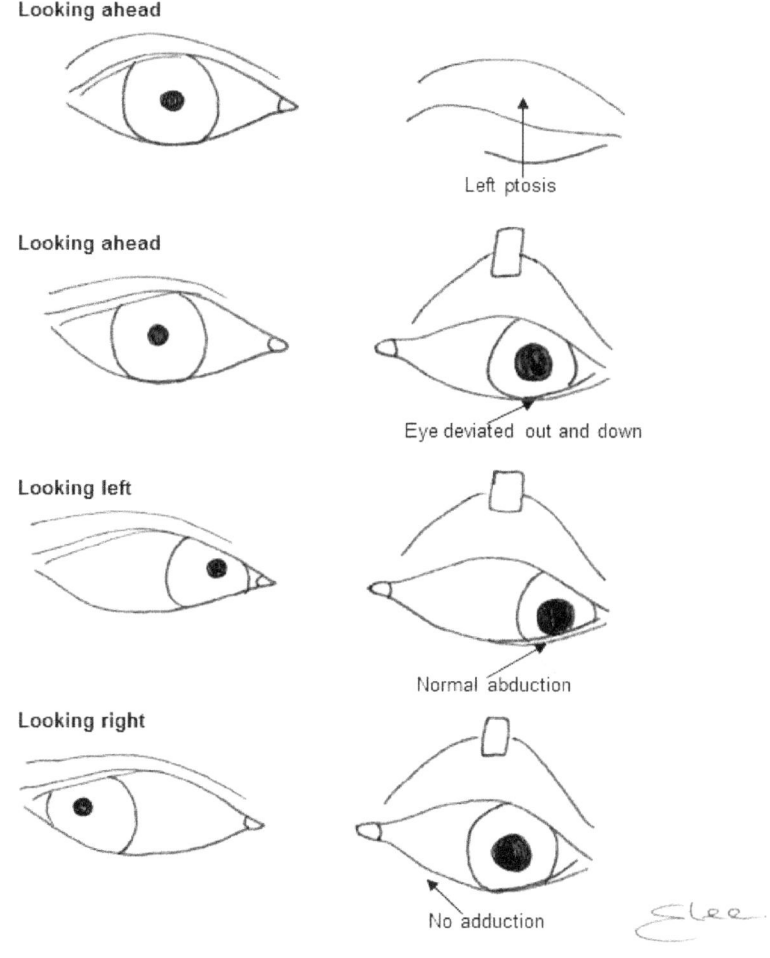

Looking ahead

Left ptosis

Looking ahead

Eye deviated out and down

Looking left

Normal abduction

Looking right

No adduction

Adapted from: McGee SR. *Saunders/Elsevier* 2007, Figure 55-5, page 681.

 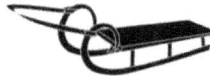

Cranial Nerve IV (Trochlear) – look in and down (superior oblique)

Midbrain paired nuclei in grey matter of aqueduct of Sylvius
↓
Fibres cross in the posterior medullary velum
↓
Around the cerebral pedicles
↓
With CN III into cavernous sinus
↓
Through superior orbital fissure
↓
Orbit, to superior oblique muscle

Cranial Nerve VI (Abducens)

Nucleus of CN VI in pons
↓
Fibres of CN VI wind around those of CN VII, which also begin in pons
↓
Cerebellopontine angle, inferior border of the pons
↓
Initially, fibres of VI are medial to those of VII

Later, fibres of VI are lateral to those of VII

Pierces dura over basilar portion of occipital bone

Beneath dura, lies on the petrous portion of the temporal bone

Cavernous sinus

Superior orbital fissure

Extraocular muscle of eye

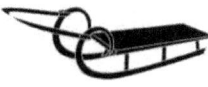

➢ Clinical

   ○ Eye movements
- With the eyes turned *laterally* – the *elevators* and depressors are the *superior* and inferior recti, respectively
- With the eyes turned *medially* – the *elevators* and depressors are the *inferior* and superior obliques, respectively
- Bilateral centres in the frontal cortices provide for voluntary eye movements through the superior oblique (CN IV) and all the other muscles through CN III.
- Nuclei for oculomotor and trachlear nerves (CNs III and IV) provide for conjugate deviation of eyes up and down.
- Nuclei for the (CN VI) in the pons provides for lateral conjugate movement through the lateral rectus muscle the medial longitudinal bundle connects the nuclei.

   ○ Diplopia caused by CN III, IV, VI disease or disease of extraocular muscles, e.g.,
- Trauma
- Tumour
- Vascular disease
- Multiple sclerosis
- Syphitis

   ○ Exophthalmos
- Inflammation (cellulitis)
- Tthrombus (cavernous sinus thrombosis)
- Bleeding or tumour behind the eye.
- Thyroid disease

Source: Burton JL. *Churchill Livingstone* 1971, page 82.

- Perform a focused physical examination for CN III palsy due to a lesion.

   ○ Brainstem (crossed paralysis)
- Ipsilateral CN III LMN hemiplegia
- Contralateral CN III UMN hemiplegia

   ○ Crus lesion, usually from thrombosis of posterior cerebral artery (aka Weber syndrome)
- Same findings as crossed paralysis from brainstem lesion

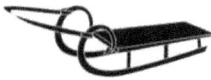

➢ Causes/associations

• Give common causes of third nerve palsy (CN III).

 o Infection
  – Encephalitis
  – Basal meningitis
  – Carcinoma at the base of the skull

 o Infiltration
  – Parasellar neoplasms
  – Meningioma at the wing of sphenoid
  – Tumours, collagen, vascular disorder, syphilis

 o Vascular
  – Opthalmoplegic migrane
  – Aneurysms of posterior communicating artery (painful opthalmoplegia)

 o Degenerative
  – Multiple sclerosis (MS)

 o Metabolic
  – Hypertension
  – Diabetes (pupil-sparing CN III palsy)

 o Trauma

Adapted from: Baliga RR. *Saunders/Elsevier* 2007, page 154.

• Give causes of **multiple cranial nerve palsies**.

 o Inherited – Arnold Chiari malformation

 o Infection – Guillain Barre syndrome (spares sensory nerves)
      – Tuberculosis
      – Sarcoidosis

 o Infiltration – Nasopharyngeal carcinoma
      – Hematological malignancy,
      – Brainstem Tumour (e.g., in the cerebellopontine angle) have similar signs

 o Vascular – Brainstem vascular disease causing crossed sensory or motor paralysis (i.e., cranial nerve signs on one side and contralateral long tract signs)

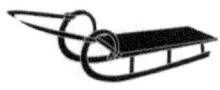

o Trauma

o Metabolic   – Paget disease
               – Mononeuritis multiplex (rarely, e.g., diabetes mellitus)

Abbreviations: LMN, lower motor neurons; MS, Multiple sclerosis; UMN, upper motor neurons

Adapted from: Talley NJ, et al. *Maclennan & Petty Pty Limited* 2003, Table 10.7, page 384.

- Give causes/associations of VI nerve palsy.
    o Hypertension
    o Diabetes
    o Raised intracranial pressure (false localizing signs)
    o Multiple sclerosis
    o Basal meningitis
    o Encephalitis
    o Nasopharyngeal carcinoma
    o Acoustic neuroma

Source: Baliga RR. *Saunders/Elsevier*, Philadelphia 2007, page 156.

Gaze Defects of CN III, IV, VI

Gaze defect	Location of lesion
o Looks down and out (including ptosis)	– CN III palsy (look for pupil involvement)
o Can't look in and down (difficultly walking downstairs)	– CN IV palsy
o Can't move affected eye laterally	– CN VI palsy
o Slow adduction of ipsilateral eye and nystagmus in abduction of contralateral eye	– Medial longitudinal fasciculus (MLF) – Internuclear ophthalmoplegia (suggests Multiple Sclerosis)

Source: Filate W, et al. *The Medical Society, Faculty of Medicine, University of Toronto* 2005, page 159.

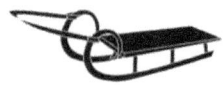

- Perform a focused physical examination of the eye muscles and nerve innervations for a CN III lesion (of the left side in this example).

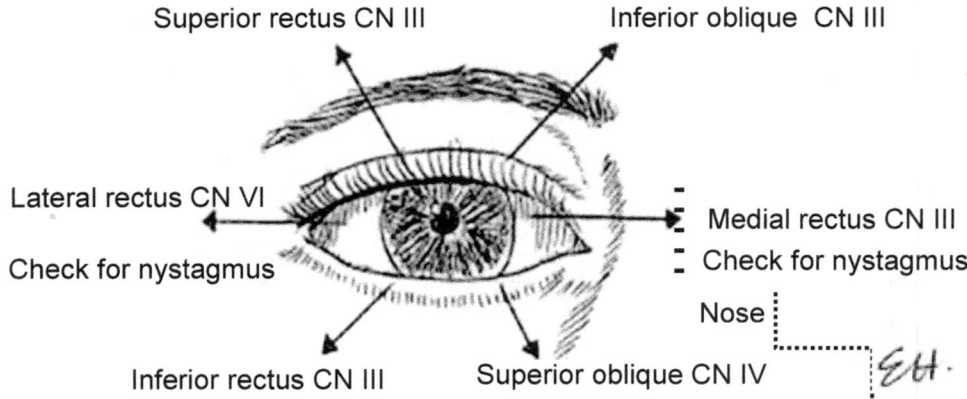

Superior rectus CN III   Inferior oblique CN III

Lateral rectus CN VI   Medial rectus CN III

Check for nystagmus   Check for nystagmus

Nose

Inferior rectus CN III   Superior oblique CN IV

Adapted from: Talley NJ, et al. *Maclennan & Petty Pty Limited* 2003, Figure 10.9, page 366.

Ptosis

- Give the neurological conditions causing ptosis
  - CN III palsy
  - Horner syndrome
  - Myasthenia gravis

Source: Mangione S. *Hanley & Belfus* 2000,

- Neuroanatomy
  - Movement : CN III → levator
  - Tone: sympathetic fibres in CN V → palpebrae superioris

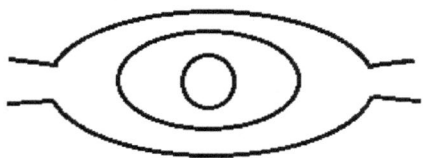

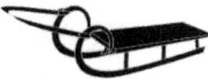

➢ Causes/associations

  o Congenital

  o Hysterical (ptosis always unilateral)

  o Muscle diseases

  o Neurological disorders
    – III
    – VI
    – Tabes dorsalis

➢ Clinical

Sign	CN VI sympathetic lesion	CN III
o Ptosis at rest	+	-
o Movement on looking upwards	+	-

  o Forehead wrinkles

  o Ptosis due to damage to CN V, in addition to ptosis, may be associated with myosis, lack of sweating or tearing (lacrimation)

• Perform a focused physical examination for the causes of unilateral or bilateral ptosis.

  o Unilateral
    – Congenital (usually bilateral)
      ▪ always partial
    – Oculomotor nerve lesion
      ▪ usually unilateral, complete, frontalis overaction
    – Cervical sympathetic lesion (Horner syndrome)
    – Myasthenia gravis
    – Myopathy (senile)
      ▪ facioscapulohumeral; dystrophia; myotonica; trauma
    – Tabes dorsalis, syphilis
    – Hysterical
      ▪ unilateral, no frontalis overactivity, complete
    – Ideopathic

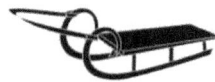

- o Bilateral
  - – Myasthenia gravis
  - – Myotonica dystrophia
  - – Ocular myopathy or oculopharyngeal dystrophy
  - – Mitochondria dystrophy
  - – Tabes dorsalis
  - – Congenital
  - – Bilateral Horner syndrome (e.g., syringomyelia)

Adapted from: Burton JL. *Churchill Livingstone* 1971, page 82 and Baliga R.R. *Saunders/Elsevier* 2007, page 127.

SO YOU WANT TO BE A NEUROLOGIST!

Nystagmus may be horizontal, vertical or rotatory, and has a quick and slow component. The rhythmic movement of the extraocular muscles may arise from disease of the cerebellum, vestibularis or oculomslor system. And so, the question.

- Give how you would determine if nystagmus is "physiological".

  - o Test for "optokinetic" nystagmus by having the person look at a rapidly rotating vertically striped drum.

SO YOU WANT TO BE A NEUROLOGIST!

- You are familiar with how to examine CN III. Perform an examination for "aberrant regeneration" of CN III.

  - o Pathogenesis
    - – After damage to the third nerve (from trauma, aneurysms, or tumours but not ischemia), regenerating fibres originally destined for the medial rectus muscle may instead reinnervate the pupillary constrictor

  - o Clinical
    - – Unilateral pupillary constriction during convergence but no reaction to light. Unlike Argyll Robertson pupils, however, this finding is unilateral
    - – Anisocoria, ptosis, and diplipia

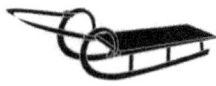

Mastering the Boards: Neurology   A.B.R. Thomson

- Perform a focused physical examination for a CN VI lesion (on the left side in this example).

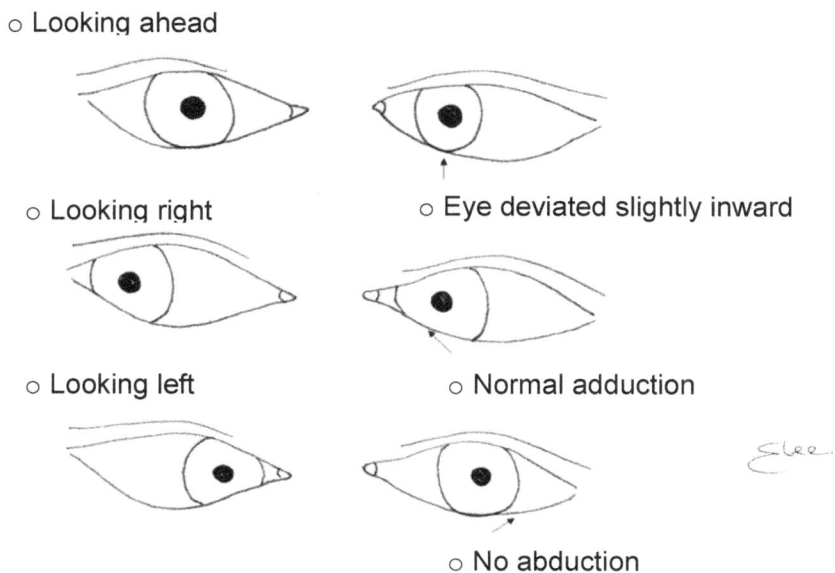

  o Looking ahead

  o Looking right

  o Eye deviated slightly inward

  o Looking left

  o Normal adduction

  o No abduction

Adapted from: Baliga RR. *Saunders/Elsevier* 2007, Figure 55-7, page 685.

- Perform a focused physical examination for a lesion in the cavernous sinus, cerebellopontine angle, jugular foramen, pseudobulbar and bulbar palsy (multiple cranial nerve palsies), and its causes.

Site	Affected Cranial Nerve
o Cavernous sinus	– Unilateral III, IV, V and VI
o Cerebellopontine angle lesion (usually a Tumour)	– Unilateral V, VII and VIII
o Jugular foramen lesion	– Unilateral IX, X and XI
o Bulbar (LMN) and pseudobulbar (UMN) palsy	– Combined bilateral X, XI and XII

 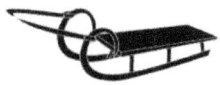

SO YOU WANT TO BE A NEUROLOGIST!

- Give the eponymous syndromes affecting CN VI.
    - o Pons Infarction
        - – Raymond syndrome: ipsilateral CN VI paralysis and contralateral paresis of extremities
        - – Millard-Gubler syndrome, in which there s ipsilateral VI and VII palsy, with contralateral hemiplegia.
        - – Foville syndrome has all the features of Millard-Gubler paralysis, plus lateral conjugate gaze palsy.
    - o Gradening syndrome
        - – Inflammation of the tip of the temporal bone, involving V and VI, as well as the greater superfacial petrosal nerve
        - – This results in unilateral paralysis of the lateral rectus, nerve, pain in the distribution of V (particularly V_1), and excessive lacrimation
    - o Others
        - – Duane syndrome: widening of the palpebral fissure on abduction, and narrowing on adduction
        - – Gerhardt syndrome: bilateral abducens palsy
        - – Mobius syndrome: paralysis of extraocular muscles, especially abducens, with paresis of facial muscles

Adapted from: Baliga RR. *Saunders/Elsevier* page 157.

Diplopia

➢ Clinical

o The main features of any ocular palsy are
- – The symptom of diplopia
- – The sign of strabismus
- – The inability to move both eyes in the same direction.

➢ When examining the patient for diplodia, determine if diplopia is present, where is it maximal, and what is the most peripheral image.

    - o Present
        - – Move the eye in the direction of the muscle which is suspected to be paralyzed

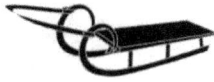

- o Maximal
  - – Move the eye in the direction of the pull of the muscle which is suspected to be paralyzed

- o Worse
  - – Worst when looking down and to the left, indicating that the weak muscle is either the left inferior rectus muscle or right superior oblique muscle.

- o Image
  - – Side-by-side images
    - ▪ Only lateral (VI) or medial (III) cranial nerves
  - – One-above-the-other
    - ▪ Superior (IV) or inferior (III) oblique, inferior rectus (III)
    - ▪ Peripheral
      - – The most peripheral of the two images from the two eyes is from the eye with the weak muscle
      - – Cover one eye, to establish which eye has the weak muscle
  - – False image
    - ▪ Pale, peripheral, poorly seen
  - – Loss of lateral image with covering one eye at point of maximum separation indicates that the covered eye is causing the diplopia.
  - – Persistence of both images with covering one eye is due to dislocated lens, astigmatism, or false reporting.

- ➢ Causes/associations

- • Perform a focused physical examination to determine the cause of diplopia.

  - o When examining the patient with suspected diplopia, look for possible causes
    - – Trauma
    - – Tumour
    - – Vascular lesion
    - – Syphilis
    - – Multiple sclerosis

Adapted from: McGee SR. *Saunders/Elsevier* 2007, pages 671 to 679.

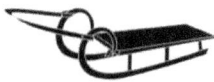

Strabismus

➢ Concomitant Strabismus

  o Slight asymmetry of corresponding ocular muscles

  o Extent of squint remains similar when eyes are looking in any direction

  o Normal ranges of movements of each eye present at rest

  o No diplopia associated

➢ Divergent (paralytic) strabismus

  o Paralysis of ocular muscles

  o Often not present at rest

  o Becomes apparent only when the eye is moved in the direction of the pull of the paralysed muscles

  o Associated diplopia

Nystagmus

  o Please also see the section on nystagmus and vertico-cranial nerve VIII

SO YOU WANT TO BE A NEUROLOGIST!

• How may you distinguish clinically between CN III palsy and exophthalmos due to a cavernous sinus thrombosis or aneurysm versus a tumour of the orbit?

  o With a tumour of the orbit
    – The CN III palsy and exophthalmos are usually bilateral
    – Associated chemosis (red, edematous conjunctive)
    – Associated papilledema

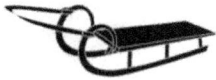

SO YOU WANT TO BE A NEUROLOGIST!

- Give conditions which may cause spasms of conjugate deviation of the eye.

    - At the beginning of a seizure
    - At the beginning of CVA
        - Early, head and eye turn away from the side of the lesion
        - Later, head and eye turn towards the side of the lesion
    - Oculogyric crisis in encephalitis lethargica
    - Hysteria

- In the context of the CN V and VI, give the meaning of the Gradenigo syndrome.

    - Gradenigo syndrome is involvement of CN V and VI, with facial pain and sixth nerve palsy, such as may occur as a complication of otitis media and periostitis of the petrous

- In the presence of increased intracranial pressure, give which two nerves provide false-localizing sign of a lower motor neuron (LMN).
    - Cranial nerves III and VI

- Give which cranial nerve (CN) is most susceptible to a transient increase in intracranial pressure, such as might occur with a subarachnoid hemorrhage.
    - CN VI

- Give the structures in close proximity to the CN VI nucleus and fascicles.

    - Facial and trigeminal nerves
    - Corticospinal tract
    - Median longitudinal fasciculus
    - Parapontine reticular formation
    - Temporal bone

Source: Baliga RR. *Saunders/Elsevier* 2007, page 151.

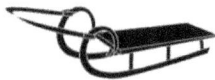

Mastering the Boards: Neurology   A.B.R. Thomson

SO YOU WANT TO BE A NEUROLOGIST!

- Give the muscle groups are supplied by the oculomotor nerve (CN III).
  - All eye muscles, except lateral rectus (LR) and superior oblique (SO)
  - Eye is rotated out by LR and down by SO
  - Levator palpebrae superioris
  - Constrictor muscle of pupils
  - Loss of constrictor muscle leads to unopposed sympathetic effects on pupil

The cranial nerves to the muscles of the eye run closely together, so then two or three may be affected by the same lesion.

- Give the lesion which damages CN IV, and usually not CN III and VI.
  - Aneurysm of PCA

- Give the difference between hyphema and hypopyon.
  - Hyphema is blood, and hypopyon is pus in the anterior chamber of the eye.

- Give the meaning of 'Fisher's one and a half syndrome'.

Horizontal eye movement is absent, and the other eye is capable only of abduction ("one and a half movements are paralysed").

  - The vertical eye movements and the pupils are mormal.
  - The cause is a lesion in the pontine region involving the medial longitudinal fasciculus and the parapontine reticular formation on the same side.
  - This results in failure of conjugate gaze to the same side, impairment of adduction of the eye, and nystagmus on abduction of the other eye.

Source: Baliga RR. *Saunders/Elsevier* 2007, page 222.

- Internuclear ophthalmoplegia

Looking left: Both eyes move normally

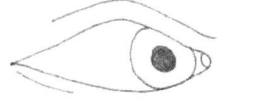 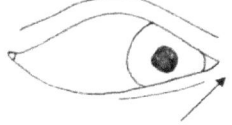

Normal abduction

Looking right: Left eye fails to adduct

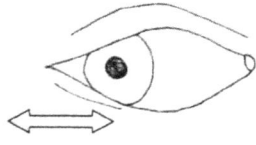 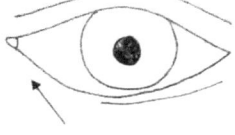 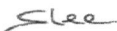

Jerk nystagmus   No abduction

- The finding is named for the side with weak adduction (i.e., in this example, a left internuclear ophthalmoplegia).
- The lesion is in the ipsilateral medial longitudinal fasciculus (i.e., left medial longitudinal fasciculus in this example).

Adapted from: McGee SR. *Saunders/Elsevier* 2007, Figure 55-4, page 678.

"When we are no longer able to change a situation, we are challenged to change ourselves."

Viktor Frankl

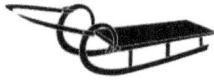

Cranial Nerve V – Trigeminal

➢ Translational Neuroanatomy

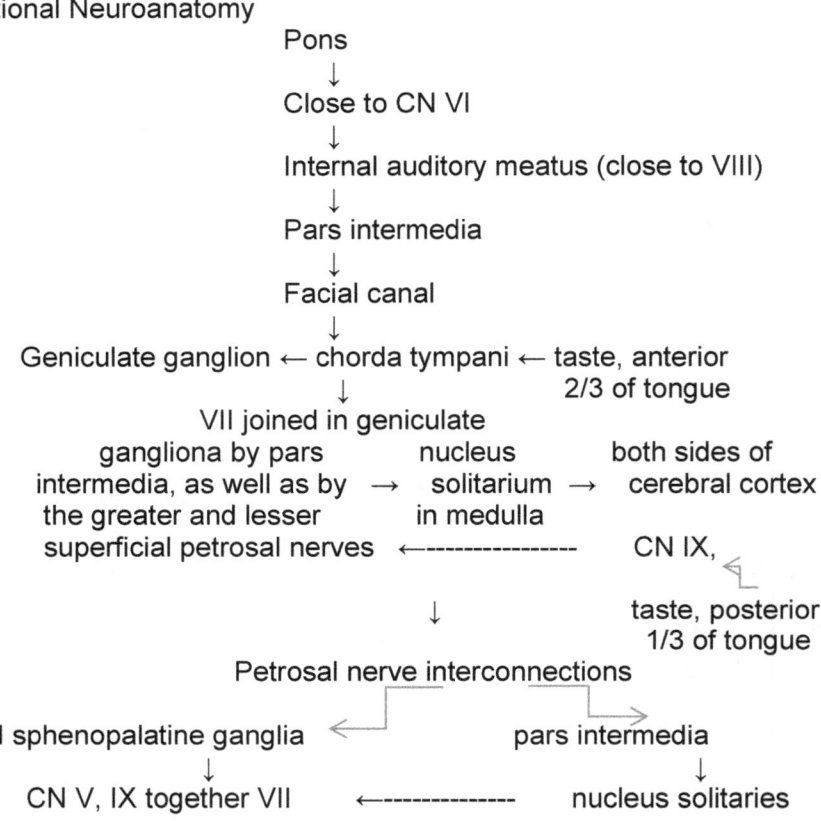

Pons
↓
Close to CN VI
↓
Internal auditory meatus (close to VIII)
↓
Pars intermedia
↓
Facial canal
↓
Geniculate ganglion ← chorda tympani ← taste, anterior
↓   2/3 of tongue
VII joined in geniculate
gangliona by pars   nucleus   both sides of
intermedia, as well as by → solitarium → cerebral cortex
the greater and lesser   in medulla
superficial petrosal nerves ←------------- CN IX,

↓   taste, posterior
                         1/3 of tongue

Petrosal nerve interconnections

Otic and sphenopalatine ganglia ←   pars intermedia
↓   ↓
CN V, IX together VII   ←--------------   nucleus solitaries

o Sensory – Pain, temperature and light touch for same side of face, cornea, sinuses, nasal mucosa, teeth, tympanic membrane, anterior 2/3 of tongue? or VII

o Motor – Mouth, open symmetrically, open against resistance, move jaw against resistance, clench teeth, chewing (masseter and lateral pterygoid muscles)

o Reflex
- Corneal reflex (afferent limb), jaw jerk (afferent and efferent limbs)
- Glabeller reflex (limb)

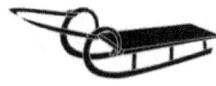

- o Asymmetry of face

  - V1= ophthalmic   Forehead and tip of nose
    Afferent limb of the corneal reflex

  - V2= maxillary   Medial aspect of cheek
    Afferent limb of jaw jerk reflex
    Chin, except angle of the jaw(C2)

  - V3= mandibular   Innervates jaw muscles

- o Eye V1 sensory, V2 motor to orbicularis oculi
- o Face
- o Nose
- o Pharynx, mouth-motor to muscle of mastication
- o Tongue – anterior 2/3, taste
- o V2 (mandibular branch)
- o Ear – fibres from lingual nerve to
- o Chorda tympani
- o Jaw

Trigeminal Neuralgia (aka "tic douloureaux")

- ➢ Clinical
  - o Recurrent, brief (1 sec to 2 min), unilateral, triggered onset of pain
    (V_1, forehead; V_2, cheek*; V_3, jaw/chin*)

- ➢ Causes/associations
  - o < 40
  - o > 40 (90%)
    - Focal demyelination of root of CN V at level of the pons from vascular compression
    - Focal demyelination leads to aberrant neural discharge

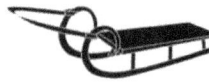

> Treatment

   o First-line   – Carbamazepine 100 mg po bid, with increasing doses, or oxcarbazepine

   o Second-line   – Baclofen
                          – Gabapentin
                          – Clonazepam

   o Consider combinations of 3 medications before pain non-responsive to medical therapy (30%

   o Surgery
     - Cranial nerve (CN) V depression or destruction
       ▪ Balloon
       ▪ Radiofrequency
       ▪ Gamma knife radiation
       ▪ Glycerol injection
       ▪ Microvascular decompression

In the context of facial nerve palsy (CN V) and external otitis (vesicles), the Weber test lateralizes to the good ear, and the Rinne test is less loud in the good ear. Sensioneural hearing loss is diagnosed, and the Ramsay Hunt syndrome due to Varicella-zoster viral infection is diagnosed.

Corneal Light Reflex

> Neuroanatomy

   o V1
     - Ophthalmic branch of the trigeminal nerve, sensory to eye, including cornea

   o V3
     - Motor branch of the trigeminal nerve
     - Innervates the orbicularis oculi
     - Orbicular oculi of each eye are innervated bilaterally

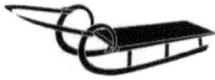

> Clinical

- o Touching the cornea of the one eye causes contraction of the orbicularis oculi of loss of cornea) reflex is an early sign of a tumour of the cerebellopontine angle.

Jaw Jerk

V1 – sensory branch of trigeminal nerve CN III

V3 – motor branch
- Bilateral innervation of jaw muscles
- Jaw muscles: masseters, pterygoids

- o Deviation of jaw
  - Fracture of jaw bone
  - Deviation of side of weakness
  - Unilateral weakness represents a LMN lesion (because V3 innervation to jaw is bilateral)

- o Weakness of jaw
  - UMN
    - Bilateral weakness
  - Associated with bilateral weakness of CN VII
  - LMN
    - Unilateral weakness of jaw
    - Unilateral deviation of jaw

- o When testing the corneal reflex, what are the expected findings with a LMN lesion of CN VII
  - Contralateral closure of eye
  - Withdrawal of the eye from the stimulus

SO YOU WANT TO BE A NEUROLOGIST!

- Cranial nerve V (trigeminal nerve) is entirely sensory, except motor to which muscle?
  - o The masseter muscle for chewing

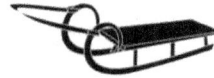

Cranial Nerve VII – Facial

➢ Anatomy

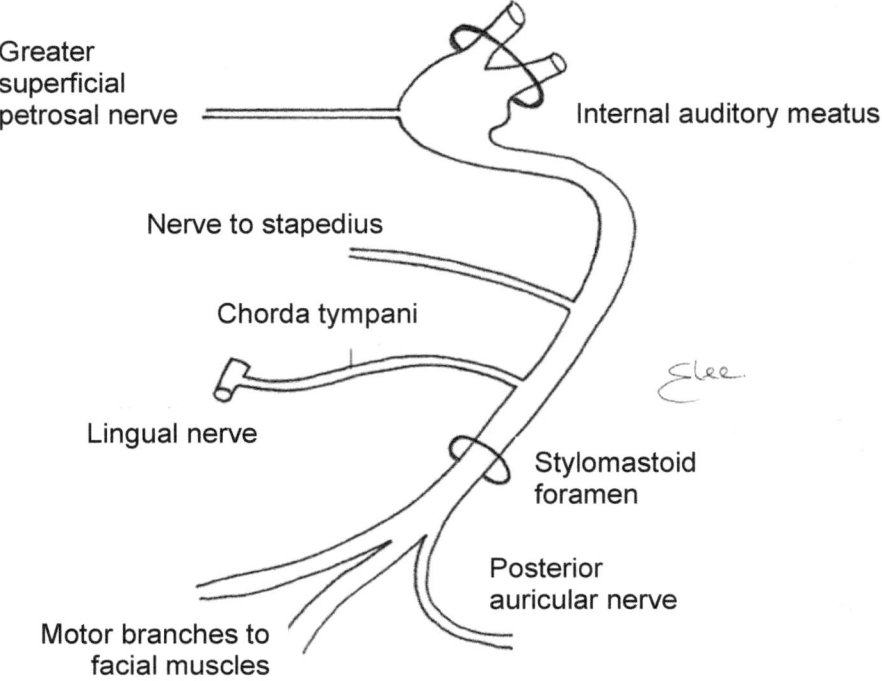

Greater superficial petrosal nerve

Internal auditory meatus

Nerve to stapedius

Chorda tympani

Lingual nerve

Stylomastoid foramen

Posterior auricular nerve

Motor branches to facial muscles

Adapted from: Burton JL. *Churchill Livingstone*, 1971, page 74.

- o Accompanies
  - – Through the cerebello-positive angle
  - – Acoustic neuroma may affect CN V, VI, VII, VIII
- o Accompanies CN V
  - – Over the temporal bone
  - – Periostitis from otitis media
- o The nervus intermedius or pars intermedia of Wrisberg is the sensory or the parasympathetic root of the facial nerve, and is lateral and inferior to the motor root.
- o Inside the internal auditory meatus it lies between the motor root and the eighth cranial nerve.
- o The sensory cells are located in the geniculate ganglion (at the bend of the facial nerve in the facial canal) and their nerve fibres enter the pons with the motor root.

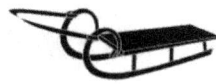

- o The geniculate ganglion is continued distally as the chorda tympani, which carries taste and preganglionic parasympathetic fibres.
- o This nerve consists of contributions from three areas:
  - – Superior salivary nucleus (in the pons) supplies secretory fibres to the glands
  - – Gustatory or solitary nucleus (in the medulla) receives taste fibres via the chorda tympani
  - – Dorsal part of the trigeminal nerve receives cutaneous sensation from the external auditory meatus and the skin behind the ear (distributed with the facial nerve proper).
- o The branches of the facial nerve
  - – Greater superficial petrosal nerve (supplies lacrimal, nasal and plantine glands)
  - – Nerve to stapedius muscle
  - – Chorda tympani (supplies taste to anterior two thirds of the tongue, submaxillary and sublingual glands)
  - – Motor branches (exit from the stylomastoid foramen)
- o Reflexes involving the facial nerve
  - – Corneal reflex
  - – Palmomental reflex
  - – Suck reflex
- o Localizing facial nerve palsy
  - – Involvement of the nuclei in the pons – associated ipsilateral sixth nerve palsy.
  - – Cerebellopontine angle lesion – associated fifth and eighth nerve involvement.
  - – Lesion in the bony canal – loss of taste (carried by the lingual nerve) and hyperacusis (due to involvement of the nerve to stapedius).

➢ VII (Facial)
- o Motor (scalp and fascial muscles of expression; all facial movements except eyelid elevation [CN III])
  - – Raise eyebrows, wrinkle forehead (all facial movements except lid elevation [CN III] or mouth and jaw movement [CN V])
  - – Open/close eyes
  - – Smile, showing teeth
  - – Puff out cheeks
  - – Phonation

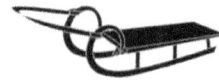

o Sensory
  - Speech, say 'PAH' (via the chorda tympani)
  - Taste, anterior 2/3 of tongue taste to (posterior 1/3 of tongue [CN IX])

o Corneal reflex (efferent limb; afferent limb, CN V)

o Glabellar reflex (efferent limb afferent limb, CN V)

o Nerve to stapedius muscle

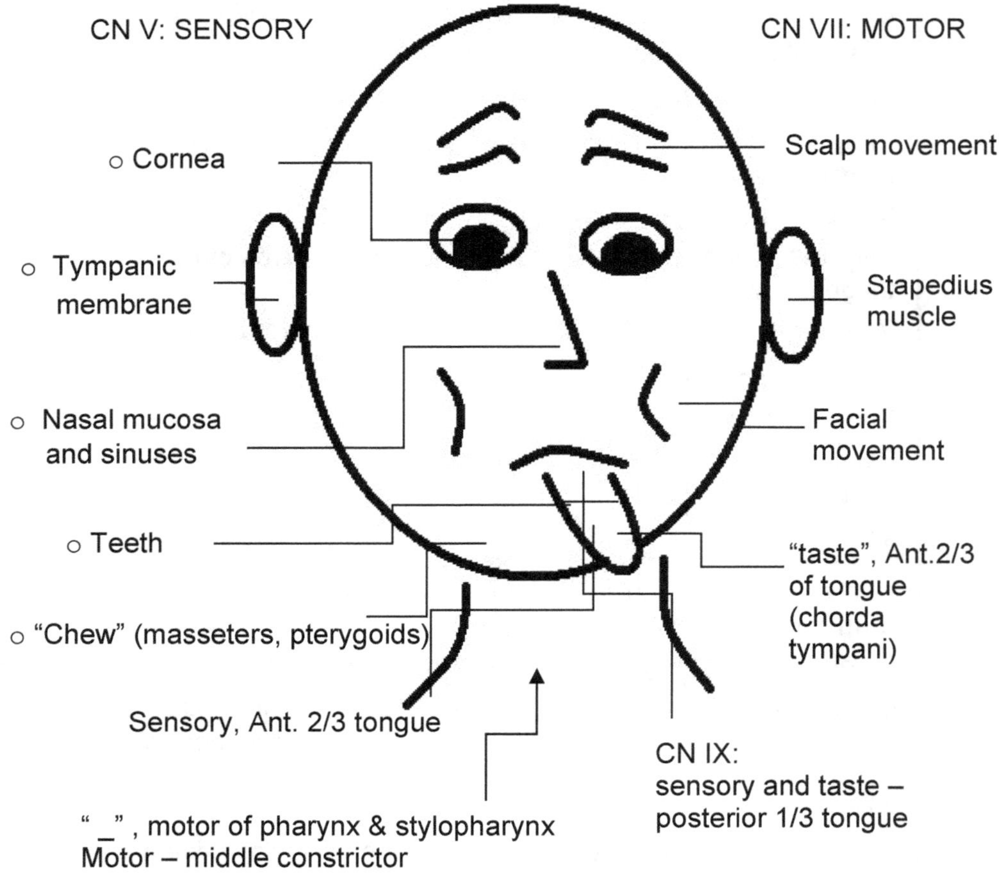

CN V: SENSORY   CN VII: MOTOR

o Cornea ─────   ──── Scalp movement

o Tympanic
  membrane ─────   ──── Stapedius
                                                      muscle

o Nasal mucosa
  and sinuses ─────   ──── Facial
                                                      movement

o Teeth ─────   "taste", Ant.2/3
                                                 of tongue
                                                 (chorda
o "Chew" (masseters, pterygoids)   tympani)

Sensory, Ant. 2/3 tongue

                                                 CN IX:
                                                 sensory and taste –
" _ " , motor of pharynx & stylopharynx   posterior 1/3 tongue
Motor – middle constrictor

CN V is sensory except for "chewing"
CN VII is motor, except for "taste", anterior 2/3 of tongue

Clinical Pearl

  o Uvula – deviates to strong side; jaw and tongue – deviate to weak side.

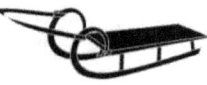

Mastering the Boards: Neurology   A.B.R. Thomson

Facial Weakness

➤ Clinical

    o Asymmetry (diminished ipsilateral)

    o Weakness of most ipsilateral facial muscles (muscles used during speaking, blinking, raising eyebrows, smiling, wrinkling the forehead, closing the eyes, showing teeth, and retracting the chin)

    o May be abnormalities of ipsilateral tearing (lacrimal gland), hearing (stapedius muscle), taste (anterior two third of the tongue), and the corneal and glabellar reflexes

➤ Types

• Central (UMN) facial weakness

    o Unilateral facial weakness may be "central" (lesions in the contralateral motor cortex or descending pyramidal tracts)

    o Weakness of lower facial muscle (wrinkling of the forehead is relatively spared in central lesions because the facial nuclei innervating these muscles receive bilateral cortical innervartion)

    o Affect voluntary movements affected but not spare emotional ones

    o May be unable to wrinkle one corner of the mouth volitionally yet can move it normally during laughter or crying (occurs because emotional input to the facial nuclei does not come from the motor cortex)

• Peripheral (LMN) facial weakness
    o Lesions in the peripheral nerve or facial nucleus in the ipsilateral pons

    o Affect upper as well as lower facial muscles

    o All facial movements on the side affected are paralyzed

Adapted from: McGee SR. *Saunders/Elsevier* 2007, page 695.

• Give the way to distinguish between a UMN and a LMN lesion of CN VII.

    o UMN (internal capsular lesion)
      – Paralysis of the lower facial muscles on one side (that part of the nucleus of CN VII which innervates the upper facial muscles is supplied by both sides of the motor cortex, and so the upper facial muscles are intact)

    o LMN (damage to the facial nerves eg, Bell palsy)
      – Paralysis of both the upper and the lower facial muscles on one side

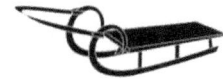

- Perform a focused physical examination for the causes of facial weakness/paralysis (CN VII lesion).

    o Supranuclear
        - Cortico-pontine tract lesions
        - Sub-thalamic and corpus striatum lesions
        - Temporal lobe lesions

    o Nuclear and infra-nuclear
        - Pontine
            ▪ Polio
            ▪ DMS
            ▪ Neoplasm
        - Cerebello-pontine angle
            ▪ Acoustic neuroma
            ▪ Meningionoma
            ▪ Basilar artery aneurysm
            ▪ Guillain-Barré syndrome
            ▪ Chordoma
            ▪ Chronic meningitis, including carcinomatous

    o Internal auditory canal
        - Acoustic neuroma
        - Geniculate herpes

    o Facial canal
        - Bell palsy
        - Chronic otitis
        - Cholesteatoma
        - Mastoidectomy
        - Head injury
        - Hypertension in children
        - Sarcoidosis
        - Leukemic infiltrate

    o Face
        - Forceps delivery
        - Stab wounds
        - Parotid tumours
        - Leprosy

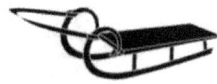

- o Unilateral
  - – UMN (sparing of forehead)
    - ▪ Melkersson-Rosenthal syndrome (facial palsy, recurrent facial edema, and pliocation of the tongue)
    - ▪ Myasthenia (may mimic bilateral facial nerve palsy)
  - – LMN lesion
    - ▪ Ideopathic (Bell palsy)
    - ▪ Herpes zoster
    - ▪ Cerebellopntine angle Tumours
    - ▪ Parotid Tumours
    - ▪ Old polio
    - ▪ Otitis media
    - ▪ Stroke (hemiplegia)
    - ▪ Skull fracture

- o Bilateral
  - – Facial nerve (VII) damage
    - ▪ Guillain-Barré syndrome
    - ▪ Sarcoidosis
    - ▪ Bilateral parotid disease
    - ▪ Lyme disease
    - ▪ Mononeuritis multiplex
  - – Muscle disease
    - ▪ Myopathy
    - ▪ Mynsthenia gravis

Abbreviations: MS, multiple sclerosis; LMN, lower motor neurons; UMN, upper motor neurons

Source: Burton JL. *Churchill Livingstone* 1971, page 75; Baliga RR. *Saunders/Elsevier* 2007, page 159.

Facial Pain

➢ Clinical

- • Perform a focused physical examination for the causes of facial pain.

  - o CNS
    - – Migrainous neuralgia ('cluster' headache)

  - o Skull/spine
    - – Cervical spondylosis, Paget disease of skull

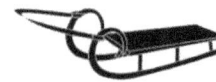

- o Disease of teeth
  - – Sinuses
  - – Ear
  - – Nose
  - – Throat

- o CN VII
  - – Post-herpetic neuralgia
  - – Trigeminal neuralgia

- o TMJ
  - – Temporo-mandibular arthritis (Costen syndrome)

- o Ear
  - – Acoustic neuroma

- o Heart
  - – Myocardial ischemia

- o Blood vessels
  - – Cranial arteritis
  - – Aneurysm of posterior communicating artery- posterior inferior cerebellar artery

- o Miscellenous
  - – Atypical facial pain – Constant, nagging deep pain not corresponding to any anatomical sensory distribution

Adapted from: Burton JL. *Churchill Livingstone* 1971, page 74.

Bell Palsy

➤ Definition
  - o "Bell palsy is a lower motor neuron paralysis of the facial nerve [CN VII], often due to herpes simplex virus -1 infection, causing inflammation and edema" (Pryse-Phillips W, et al. Chapter 19. In: Therapeutic Choices. Grey J, Ed. 6th Edition, *Canadian Pharmacists Association*: Otttawa, ON, 2011, page 258).
  - o Compression of cranial nerve V (facial nerve) causing of the facial muscles on the same side (forehead, face, jaw [orbicularis oculi] → periorbital difficulty closing eyes and raising eyebrows)

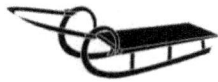

- ➢ Cause
  - ○ Idiopathic
  - ○ Infection
    - – Epstein Barr Virus (infections mononucleosis)
    - – Guillain-Barr'e syndrome
  - ○ Infiltration
    - – Tumour of cerebellopontine angle
  - ○ Metabolic
    - – Diabetes
    - – Hypertension
    - – Pregnancy

- ➢ Clinical
  - ○ May be associated losses
    - – ↓ taste
    - – Dry mouth
    - – Hyperacusis

Good Party Trick

- ○ Someone winks at you while they smile. This is a complication of what neurological disorder?
  - - In Bell palsy (cranial nerve V mononeuropathy), some patients do not recover but instead develop aberrant re-innervation → synkinesis, such as involuntary eye closure when they smile.

SO YOU WANT TO BE A NEUROLOGIST!

- • Give the reason why the patient with Bell palsy not wrinkle their foreheads.

  - ○ Bell palsy is a peripheral mononeuropathy of CN VII.
  - ○ Their peripheral nerve damage causes paralysis of both UMN and LMN, so the motor function of both upper and lower portions of the face are affected.
  - ○ The eyelid of the affected side cannot be closed.

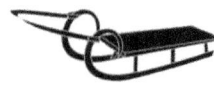

SO YOU WANT TO BE A NEUROLOGIST!

- Give the neuroanatomical basis for only the tongue and lower face being affected in UMN-associated hemiplegia.

All cranial nerves are innervated bilaterally, except the lower half of the face and tongue.

  o Thus all muscles except the tongue and lower face escape in UMN hemiplegia

- Give the neuroanatomy which explains the corneal reflex.

  o The sensory fibres of the CN V (touch, proprioception) enter the brainstem and cross the midline to ascent in the medial lemniscus to the thalamus and cerebral cortex
  o Sensory nuclei in pons CN V → brainstem → decussate → medial lemniscus → thalamus and cerebral cortex
  o Sensory and motor V → leave the pons V cross the cerebellopontine angle → sensory root in a large ganglion at the apex of the petrous temporal bone → sensory V accompanies CN III, IV, and VI in the cavernous sinus

SO YOU WANT TO BE A NEUROLOGIST!

- In the patient with Bell palsy, what is the Bell phenomenon?

  o Bell palsy is a peripheral mononeuropathy of CN VII which affects the peripheral nerve and results in both UMN and LMN lesions.

  o In a person with lower (peripheral) CN VII damage, the eyelid of the affected side cannot be closed, so the eyeball on that side moves upwards when the person closes the eyelid of the unaffected side (synkinesis), using the intact orbicularis muscle contraction on that side.

Source: Mangione S. *Hanley & Belfus* 2000, page 410.

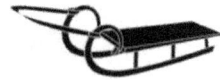

> Differential diagnosis

- Give the differential diagnosis of unilateral Bell Palsy.
    - o Ramsay Hunt syndrome (herpes zoster infection of geniculate ganglion; vesicles in the ear or throat)
    - o Pain in ear and mastoid region
    - o Facial paresis or spasm
    - o Deafness, dizziness or hyperacusis
    - o Vesicles on auricle or anterior fauces
    - o Ipsilateral taste loss in anterior two-thirds tongue
    - o Facial nerve Tumours (usually painless; examine for neurofibromatosis)
    - o Cerebellopontine angle Tumours (added neurologic signs)
    - o Parotid Tumours (clinical examination)
    - o Mastoiditis (deafness, discharge)
    - o Lyme disease (skin and joint signs)
    - o Neurosarcoidosis (chest x-ray)
    - o Brainstem lesions, such as multiple sclerosis

Reproduced with permission: Therapeutics Choices. Sixth Edition. Ottawa, Canada: *Canadian Pharmacist Association* 2012, Table 1, page 259; Burton JL. *Churchill Livingstone* 1971, page 74.

- Take a directed history and perform a focused physical examination for a **lesion at the cerebellopontine angle**.

> Definition
    - o Symptoms and signs related to cranial nerves VIII and IX.
    - o The cerebellopontine angle is the shallow triangular fossa lying between the cerebellum, lateral pons and the inner third of the petrous temporal bone.
    - o This angle extends from the trigeminal nerve (above) to the glossopharyngeal nerve (below).
    - o The abducens nerve runs along the medial edge, whereas
    - o Facial and auditory cranial nerves transverse the angle, to enter the internal auditory meatus.

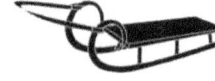

➢ Causes
  o Infection
    – Local meningeal involvement
    – Syphilis
    – Tuberculosis
  o Infiltration
    – Acoustic neuroma
    – Meningioma
    – Cholesteatoma
    – Hemangioblastoma
    – Pontine glioma
    – Medulloblastoma and astrocytoma of the cerebellum
    – Carcinoma of the nasopharynx
  o Vascular
    - Aneurysm of the basilar artery

Adapted from: Baliga RR. *Saunders/Elsevier* 2007, pages 222 and 223.

SO YOU WANT TO BE A NEUROLOGIST!

• Give the component of the facial nerve (CN VII) which is sensory, and state what does it supply.
  o The nervus intermedius of Wrisberg
  o Taste sensation from the anterio two thirds of the tongue
  o Probably, cutaneous impulse from the anterio wall of the external auditory canal.

Source: Baliga RR. *Saunders/Elsevier* 2007, page 159 and 160.

• Give how to localize the site of the facial nerve palsy.
  o Involvement of the nuclei in pons – associated ipsilateral sixth nerve palsy.
  o Cerebellopontine angle lesion – associated fifth and eighth nerve involvement.
  o Lesion in the bony canal – loss of taste (carried by the lingual nerve) and hyperacusis (due to involvement of the nerve to stapedius).

• Give the reflexes that involve the facial nerve.
  o Corneal reflex
  o Palmomental reflex
  o Suck reflex

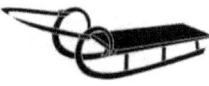

SO YOU WANT TO BE A NEUROLOGIST!

- Why can the patient with central damage to CN VII wrinkle their foreheads?
    - Both sides of the cortex supply the LMN innervation of the upper half of the face.

SO YOU WANT TO BE A NEUROLOGIST!

- In the context of CN VII, what is the Raeder paratrigeminal syndrome, and the superior orbital fissure syndrome?
    - Raeder paratrigeminal syndrome – severe retro-orbital pain succeeded by ipsilateral miosis and ptosis
    - Superior orbital fissure syndrome – boring retro-orbital pain and paresis or cranial nerves III, IV, V and VI

SO YOU WANT TO BE A NEUROLOGIST!

- Give the epomous syndrome in which the third cranial nerve (CN III) is involved.
    - Weber syndrome:
        - Ipsilateral third nerve palsy with contralateral hemiplegia.
        - The lesion is in the midbrain.
    - Benedikt syndrome:
        - Ipsilateral third nerve palsy with contralateral involuntary movement
        - Due to a lesion of the red nucleus in the midbrain.
    - Claude syndrome: ipsilateral oculomotor paresis with contralateral ataxia and tremor.
        - Due to a lesion of the third nerve and red nucleus.
    - Nothnagel syndrome:
        - Unilateral oculomotor paralysis combined with ipsilateral cerebellar ataxia.

Source: Baliga RR. *Saunders/Elsevier* 2007, page 155.

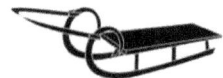

➢ Treatment
  o Spontaneous recovery, 70%
  o patch eye, use eye drops
  o Prednisone po for 3 d (↑ recovery)
  o No role for anti-HSV therapy

Ear: Cranial Nerve VIII

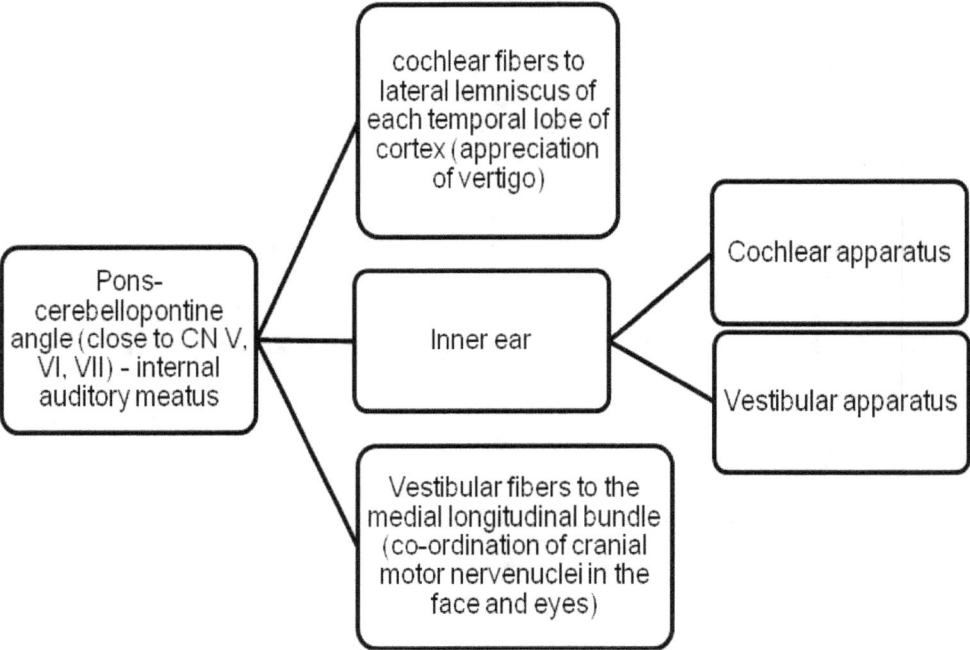

  o VIII (Vestibulo-cochlear) – auditory and vestibular components (sensory)
    – Hearing (whisper test)
    – Local sound and vibration (S12 Hz tuning fork)

  o Auditory Nerve CN VIII

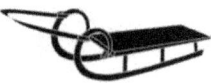

➢Translational Neuroanatomy

CN VIII, cochlear (hearing) branch
↓
End organs of Corti
↓
Spiral ganglion
↓
Joined by CN VII vertibular branch ←———
↓
Facial canal
↓
Internal auditory meatis
↓
Cerebellopontine angle

CN VIII, vestibular (balance) branch
endolymph, and otolith system
↓
Crista acoustica in horizontal, anterior
and posterior semicircular canals
↓
Vestibular nerve
↓
Vestibular ganglion

    Cochlear fibres   Vestibular fibres
    ↓   ↓
    Caudal portion   Vestibular nuclei
      of pons
    ↓   Cerebellum: restiform Spine: vestibula-spinal   Midbrain posterior
Dorsal and   body   tract (extrapyramidal)
    longitudinum bundle
Ventral nuclei
of cochlea   ←------- Corpus trapezium and dorsal nuclei
↓
Luteral lemniscus
↓
Medial geniculate body and inferior corpus quadrigemina
↓
Acoutic radiation
↓
Internal capsule, posterior limb
↓
Temporal cortex

Cranial Nerve VIII, acoustic branch

➢   Clinical

   A tuning fork is normally heard longer with air conduction (AC) than with
   bone conduction (BC; mastoid bone) (Rinne test)
     AC > BC   Normal
     AC < BC or BC > AC   Conductive deafness
     AC = BC   Sensorineural deafness

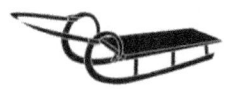

- Perform a focused physical examination for labyrinth disease.

    o Vertigo

    o Nystagmus

    o Postural defect (inability to maintain the position of an outstretched arm when the eyes are open)

    o Past-pointing

- Take a directed history and perform a focus physical examination to distinguish between cerebral, psychogenic and hypertensive vertigo.

    o Cerebral vertigo
      – Associated with
        ▪ Epilepsy
        ▪ Migraine
        ▪ ↑ intracerebral pressure

    o Psychogenic vertigo
      – Often associated with parathesine of lower limbs

    o Hypertensive vertigo
      – Comes on with or worsens on stooping

- Give the causes of the external otitis.

    o Malignant external otitis   -   Pseudomonas aeruginosa infection in diabetic or immune compromised patient becomes systemic

    o Acute myringitis   -   Mycoplasma or viral infection causing hemorrhagic bullae on lateral surface of tympanic membrane

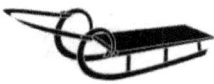

Deafness

➤ Causes

    o Conduction deafness
       - Middle ear
          ▪ Otitis media
          ▪ Otosclerosis
       - Bone conduction > air conduction

    o Nerve deafness
       - Cochlear
          ▪ Infection –mumps
          ▪ Idiopathic – Meniere disease
          ▪ Drugs

➤ Tests

    o Rinne – normal: air > Bone conduction ([BC], conduction hearing loss)

    o Weber – lateralizes to good ear – neurosensory loss; lateralizes to bad ear – conductive loss

    o Vestibulo-ocular reflex (vestibular component)

		Nerve	Middle ear
o	Rinne	– AC> BC	▪ AC= AC; ACb, BCb
o	Weber	– Normal ear louder	▪ Abnormal ear louder

Abbreviations: AC, air conduction; BC, bone conduction; C, conductive; CN cranial nerves

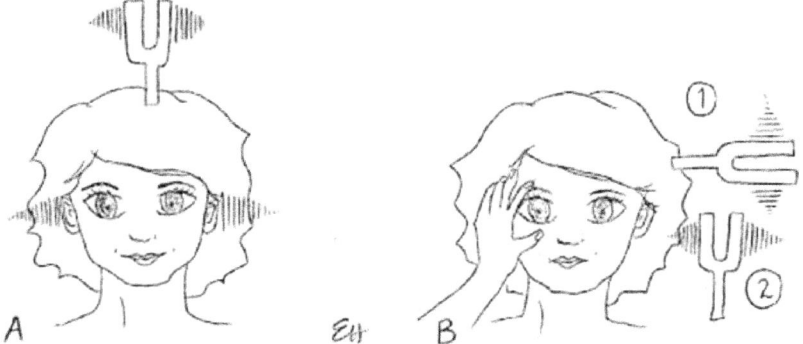

A   *EH*   B

Adapted from: Mangione S. *Hanley & Belfus* 2000, page 113; McGee SR. *Saunders/Elsevier* 2007, Figure. 21, page 245; Filate W, et al. *The Medical Society, Faculty of Medicine, University of Toronto* 2005, pages 153 to154, and 157 to158.

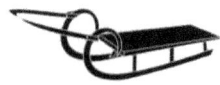

Weber Test	Rinne Test	Possible Interpretations
o Midline	– AC> BC, bilateral	• Normal hearing, bilateral • Neurosensory loss, bilateral
o Louder in left	– BC> AC, left – AC> BC, right	• Conductive loss, left
o Louder in left	– AC> BC, bilateral	• Normal hearing, bilateral • Neurosensory loss, worse on right
o Louder in right	– BC> AC, bilateral	• Conductive loss, bilateral but worse on right • Conductive loss on right and severe neurosensory loss on left

Adapted from: Filate W, et al. *The Medical Society, Faculty of Medicine, University of Toronto* 2005, page 162; Baliga RR. *Saunders/Elsevier* 2007, page 107; McGee SR. *Saunders/Elsevier* 2007, Table 21-1, page 246.

- Give the performance characteristics of hearing and conduction tests of CN VIII.

Finding	Sensitivity (%)	Specificity (%)	PLR	NLR
o Hearing tests				
– Abnormal whispered voice test	90-99	80-87	6.0	0.03
o Tuning fork tests (patients with unilateral hearing loss)				
– Rinne test, detecting conductive hearing loss	60-90	95-98	16.8	0.2
– Weber test, lateralizes to good ear, detecting neurosensory loss	58	79	2.7	NS
– Weber test lateralizes to bad ear, detecting conductive loss	54	92	NS	0.5

 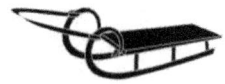

Probability						
Decrease			Increase			
-45%	-30%	-15%		+15%	+30%	+45%
0.1	0.2	0.5	1	2	5	10

NLR   PLR

- o Sen N out – <u>Sen</u>sitive test; when negative, rules <u>out</u> disease

- o Sp P in – <u>Sp</u>ecific test; when positive, rules <u>in</u> disease

Abbreviation: NLR, negative likelihood ratio; NS, not significant; PLR, positive likelihood ratio
Source: McGee SR. *Saunders/Elsevier* 2007, Box 21-1, page 247.

SO YOU WANT TO BE A NEUROLOGIST!

- • Give what structural damage causes Nystagmus.

  - o Nystagmus is the involuntary oscillation of the eye. It is caused by damage to the mechanisms in the brain or brainstem for the coordination of eye movements (not due to damage to CN III, IV, VI).

Articulation: Cranial Nerves IX, X, XII

- ➢ Translational Neuroanatomy of IX, X, XI

  - o Interconnected nuclei of IX, X, XI
  - o All three situated in the dorsum of the open medulla in the floor of the forth ventricle
  - o Ventral nucleus solitaries
    - – Motor

  - o Dorsal nucleus and solitaries
    - – Sensory
    - – Autonomic

  - o Bilateral representation
    - – No unilateral UMN lesion
    - – Only bilateral UMN lesion

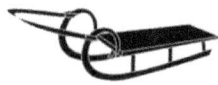

- o Unilateral LMN lesion
  - – Jugular foramen syndrome
    - ▪ Cancer of nasopharynx
    - ▪ Fracture of base of skill
    - ▪ Paget's disease
    - ▪ Basal meningistis
    - ▪ Jugular vein thrombosis

  - – Unilateral LMN lesion isolated to trapezius and sternomastoid
    - ▪ Injury to neck
- o CN X – Sensory and motor supply to larynx

- o X (Vagus)
  - – Motor
    - ▪ Gag reflex (afferent limb, IX; efferent limb, X)
    - ▪ Soft palate, larynx, pharynx (nucleus ambiguus)
    - ▪ Ipselateral palate elevation (with CN IX)
    - ▪ Swallowing, phonation
  - – Reflex
    - ▪ Gag reflex (afferent limb, IX; efferent limb, X)
  - – Secretory
    - ▪ Parotid gland
    - ▪ Afferent and efferent pathways to heart, lung and GI tract (nucleus solitaries)

- o XI (Spinal accessory) (motor)
  - – Rotate head against resistance (sternocleidomastoid muscle)
  - – Shrug shoulders (trapezius muscle)
  - – Necessary fibres to vagus nerve

- o XII (Hypoglossal)
  - – Motor to tongue and hyoid bone depressors
  - – Tongue movement (deviation, fasciculation, atrophy, pushing tongue against teeth)
  - – Speech – say 'AH' (dysarthria)

- o Multiple Cranial nerve abnormalities

CN Combination	Common cause
– Unilateral III, IV, V1, VI	▪ Cavernous sinus lesion
– Unilateral V, VII, VIII	▪ Cerebellopontine angle lesion
– Unilateral IX, X, XI	▪ Jugular foramen syndrome
– Bilateral X, XI, XII	▪ Bulbar palsy (LMN), pseudobulbar palsy (UMN)

Adapted from: Filate W, et al. *The Medical Society, Faculty of Medicine, University of Toronto* 2005, page162.

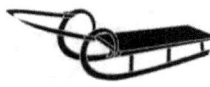

Cranial Nerve (CN) IX

- ➤ IX (Glosopharyngeal)
  - ○ Sensory – posterior third of tongue, pharynx, nasopharynx, middle ear; voice-hoarse, nasal, taste; phonation
  - ○ Motor
    - – Initiate swallow (middle constrictor of pharynx, and stylopharyngeus)
    - – Gag reflex (afferent limb, IX; efferent limb, X)
    - – Ipselateral palate elevation (with CN X)
    - – Soft palate, larynx, pharynx (nucleus ambiguus)

- ➤ Sensation (including taste) to
  - ○ Back of tongue
  - ○ Fauces
  - ○ Palate
  - ○ Secretory fibres to papratid gland
  - ○ Motor fibres to
    - – Stylo – pharyngeus
    - – Palate – palato – pharyngeus
    - – Palato – glasses

- ➤ Weakness of the sternomastoids is not a reliable sign for CN XI damage: instead, look for wasting of sternomustoid muscles

- ➤ Clinical

- • Perform a focused physical examination to determine the site of defect and the causes of dysarthria (disorder of articulation).

Site of defect	Causes	Characteristics of speech
○ Supra-nuclear (pseudo-bulbar palsy) – UMN lesions of CN IX, X or XII)	– CVA – MND – MS	▪ Monotonous ▪ High-pitched ▪ "Hot potato" speech
○ Nuclear (bulbar pasy, LMN lesions of CN IX, X or XII)	– MND – Guillain-Barré syndrome – Tumour of medulla – Bulbar polio – Syringobulbia	

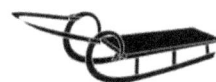

Site of Defect	Causes	Characteristics of Speech
o Basal ganglia	– Parkinsonism – Choreoathetosis	▪ Slow ▪ Slurred ▪ Monotonous
o Cerebellum	– MS – Tumour – Drugs and toxins (alcohol)	▪ Staccato ▪ Scanning
o Muscle	– Myasthenia gravis – Muscular dystrophy	
o Mouth	– False teeth – Cleft palate – Stuttering	

Abbreviations: CN, cranial nerve; CVA, cerebrovascluar accident; LMN, lower motor neuron; MND, motor neuron disease; MS, multiple sclerosis; UMN, upper motor disease

Adapted from: Burton JL. *Churchill Livingstone* 1971, page 170; Baliga RR. *Saunders/Elsevier* 2007, pages 149 and 153

SO YOU WANT TO BE A NEUROLOGIST!

- In the context of looking at the anatomy of the oropharynx, give the abnormalities you are looking for in the uvula.

  - o Absence
    - – Congenital
    - – Surgical - UPPP (uvulopalatinopharyngoplasty) for obstructive sleep apnea

  - o Bifid
    - – Occult cleft palate
    - – Normal variant

- In the context of examining the uvula, give the meaning of Mueller sign.

  - o Rhythmic pulsatile movement of uvula seen in chronic aortic regurgitation

Adapted from: Mangione S. *Hanley & Belfus* 2000, page 123.

 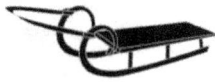

Clinical Gems: Uvula – deviates to strong side; jaw and tongue – deviate to weak side

o In the absence of wasting of the tongue, then even if there is fibrillation or deviation of the tongue, a CN XII LMN cannot be diagnosed.

o In the absence of an UMN lesion causing hemiplegia, an UMN lesion of tongue cannot be diagnosed (in the absence of pyramidal UMN lesion of area or leg there cannot be a pyramidal lesion of the tongue).

o Bilateral lesion of tongue
   – UMN – pseudobulbar palsy
   – LMN – bulbar palsy

SO YOU WANT TO BE A NEUROLOGIST!

- When you ask the patient to say "Ahh", give the structures you are looking at?

Anatomy of the oropharynx

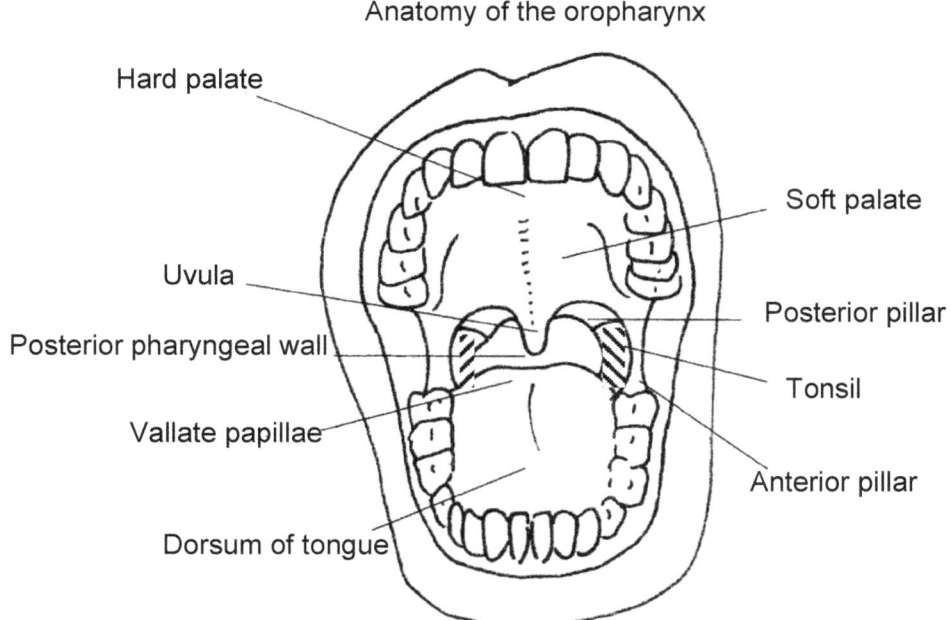

Adapted from: Mangione S. *Hanley & Belfus* 2000, page 123.

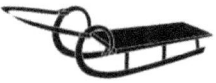

Mastering the Boards: Neurology   A.B.R. Thomson

Jugular Foramen Syndrome (Posterior Fossa Syndrome)

➢ Definition

 o Symptoms/signs from impaired function of cranial nerves IX, X and XI.

 o The jugular foramen is beated between the lateral part of the occipital bone and the petrous protion of the temporal bones.

➢ Clinical

• Perform a focused physical examination for a lesion in the posterior fossa (jugular foramen syndrome).

 o Glossopharyngeal nerve, CN X
  - Nucleus ambiguous (motor branch)
    ▪ Taste, posterior 1/3 of tongue
    ▪ Sensation of the inside of the mouth

 o Accessary nerve, CN XI
  - Motor
    ▪ Trapezius and sternomastoid muscles
    ▪ Accessary nerve is joined by a branch of the upper cervical spine

 o Hypoglossal, CN XII

• Take a directed history and perform a focused physical examination for the jugular foramen syndrome.

 o Eye
  - Ptosis (due to Horner syndrome).

 o Ear
  - Pain in and around the ear (due to damage of the ninth and tenth cranial nerves which carry sensation to the external auditory meatus and behind the ear).

 o Head
  - Headache

 o Voice
  - Hoarseness of voice
  - Nasal quality to the speech

 o Throat
  - Nasal regurgitation and dysphagia
  - Aspiration of food with choking attacks
  - Sluggish movement of the palate on the affected side when the patient says 'aah'
  - Absent gag reflex on the same side

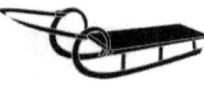

- o Tongue
  - Wasting of the tongue (often noticed by the dentist)
- o Neck
  - Weakness of the sternomastoids and trapezii
  - Flattening of the shoulder on the same side
  - Wasting of the sternomastoid
  - Difficulty in shrugging the shoulder on the same side
- o Chin
  - Weakness when the patient moves her chin to the opposite side

➢ Causes
- o Infection
  - Basal meningitis
- o infiltration
  - Carcinoma (of the pharynx is the commonest cause)
  - Neurofibroma or any tumour
- o Vascular
  - Thrombosis of jugular vein
- o Trauma
  - Fractured base of the skull
- o Metabolic
  - Paget's disease

Adapted from: Baliga RR. *Saunders/Elsevier* 2007, pages 224 and 225.

- Give the reason why the hypoclossal nerve (CN XII) is not part of the jugular foramen syndrome.

  - o CN XII leaves through the anterior condylar foramen

Source: Baliga RR. *Saunders/Elsevier* 2007, pages 224 and 225.

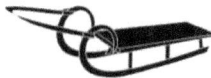

Mastering the Boards: Neurology   A.B.R. Thomson

- Give examples of syndromes that result from abnormalities of groups of cranial nerves.

    o Unilateral III, IV, V and VI
      - Suggests a lesion in the cavernous sinus

    o Unilateral V, VII, and VIII
      - Suggests a cerebellopontine angle lesion (usually a tumour)

    o Unilateral IX, X AND XI
      - Suggests a jugular foramen lesion

    o Combined bilateral X, XI, XII suggests bulbar palsy if lower motor neurone changes are present, and psudobulbar palsy if there are upper motor neurone signs.

Posterior Inferior Cerebellar Artery Thrombosis

➢ Clinical

- Perform a focused physical examination for posterior inferior cerebellar artery thrombosis.
    o V-Ipsilateral loss
    o VI, VII, VIII – (Often transient)
    o IX, X, XII – (Bulbar palsy)
    o Cerebellum – ataxia, with nystagmus to the side of the lesion
    o Lateral spinothalamic pathway – (often transient)
    o Homolateral Horner syndrome
    o Bulbar palsy affects motor nuclei.

Adapted from: Burton JL. *Churchill Livingstone* 1971, page 78.

- Perform a focused physical examination for a disorder of CN IX/X.

    o Absent pharyngeal sensation (tested with a cotton applicator stick touching the posterior oropharynx)

    o Diminished velar movement (reduced elevation of the soft palate as the patient vocalizes a prolonged "ah")

    o Abnormal gag reflex (diminished, absent, hyperactive or asymmetric)

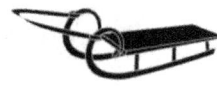

➢ Causes/associations

    o Bilateral cerebral hemispheric disease (Unilateral cerebral hemispheric disease does not ordinarily cause palatal weakness because each nucleus of these nerves receives bilateral corticobulbar innervation)

    o Ipsilateral medulla or peripheral nerves (i.e., cranial nerves IX and X)

Adapted from: McGee SR. *Saunders/Elsevier* 2007, page 697.

- Perform a focused physical examination of the tongue to distinguish between a lower motor neuron (LMN) lesion, bulbar palsy, and pseudobulabr/bilateral upper motor neuron (UMN) lesion.

    o LMN
- Atrophy on half of the tongue
- With mouth, tongue deviates away towards the weak side
- Protruding tongue from the mouth, tongue deviates away towards the weak side

    o Bulbar
- Bilateral wasting of tongue (bilateral LMN)

    o Pseudobulbar
- Bilateral UMN
- Tongue is stiff, opestic
- No atrophy
- Patient has difficulty protruding tongue

- Give causes of absent knee and ankle jerks, with an extensor plantar response.

    o Sub-acute combined degeneration

    o Syphilitic tabo-paresis

    o Friedreich ataxia

    o Motor neurone disease

Source: Burton JL. *Churchill Livingstone* 1971, page 88.

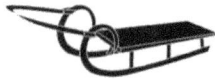

Speech

- ➤ Components
    - ○ Phonation: abnormality is called dysphonia.
    - ○ Articulation: abnormality is called dysarthria.
    - ○ Language: abnormality is called dysphasia.

Source: McGee S. R. *Saunders/Elsevier* 2007, page 149.

- ➤ Speaking of speech – **terminology**
    - ○ Agnosia
        - – Failure to recognise, whether visual, auditory or tactile
        - – Related to receptive dysplasia
    - ○ Apraxia
        - – Inability to carry out purposive movements in absence of motor paralysis, sensory loss or ataxia
        - – Related to expressive dysplasia
    - ○ Dysarthria
        - – Disorder of articulation
    - ○ Dysphasia
        - – Disorder in use of symbols for communication, whether spoken, written or read
    - ○ Echolalia
        - – Parrot-like repetition by the subject of statements or acts made before them
    - ○ Epilepsy
        - – A paroxysmal transitory disturbance of brain function, ceasing spontaneously, with a tendency to recurrence
    - ○ Expressive
    - ○ Myoclonus
        - – A brief shock-like contraction of a number of muscle fibres, a whole muscle or several muscles, either simultaneously or successively
    - ○ Perseveration
        - – Continuation or recurrence of an activity without appropriate stimulus
    - ○ Receptive
    - ○ Verbigeration
        - – Meaningless repetition of words or sentences

Adapted from: Burton JL. *Churchill Livingstone* 1971, page 69.

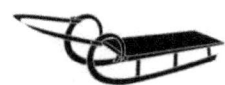

Mastering the Boards: Neurology   A.B.R. Thomson

SO YOU WANT TO BE A NEUROLOGIST!

- Give the differences between receptive and expressive aphasia.

  o Aphasia is an acquired disturbance of language

  o Receptive aphasia (sensory, fluent or Wernicke aphasia)
    - Lesion in temporal or parietal lobe
    - Jumbled words
    - Difficulty naming objects
    - Poor comprehension of spoken or written words

  o Expressive aphasia (motor, nonfluent or Brocca aphasia)
    - Lesion in frontal lobe
    - Good comprehension of spoken or written words
    - Slow, monosyllabic sentences

- Give the meaning of dysarthria, and its causes.

  o Dysarthria is the poor articulation of words
  o Causes
    - Brain
      Injury
    - Muscles of phonation
      Paralysis
      Spasticity
    - Emotional stress

- Canada is a multicultural country, and many different languages are spoken. When asking the patient to "say something" for you to access if there are abnormally transmitted voice sounds, give what you can ask the non-English language speakers to say.

  o All five vowel sounds (A, E, I, O, U) become "a", so pick words with vowels.

Source: Mangione S. *Hanley & Belfus* 2000, page 331.

- Give the meaning of cerebellar speech.
  o Slow irregular speech, with sudden changes in speed and volume

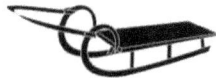

Dysphasia

➢ Definition

    o A disorder in the use of symbols for communication, whether spoken, written, or read.

➢ Anatomy

    o Cortex
- Grey matter
  - Dementia
- Precentral gyrus
  - Expressive
- Postcentral gyrus
  - Receptive

Dysphasia (aphasia is often associated with acalculia and agraphia)

➢ Clinical

• Perform a focused examination of a patient with dysphasia.

Fluent speech	Nominal	Conductive	Receptive	Expressive no Fluent
o Name object	↓	↓	↓	↓
o Repetition	-	↓	↓	+/-
o Comprehension	-	-	↓	-
o Reading (dyslexia)		✓	✓	✓
o Dysgraphic (writing)		✓	✓ abnormal content	✓

• Take a directed history and perform a focused physical examination for a **speech disorder**.

    o Usually follows a lesion of the dominant cortex:

    o Expressive (motor), nominal dysphasia or motor dysphasia

    o The patient understands, but cannot answer appropriately

    o Speech is non-fluent

    o This occurs with a lesion in the posterior part of the dominant third frontal gyrus (Broca)

    o Sensory or receptive dysphasia
- The site of the lesion is the superior temporal lobe (Wernicke area)

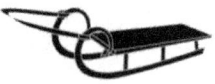

- ➢ Nominal dysphasia: all types of dysphasia
  - o Is also a specific type of nominal dysphasia.
  - o Objects cannot be named (e.g., the nib of a pen) but other aspects of speech are normal.
  - o The patient may use long sentences to overcome failure to find the correct word (circumlocution).
  - o It occurs with a lesion of the dominant posterior temporoparietal area.
  - o Certain types of speech may be retained by these patients. These include automatic speech. The patient may be able to recite word series such as the days of the week or letters of the alphabet.
  - o Emotional speech may be preserved so that when frustrated or upset the patient may be able to swear fluently.
  - o The patient may be able to sing familiar songs while unable to speak the words.
  - o Unless the lesion responsible for these defects is very large there may be no reduction in the patient's higher intellectual functions, memory or judgement.
  - o Some of these patients may incorrectly be considered psychotic, because of their disorganised speech.
  - o Other causes include
    - – Encephalopathy or the intracranial pressure effects of a distinct space-occupying lesion;
    - – It may also occur in the recovery phase from any dysphasia.

- ➢ Conductive dysphasia
  - o Repeat statements and name objects poorly, but can follow commands.
  - o Caused by a lesion of the arcuate fasciculus and/or other fibres linking the Wernicke and Broca areas.

- ➢ Fluent speech (receptive, conductive or nominal aphasia, usually)
  - o Name object — patients with nominal, conductive or receptive aphasia will name objects poorly
  - o Repetition — cannot repeat 'no ifs, ands or buts'.
  - o Comprehension — follow commands (verbal or written): 'Touch your nose, then your chin and then your ear.'
  - o Reading — dyslexia
  - o Writing — writing (dysgraphia)

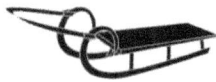

➤ Non-fluent speech (expressive aphasia, usually)

    o Naming of objects — this is poor, but may be better than spontaneous speech

    o Repetition — may be possible with great effort. Phrase repetition (e.g., 'no ifs, ands or buts') is poor.

    o Comprehension — often mildly impaired despite popular belief, but written and verbal commands are followed

    o Reading — patients may have dyslexia

    o Writing — dysgraphia may be present

Adapted from: Talley N. J., et al. Maclennan & Petty Pty Limited 2003, page 351.

    o Remember

        – There are two speech centres, one sensory (receptive) and one motor

        – These speech centres are in the dominant hemisphere

"Science is never cast in stone and ideas are written with a finger on shifting sand."

Anonymous

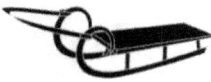

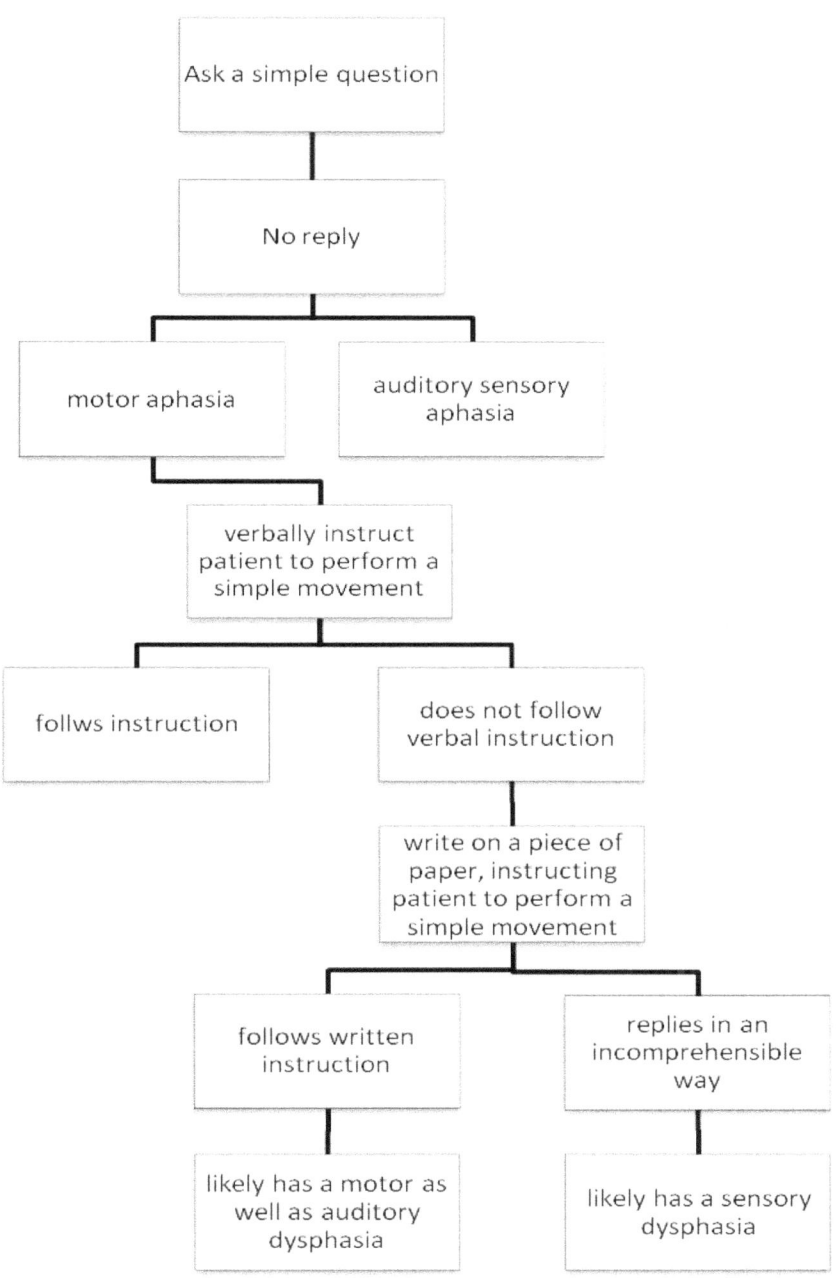

Dysarthria

➢ Definition

    o An inability to articulate properly

    o Because of local lesions in the mouth, or

    o Disorders of speech muscles or their connections (there is no disorder of the content of speech)

➢ Causes/associations

    o Stutter, stammer: psychological origin

    o Paralysis of cranial nerves – Bell palsy, CN IX, X, XI

    o Cerebellar disease – staccato, scanning speech

    o Signs of cerebellar dysfunction

    o Parkinson speech – slow, quiet, slurred, monotonous

    o Pseudobullar palsy – monotonous, high-pitched 'hot potato' speech

    o Look for bilateral paralysis of lips, tongue, soft palate

    o Progressive bulbar palsy – nasal

➢ Clinical

    o Testing for dysarthria – lips, tongue, palate (VII, IX, X) (Say "The True Methodist Episcopal Church")

    o Expressive or motor dysphasia – understands spoken words and can obey commands; lesions of posterior inferior 3rd frontal convolution

    o Cranial nerve VII, IX, X

        – Disordered function of lips, tongue and soft palate

            ▪ Dysarthria

        – Dysphonia

            ▪ Disordered function of laryngeal muscles

    o Disorders affecting the motor function of cranial nerves VII, IX and X may be caused by disease of the following site:

        – Abnormalities of upper motor neurone lesions of the cranial nerves, extrapyramidal conditions (e.g., Parkinson's disease) and cerebellar lesions cause disturbances to the rhythm of speech.

        – LMN lesion cranial nerve VII, IX, X, XII

        – Bilateral papralysis of lips, tongue and soft palate

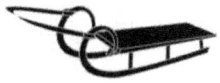

- Bulbar
  - Sounds like the voice of the cartoon character, Donald Duck
- Cerebral cortices
  - Both R and L internal capsules affected
  - "pseudo-bulbar palsy"
- Pseudobulbar palsy is an upper motor neurone weakness which causes spastic dysarthria (it sounds as if the patient is trying to squeeze out words from tight lips)
- Cerebrum
  - Signs of cerebellar dysfunction
  - Jerky, monotomous speech, like talking with your mouth full of food
- Extrapyramidal fibres
  - Monotonous speech
  - Festinations (labial, lingual, palatal and laryngeal
- Disease of muscle
  - Myopathy
  - Myasthenia gravis
- Syphilis
  - GPI (general paralysis of the insane)
  - Sounds like "baby talk"
- Ask the patient to say a phrase such as 'British Constitution' or 'Peter Piper picked a peck of pickled peppers'.
  - Mouth ulceration or disease may mimic dysarthria

Other Disorders of Speech

- Bulbar palsies cause a nasal speech
- Facial muscle weakness causes slurred speech
- Extrapyramidial disease
  - Monotonous speech (bradykinesia and muscular rigidity)
  - Other causes of alcohol intoxication and cerebellar disease
  - Loss of co-ordination and slow, slurred and often explosive speech, or speech broken up into syllables called scanning speech

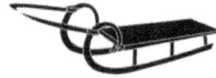

- o Dysphonia
  - – Alteration of the sound of the voice such as huskiness of the voice with decreased volume
  - – May be due to laryngeal disease (e.g., following a viral infection or a tumour of the vocal cord), or to recurrent laryngeal nerve palsy, but occasionally may be hysterical

Adapted from: McGee SR. *Saunders/Elsevier* 2007, page 149.

WHY WOULD ANYONE IN THEIR RIGHT MIND WANT TO BE A NEUROLOGIST IF YOU HAVE TO REMEMBER TRIVIA LIKE THIS?

- • What are the eponymous syndromes of the lower cranial nerves (CN)?
  - o IX, X and XI   – Vernet syndrome
    - ▪ Paresis due to extension of tumour into the jugular foramen.
  - o IX to XII   – Collet-Sicard syndrome
    - ▪ Fracture of the floor of the posterior cranial fossa.
  - o IX to XII   – Villaret syndrome
    - ▪ Ipsilateral paralysis of the last four cranial nerves and cervical sympathetic.
  - o X , XI   – Schmidt Syndrome
  - o XI, XII   – Hughlings Jackson Syndrome

Nystagmus

- ➤ Definition
  - o A series of involuntary, rythmic oscillation of one or both eyes
  - o May be horizontal, vertical or rotary
  - o Slow drifting of eye, then rapid correcting movement
  - o The direction of the rapid correcting movement is the direction used to describe the nystagmus
  - o Ascentuate nystagmus by looking away from the straight-ahead or middle line
  - o Lesions of vestibular apparatus, cerebellum, toxins (alcohol)

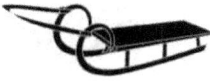

➤ Types of nystagmus

- o Phasic nystagmus
  – Slow and fast component of eye movement is in horizontal or vertical direction
  – Named according to the direction of the fast component

- o Vertical nystagmus
  – Often caused by brain-stem lesions

- o Rotatory nystagmus
  – Often present with forward gaze
  – Due to defective vision (often from defective development of visual purple)
    ▪ Lens
    ▪ Cornea
    ▪ Myopia
    ▪ Optic nerve atrophy
    ▪ Albinos
    ▪ Miners (not minors!)

➤ Causes/associations

- o Physiological e.g., opto-kinetic
- o Eye
  – Errors of refraction and macular lesions
  – Weakness of ocular muscles (Lesion of CN III, IV or VI)

- o Lesions of vestibular apparatus, cerebellum, brain stem

Source: Burton JL. *Churchill Livingstone* 1971, page 76.

➤ Clinical

• Perform a focused physical examination to determine the site of the lesion causing nystagmus.

- o Eye
  – Both phase of nystagmus are the same speed
  – Associated vision defect

- o Vestibular system
  – With lesions of the labyrinth nerve or vestibular nerve there is usually associated deafness, tinnitus and vertigo
  – The excusions back and forth are larger when looking in the direction of the fast phase, and are smaller when looking in the direction of the slow phase (i.e., the side of the lesion)

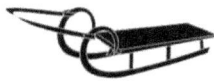

- o Central lesions (brain stem, cerebellum)
  - – No associated visual changes, deafness, tinnitus or vertigo
  - – Slow phase towards rest position of eye
  - – Slow and fast phases change with full excursion of the eyes

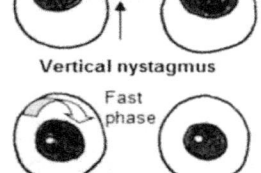

Vertical nystagmus

Rotational nystagmus

- ➢ Peripheral lesions
  - o Severe vertigo + nausea/vomiting in acute phase
  - o Lying still, fixing eyes on bright objects helps symptoms

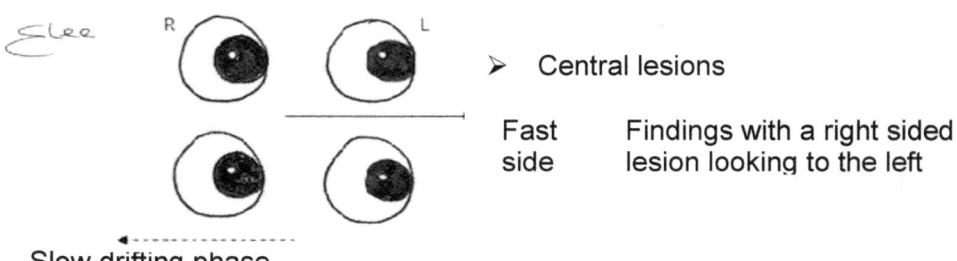

- ➢ Central lesions

| Fast side | Findings with a right sided lesion looking to the left |

Slow drifting phase

- • Perform a focused physical examination for the causes of nystagmus/vertigo.
  - o Eyes (nystagmus)
    - – Physiological, e.g., opto-kinetic
    - – Errors of refraction and macular lesions
    - – Weakness of ocular muscles
    - – Lesion of cranial nerves III, IV or VI
  - o Brainstem lesions, cerebellum, temporal cortex lesions

- ➢ Vestibular nystagmus

	Central (vestibular nuclei)	Peripheral (labyrinth or vestibular nerve)
o Vertigo	Rare	Yes
o Auditory symptoms	No	Yes
o Lying still, fixing eyes on bright objects helpful	No	Yes

Adapted from: Davey P. *Wiley-Blackwell* 2006, page 90.

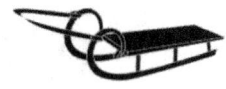

- Give the site of the lesion in vestibular nystagmus.

  - Central (affecting vestibular nuclei), as in
    - Cause
      - CVA
      - MS
      - Tumour
      - Alcoholism

  - Peripheral (labyrinth or vestibular nerve)
    - Meniere syndrome
    - Acoustic neuroma
    - Otitis media
    - Head injury

Adapted from: Baliga R.R. *Saunders/Elsevier* 2007, page 147.

High Cervical Cord Diseases/Disorders
  - Vestibular lesions
    - Physiological
    - Labrinthitis
    - Menière
    - Bledding, in leukemia
    - Drugs, e.g., quinine, salicylates, alcohol
    - Otitis media
    - Motion sickness

  - Vestibular nerve lesions
    - Acoustic neuroma
    - Drugs, e.g., streptomycin
    - Vestibular neuronitis

  - Brain stem, cerebellar or temporal cortical lesions
    - Pontine infarction or hemorrhage
    - Vertebro-basilar insufficiency
    - Basilar artery migraine
    - Temporal lobe epilepsy
    - Disseminated sclerosis
    - Tumours
    - Benign post-traumatic positional vertigo

Adapted from: Burton JL. *Churchill Livingstone* 1971, page 76.

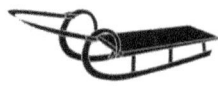

HEADACHE
- o Headaches are common, and there are many causes
- o >90% of headaches are due to
  - – Migrane (commonest)
  - – Tension type
  - – Cluster
  - – Rebound

- ➢ Types
  - o Primary — Defined by symptom complex, such as migraine, tension-type, cluster (trigeminal autonomic cephalgias)
  - o Secondary — Defined by cause, in which an anatomical approach to classification is a practical approach.

- ➢ Causes/associations
- • Give mechanisms of headache production.
  - o Muscle — Skeletal muscle contraction (e.g., "tension" headache)
  - o ENT — Referred pain, e.g., disease of eyes, ears, sinuses, teeth, cervical spine
  - o Arteries — Systemic hypertension
    - – Arterial dilatation
      - ▪ Intra-cranial
        - – systemic infections
        - – hypertension
        - – nitrites
        - – postictal
        - – concussion
      - ▪ Extracranial (e.g., migraines)
    - – Traction on arteries e.g., raised intracranial pressure
  - o Veins — Dilatation or traction on venous sinuses e.g., post lumbar puncture
    - – Analgesics
    - – Oral contraceptive pill
  - o Inflammation — Intra-cranial (e.g., meningitis)
    - – Extra cranial (e.g., giant cell arteritis)
  - o Psychogenic

Adapted from: Burton JL. *Churchill Livingstone* 1971, page 72.

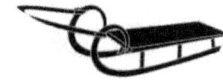

➢ Clinical

Type	Duration	Frequency	Quality	Unilateral	Nausea	AUBS	Other symptoms
Migraine	4-72 h`	Variable	Severe	/	/	20%	
Tension-type	30 min – 7 d		Tight pressure	Bilateral	-	-	
Cluster	20-60 min	3 – 6 d	Periorbital	/	-	-	Teras rhinorrhea

• Give the clinical features of headache which raise the suspicion of a secondary cause.

   o History of headache
   - New < 5 or > 50 yr
   - First or worse
   - Sudden and severe
   - Change in LOD (level of consciousness)
   - Progression or change
   - Lasts > 1 hr
   - Triggered by exertion or straining
   - Comorbidities, e.g.,
     ▪ Pregnancy
     ▪ Cancer
     ▪ Immunosuppression

   o Physical examination
   - Abnormal findings

   o Starting investigation
   - MRI ± angiography

• Take a directed history for headache.

   o Character of headache
   - Quality of pain: Is it steady/throbbing, constant/remittent, sharp/dull, superficial/deep?
   - Location of pain regional or diffuse

   o Severity of pain: Try to quantify this if possible:
   - Ask "on a scale of 1 to 10, 10 being "the worst pain you have ever had and 1 being pain free, what number would you give the pain?

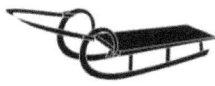

- o Temporal relationships
  - – Age of patient and age of onset of first episode, relationship to time of day, weekends, menses
  - – Clustering or chronicity
  - – Rapidity of onset and duration of episodes

- o Palliating and provocative factors
  - – Changes with position
  - – Neck movement
  - – Chewing
  - – Foods
  - – Alcohol
  - – Menses
  - – Cough/straining
  - – Stressors
  - – Eyestrain
  - – Massage
  - – Sleep

- o Associated symptoms:
  - – Scalp
    - ▪ Scalp tenderness
  - – CNS
    - ▪ Depression/change in mentation or personality
    - ▪ Aura
    - ▪ Psychiatric disease
  - – Blood vessels
    - ▪ Temporal tenderness
    - ▪ Temporal arteritis
    - ▪ Cluster headache
    - ▪ Aneurysm of the internal carotid or posterior communicating artery
  - – Eye
    - ▪ Glaucoma
    - ▪ Superior orbital fissure syndrome
    - ▪ Scintillating scotomas
    - ▪ Neurovisual disturbances
    - ▪ Photophobia/photophonia
  - – Nose
    - ▪ Lacrimation
    - ▪ Stuffy nose

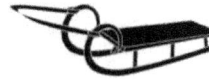

- Face
  - Flushing
  - Trigeminal neuralgia
- Jaw
  - Arthritis
  - Jaw claudications
  - Myalgias and stiffness
- GI
  - Nausea/vomiting
  - Diarrhea
- CVS.
  - Palpitations
- Systemic disease
  - Systemic illness/infection
  - Weight loss
  - Hypertension
  - Smoking
  - Diabetes mellitus
  - Hyperlipidemia
  - Atrial fibrillation
  - Bacterial endocarditis
  - Myocardial infarction (emboli)
  - Hematological disease
  - Family history of stroke

o Medications used
  - Include
    - Birth control pill (BCP)
    - Analgesics
    - Alcohol
    - "Street" drugs

o Past Medical History
  - Commonly missed on history taking. It should include prior history of headache/ investigations/diagnosis/ treatment. Hypertension, seizures, sinusitis, head injury, glaucoma, problems with refractive error, temporal arteritis, dental or ENT problems.

o Family history:
  - Frequently missed and should include migraine, subarachnoid hemorrhage or stroke at an early age.

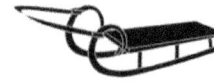

- Give the features of headache which suggest an ominous cause.
  - ○ Worst headache of patient's life, especially if rapid onset
  - ○ Exacerbation of headache with coughing, sneezing, or bending down
  - ○ Headache with seizures, reduced level of consciousness, confusion focal neurological findings
  - ○ New or progressive headache persisting for days
  - ○ New-onset headache in middle age or older
  - ○ Change in frequency, severity, or clinical features of the usual headache pattern
  - ○ Presence of systemic symptoms including fever, myalgia, malaise, weight loss, scalp tenderness, or jaw claudication

Abbreviations: BCP, birth control pill, aka OCA (oral contraceptive agent)

Reproduced with the permission of Dr.B.Fisher, U of A; Jugovic PJ, et al. *Saunders/ Elsevier* 2004, pages 42 and 43.

➢ Differential diagnosis
  - ○ Daily frequency
    - – Chronic migraine
    - – Tension type
    - – Rebound

  - ○ Unilateral
    - – Migraine
    - – Cluster
    - – Frontal
    - – Trigominal

  - ○ Nausea, vomiting; AURD
    - – Migraine

  - ○ ENT symptoms
    - – Cluster, frontal

Diagnostic Alert

Tension-or sinks type headaches are often misdiagnosed, and are migraine.

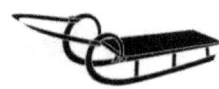

- ➢ Investigation
    - ○ MRI- in trigeminal neurologia – associated headaches exclude multiple sclerosis (MS)
    - ○ Doppler (duplex) ultrasound, or ⎫ suspected dissection of carotid artery,
    - ○ MR angiogtraphy (MRA) ⎭ presenting as migrane, stroke

- ➢ Treatment
    - ○ Acute
        - – Mild/moderate
        - – Acetaminoplan
        - – NSAID
        - – ASA (aspirin)
    - ○ Migraine
        - – Severe
            - ▪ Codaine
            - ▪ Hydrocodone
            - ▪ Oxycodone
        - – Prophylaxis (>2/wk, or 28/mon)
            - ▪ Amitryptyline
            - ▪ Metoprolol
            - ▪ Propranolol
            - ▪ Timolol
            - ▪ Topramate
            - ▪ Valproic acid
    - ○ Tension-type
        - – Acute
            - ▪ NSAID
        - – Prophylasis
            - ▪ TCA tricyclic antidepressant

Therapy Alert

Do **not** use Tripton in patient with Coronary Heart Disease.

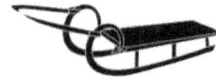

- o Cluster
  - – Acute
    - ▪ Triptan
    - ▪ O_2 therapy
    - ▪ Corticosteroids
  - – Prophylaxis
    - ▪ Verapamil

- o Frontal (sinus)
  - – Decongestants
    - ▪ Antibiotics
      - >7 days,or
      - Severe systemic symptoms

- o Trigemeral neuralyia
  - – Carbamazepine

SO YOU WANT TO BE A NEUROLOGIST!

- In the patient who presents with a migraine headache or symptoms/signs to suggest a stroke, give the clinical features which would raise the possibility of a dissection of the carotid artery, and require investigation with dopper ultrasound or MR angiography.

  - o Sitting trauma to head/neck

  - o Ipoclateral
    - – Visual symptoms
      - ▪ One eye
      - ▪ Horner syndrome
    - – Pain, throbbing
      - ▪ Eye
      - ▪ Head
      - ▪ Neck

  - o Contraleteral
    - – Numbness
    - – Weakness

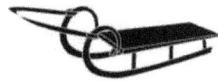

Mastering the Boards: Neurology   A.B.R. Thomson

Therapy Alert

- o Migraine in a woman
    - – Any age aura no EP OCA
    - – ≥ 35 no aura no EP OCA

Abbreviation: EP OCA, estrogen-progestin combination oral contraceptive agent

Thunderclap Headaches

- o Acute, severe, 'thunderclap'
- o Localized generalized headache, sudden onset, neck stiffness
- o May have neurologic deficits or changes in level of consciousness
- o Subarachanoid hemorrhage
    - – Instantaneous onset
    - – Severe pain
    - – Photophobia
    - – Stiff neck

- • In the context of a thunderclap headache, give a definition of the Call-Fleming syndrome, and give the non-evidence based suggested therapy.

    - o Definition: "…… a group of disorders characterized by recurrent thunderclap headache associated with transient segmental [multifocal] cerebral vasoconstriction …… that completely resolves within 12 weeks" and is associated with acute infarction in half of sufferers.

    - o Treatment
        - – CCB (calcium channel blocker verapamil or nimodipine), or
        - – Corticosteroids
        - – IV magnesium (in pregnancy setting of pre-/eclampsia)

Clinical Caution

- o "Thunderclap" headache
    - – Even though there are many conditions in which the headache may be sudden or severe, always think of SAH (subarachnoid hemorrhage)

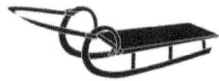

Clinical Quiz

A patient with a sudden severe headache has a normal CT head. The ER physician reassures the patient and sends them home. The patient returns in 8 hr when the headache continues and worsens.

- Give the investigation which should now be performed.
  - The patient with a SAH who is seen early may have a normal CT head
  - LP (lumbar puncture should be performed on the CSF examined for RBCs and for xanthochromia).

- A 40 yr old patient develops recurrent episodes of sudden of consciousness. Previous MR angiography demonstrated cerebral artery vasoconstriction, give the appropriate management.
  - The patient likely has thunder clap headache from reversible cerebral vasoconstriction syndrome
  - About half of these patients have an underlying disorder
  - If an underlying disorder such as SAH (subarachinoid hemorrhage) is excluded, indomethacin may be used.

Tension Headaches

➤ Types

		Frequency		1 yr prevalence
		per mon	per yr	
o	Episodic	< 15 d	< 180 d	40%
o	Chronic	> 15 d	> 180 d	~ 3%

- o Quality
  - Lasts 30 min – 7 days
  - Not pulsating, mild/moderate in intensity, bilateral
  - Not aggravated by exertion, not associated with nausea/vomiting, or sensitivity to light, sound, or smell
  - Episodic or chronic, bilateral frontal/occipital/frontal arga, not awakening person at night, with no vomiting, no photophobia or stiff neck

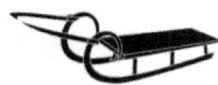

- ➢ Clinical diagnosis-based on absence of characteristics of
  - o Migraine
  - o Secondary headache
  - o Mange triggers such as disruption of sleep, and stress

- ➢ Treatment
  - o Manage triggers such as disruption of sleep and stress
  - o ASA or NSAIDs +/- caffeine
  - o Behavioural therapy
    - – Biofeedback
    - – Relaxation therapy
    - – CBT (cognitive behaviour techniques)
  - o Note
    - – Manipulation of neck and TCAs of no benefit

SO YOU WANT TO BE A NEUROLOGIST!

In the context of headache, give the meaning of the SUNCT (<u>s</u>hort-lasting <u>u</u>nilateral <u>n</u>euralgiform headache with <u>c</u>onjunctival injection and <u>t</u>earing) syndrome.

Cluster Headaches

- ➢ Definition
  - o Severe, temporal/periorbital headache 1 to 8 per day, 15 to 180 each, with clusters lasting weeks to months often triggered by smoking or alcohol
  - o Unilateral periorbital pain occurring several times a day for 30-60 min, several days per week, then stops only to recur months/years later

- ➢ Clinical
  - o Often associated with
    - – Eye
      - ▪ Ptosis
      - ▪ Lacrimation
      - ▪ Red conjuctive
    - – Nose
      - ▪ Congestion
      - ▪ Rhinorrhea

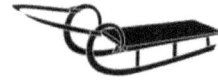

Features	Name	Mean duration, min	Frequency, per day	Treatment
o Severe trigeminal pain	– Chronic paroxysmal hemicranias	15	8 to 40	Indomethacin
o Cranial autonomic features	– Short-lasting unilateral neuralgiform headache with conjunction injection and tearing (SUNCT)	1	1 to 30	lamotrigine

- o Usually with pain over one eye with tears, runny nose, and flushing of the forehead lasting minutes to hours, in bouts lasting several weeks, and coming a few times a year.
- o Lasts 15-180 min, occurs up to 8 times per day
- o Severe, unilateral, located periorbitally and or temporally
- o Associated with at least one of: tearing, red eye, stuffy nose, facial sweating, ptosis, miosis

- ➢ Diagnosis
    - o Investigate with brain MRI

- ➢ Treatment
    - o Acute
        - – O_2 by face mask, 6 to 12 L / min for 10 min
        - – Sumatriptan SC, 25 to 100 mg
        - – Zolmitriptan nasal, 5 mg sniffs
    - o Transitional
        - – Corticosteroids
        - – Occipital nerve block
    - o Maintenance
        - – Prophylaxis
        - – CCB (calcium channel blocker), eg. high dose verapamil
        - – Lithium
        - – Melatonin
    - o Refractory (experimental)
        - – Surgery, stimulators
        - – Occipital nerve
        - – Deep brain

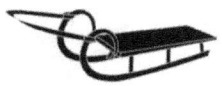

A patient with episodic cluster headaches continues to have symptoms despite the use of sumatriptan and smoking cessation.

- Give the effective management.

    - O_2 by mask, 10 L/min for 10 min

Trigeminal Autonomic Cephalagias

- Give the types of sharp, severe, penetrating headache in the CN (cranial nerve) V1 distribution which may occur as part of trigeminal autonomic cephalagias – trigeminal nerve-mediated pain plus ipsilateral autonomic associated symptoms.

    - Eye
        - Lacrimation
        - Ptosis
        - Conjuctival redness

    - Nose
        - Rhinorrhea
        - Congestion

o Clinical	Cluster headaches	Chronic paroxysmal hemicranias	SUNCT syndrome
– Frequency/ day	1-8	8-40	12-100s
– Duration, min	15-80	15	Sec to min
– Treatment	Face mask O_2 SC sumatriptan Nasal zolmitriptan	Indomethacin	None

Abbreviations: SUNCT, short-lasting unilateral neuralgiform headache with conjunctival injection and tearing

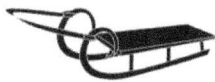

Mastering the Boards: Neurology   A.B.R. Thomson

Migraine with Aura

➢ Definition

- o Typically a migraine episode consists of "… a unilateral, throbbing headache accompanied by photophobia, phonophobia, and nausea", often triggered e.g., activity, vomiting, initially episodic and transforming into chronic headache at ~ 5% per year (Source: MKSAP 16 2012, Neurology, page 5).

- o See clinical details below which stress the limitations in the above definition because of the wide variability in clinical presentation (e.g., +/- aura, differences in frequency), and lack of specific diagnostic tests.

➢ Demography

- o 13% of adults affected, F > M

- o Commonest cause of severe headache (SAH [subarachnoid hemorrhage] is close second)

➢ Clinical
- o "POUND" (diagnosis ≥ 3 features)
  - – Pulsatile quality
  - – O "about" one-day duration (actually 4 to 72 hr)
  - – Unilateral
  - – Nausea/vomiting
  - – Disabling

- o Aura

  - – Because 20% of migraine patients have an associated aura, perhaps a better mnemonic would be "A POUND", "A" standing for "aura"
- o Aura   -   Eyes
  (typical)   -   Speech

                  -    Senses

                  -    Onset > 5 min

                  -    Duration < 60 min

- o Other symptoms

  - – Brain   ▪ Confusion
                 ▪ Hallucination
  - – Eyes   ▪ ↓ vision
                 ▪ Flashing lights
  - – Periphery   ▪ Numbness
                     ▪ Tingling
                     ▪ Weakness

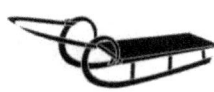

Mastering the Boards: Neurology   A.B.R. Thomson

- o Quality
  - Unilateral headache preceded by flashing light or zig-zag lines, associated with photophobia
  - Lasts 4-72 hrs
  - Throbbing, moderate/severe intensity, unilateral (not always the same side)
  - Worse with exertion
  - Associated with photophobia, phonophobia, nausea/vomiting
  - May be preceded by short prodromal period of depression, irritability, restlessness, or anorexia, 10-20% occurrences associated with an aura- transient, reversible neurologic visual, somatosensory, motor, and/or language deficit – usually precedes headache by no>1 h, can be concurrent
  - Diagnosis of migraine without aura plus neurological dysfunction sensed before or during an attack

➢ Diagnostic (neuro) imaging

- o May be necessary if a secondary cause of headache is suspected, such as brain Tumour, subarachnoid hemorrhage, sinusitis, meningitis/ encephalitis, BIH (benign intracranial hypertension).

o Note: Investigate	- Hemiplegic migraine	
	Focal motor weakness	
	- Basilar migraine	
	▪ Eyes	- Diplopia
	▪ Speech	- Dysarthria
	▪ CNS	- Ataxia
		- Vertigo
		- Dysphagia
		- Synchronous bilateral
		- Sensory dysfunction
o Frequent	- Episodic > 15 per mon	
	- Chronic ("transformed") > 15 per mon	

Please see: Headache Classification Subcommittee of the International Headache Society. The International Classification of Headache Disorders: 2nd Edition. Cephalalgia 2004; 24(suppl 1): 24-27 [PMID: 14979299]. Copyright 2004 International Headache Society.

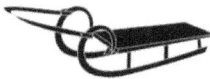

- In the context of migraine headaches, give the meaning of the term **"medication overuse** headache" (aka rebound headache)

  o About 80% of persons with chronic migraines have medication overuse headache

  o Overuse of certain drugs/chemicals/toxins used by a person with headaches may cause "rebound" headache.

  o The ↑ transformation from episodic to chronic migraine in users of treatment in excess duration, such as opiates > 8 days per month, or barbiturates > 5 days per month

  o These substances might be analgesics taken for headache (NSAIDs, narcotics, triptans), or simply coffee/tea/cola (caffeine)

  o Taper, then stop offending substance

- ➤ Treatment
  - o Acute therapy
    - – Principle
      - ▪ Early intervention
      - ▪ Use < 10 d per month
      - ▪ Avoid opiates and barbiturates
      - ▪ Minimize trigger
      - ▪ Progression from NSAIDs to triptans PO / SC bid, to dihydroereptamine

  - o Acute
    - – Acetaminophen
    - – NSAIDs
    - – ASA

  - o Rescue
    - – Triptan
    - – Codeine
    - – Oxycodone
    - – Hydrocodane

  - o Prophylaxis
    - – When migraine occurs > 2 / week or > 8 / mon
      - ▪ β-blocker
        - - Propranolol
        - - Metoprolol
        - - Timolol
      - ▪ TCA
        - - Amitriptyline
      - ▪ Valproic acid
      - ▪ Topiramate

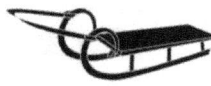

- Give **contraindications** to the use of triptans for migraine disorders.
    - Vascular disorders
        - Vasospastic
        - Ischemic
    - Hypertension, uncontrolled
    - Subtypes
        - Hemiplegic migraine
        - Basilar migraine
        - Status migrainous

Refractory Migraine

- Definition
    - Refractory migraine, single severe attack lasting > 72 h, not having responded to NSAIDs or triptans.

- Treatment (IV)
    - Hydration
    - Dopamine antagonists, +/- dihydroergotamine
    - Diphenhydramine
    - Corticosteroids, 1 dose
    - Ketorolac
    - Valproic acid

- Give the **contraindication** for the parenteral use of dihydroergotamine to treat refractory migraine.
    - Use of triptans or ergots within past 24 h

- Give the indications for use of pharmacologic agents for migraine.
    - Frequency
        - > 2 d per week or 8 d per mon
            - Headache
            - Headache medication
    - Severity
        - Disability
    - Aura
        - > 1 hr
        - Complex
            - Hemiplegic
            - Basilar
    - Failure to standard therapy (NSAIDs, triptans)
    - Patient preference

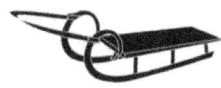

- ➢ Prevention
  - o Patient education
  - o Life-style modification, including triggers
  - o Natural/alternate product
    - Herb
      - Fever few
      - Butter bur root

  - o Behavioural therapy
    - Biofeedback
    - Relaxation
    - CBT (cognitive behaviour therapy)
    - Mineral
      - Magnesium
    - Vitamin
      - Riboflavin
    - Anti-oxidant
      - Co-enzyme Q10
      - α-lipoic acid

  - o Pharmaceuticals
    - Principles
      - Titrate upwards for 8 wk
      - Do not use > 10 d / mon
        - Acute headache
        - Opiates or barbiturates
        - Decongestants
        - Stimulants
      - When > 50% ↓ frequency of migraine is achieved, continue for 6 to 12 mon
      - To piramate 100-200 mg PO/d (ensure ↑ hydration to ↓ risk of renal calculi
      - On a botulinum toxin A SC
    - Some evidence for
      - β-blockers
      - TCAs (tricyclic anti-depressants)
      - CCBs (calcium channel blockers)
      - SSRIs (selective serotonin reuptake inhibitors)
      - Anti-convulsants

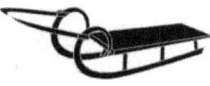

Management of Migraine Under Special Circumstances
- o Menstruation
- o Pregnancy
- o Perimenopause

- ➢ Migraine and menstruation
  - o ↑ frequency and ↑ severity
  - o Triptans, including SC / IM sumatriptan, +/- NSAIDs
  - o Premenstrual prophylaxis
    - TC(transcutaneous) estradiol
    - Frovatriptan PO
    - Naratriptin
  - o HRT (hormone replacement therapy) plus monophasic progestin – only OCAs) oral contraceptive agents)
  - o Warning
    - Migraine and ↑ risk of ischemic strokes

Population	Risk of ischemic stroke, per 10^5 per 10 yr
– Baseline	27
– Migraine + aura	110
– Migraine +aura + OCA	230

  - o Rather than using OCA with < 50 mcg estrogen, use progestin-only OCA, or IUD (intrauterine device), copper plus progesterone
  - o Don't forget to advise patient with ↑ risk of stroke from estrogen
    - To stop smoking
    - Maternal risk
    - Fetal risk
      - ▪ ↓ birth weight
      - ▪ Premature delivery
      - ▪ ↑ risk of adverse outcome of pregnancy

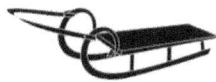

- ➢ Migraine and pregnancy
  - o In 2/3 women with migraine, ↓ attacks in T (trimester) 2 and T3, because of ↑ estrogen concentrations
  - o NSAIDs
    - Class B, but
    - Stop at week 32 (↑ risk of fetal PDA [patient ductus arteriosus])
  - o Triptans
    - Class C
  - o Prednisone
    - Class B
  - o Consider
    - ↓ / D/C prophylactic medications during pregnancy, or using
    - β-blockers (e.g., metoprolol, propranolol)
      - Class C
      - Stop 2 wk before delivery to ↓ risk of fetal bradycardia

- ➢ Migraine and perimenopausal period
  - o More aggressive therapy may be needed if ↑ frequency/severity of headaches because of perimenopausal variations of female hormone
  - o HRT (hormone replacement therapy)

Migraine Without Aura

- o A diagnosis of migraines without aura requires each of the following:
  - Minimum of 5 attacks
  - Duration of headache is 2-72 h (with or without therapy)
  - 2 of the following are present: unilateral pain, pulsing or throbbing quality to pain, moderate-to-severe intensity preventing daily activities, or pain provoked by routine physical activity
  - One of the following is present: nausea, vomiting, photophobia, phonophobia, or osmophobia
  - No evidence of other causes of headache

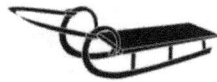

Migraine

Stimulus
- Stress
- Relief from stress
- Periods, 'the OCP'
- Infection, fever
- Bright light
- Possibly foods

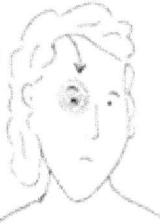

Typical migraine
- Unilateral
- Frontoparietal
- Throbbing
- Nausea

Orbital migraine
- Throbbing (less usual)
- One or botheyes
- Deep nagging pain/ stabbing

Common variations

Occipito orbital migraine
- Starts in occiput
- Moves to behind eye
- May last several days
- Can be bilateral

Adapted from: Davey P. *Wiley-Blackwell* 2006, page 106.

A young man working in IT is diagnosed with tension headache. He fails to respond to a tricyclic anti-depressant. He has no aura or photophobia. He fails benzodiazepines therapy. He goes online and discovers that while he was properly diagnosed, he was not correctly treated.

- Give the first and second-line treatment of tension headaches.

    o Ibuprofen, naproxen

    o ASA, acetaminophen

Clinical Gem

   o Sudden onset of severe headache or pain around the eye, face or neck suggests dissection of the carotid or vertebral arteries.
     - A common association is Horner syndrome.

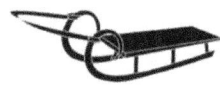

Temporal Arteritis

➢ Clinical

- o Systemic
  - – Fever, weight loss, fatigue, anorexia

- o Head
  - – Scalp tenderness
  - – Temporal headache
  - – Ocular symptoms: Blindness, DIplopia
  - – Ptosis
  - – Jaw or tongue claudication
  - – Mononeuritis multiplex

- o Skin lesions
  - – Palpable purpura
  - – Necrotic ulcers
  - – Livedo reticularis
  - – Urticaria
  - – Nodules and digital infarcts
  - – Acute/chronic necrotizing angiitis
  - – Erythema nodosum
  - – Nodular vasculitis

- o MSK
  - – Anthralgia or arthritis (e.g., rheumatoid arthritis, Sjogren's, DS, SLE, scleroderma)
  - – Myalgia or prominent fibrositis
    - ▪ Polymyalgia rheumatico
    - ▪ Dermatomyositis
    - ▪ Polyarteritis nodosa
    - ▪ Wegener granuloma
    - ▪ Aortic arch syndrome

- o Cardiac
  - – Hypertension

- o Infection
  - – Extension of inflammation from cellulitis, abscess
  - – Sepsis, septic emboli
  - – Cutaneous arteritis during infective rash (meningococcemia, typhus)
  - – Syphilis
  - – Tuberculosis

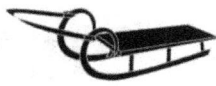

- o Pulmonary abnormalities
  - – Pulmonary hemorrhage
  - – Pulmonary nodules with cavities
  - – Dry cough

- o GI/GU
  - – Abdominal pain
  - – Intestinal hemorrhage
  - – High liver enzymes, low serum albumin
  - – Abnormal renal sediment

Adapted from: Ghosh AK. *Mayo Clinic Scientific Press* 2008, Table 24-14, page 988.

- ➢ Diagnosis
  - o Four of the 5 following criteria for diagnosis
    - – Tender, swollen temporal artery
    - – Blindness
    - – Jaw claudication
    - – Polymyalgia rheumatica symptoms
    - – Rapid response to corticosteroids

  - o Nonspecific indicators of inflammation
    - – Anemia, eosinophilia, thrombocytosis, low levels of albumin, elevated erythrocyte sedimentation rate (ESR)

Adapted from: Ghosh AK. *Mayo Clinic Scientific Press* 2008, page 988.

A Little Tip

- o The four features of a headache which increase the possibility of temporal arteritis are a temporal location of any headache in a Caucasian with any abnormality of the temporal artery (large, absent, tender) plus and ↑ ESR.

Source: Simel DL, et al. *JAMA* 2009, page 648-9.

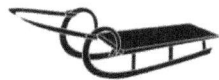

- Take a directed history for arteritis.

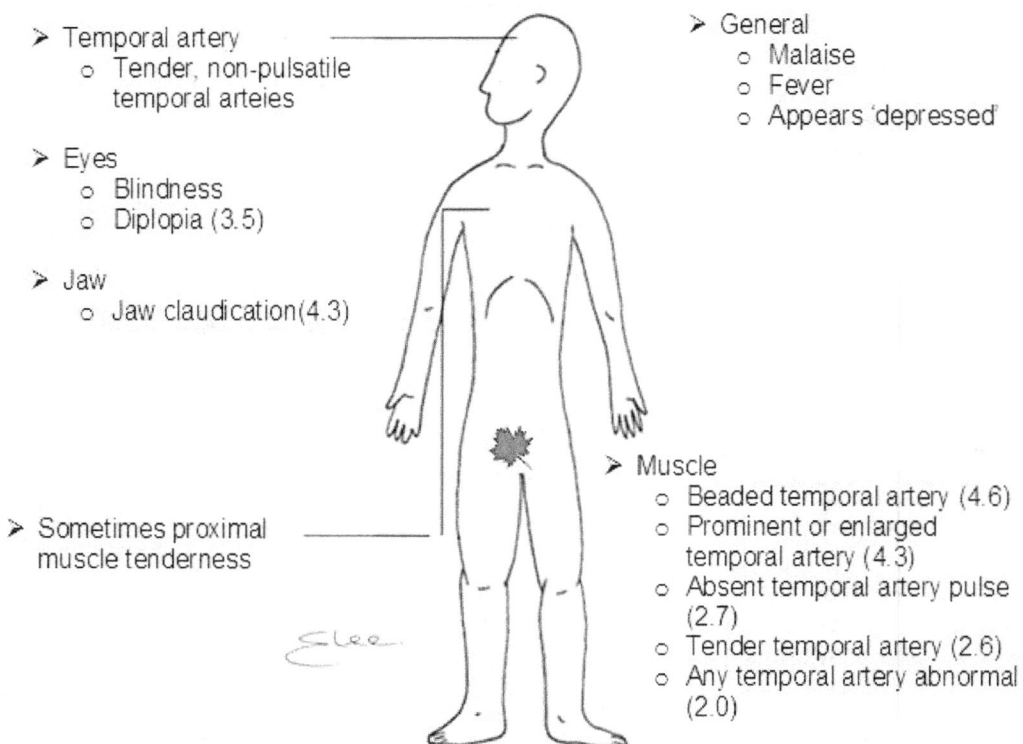

> Temporal artery
  o Tender, non-pulsatile temporal arteies

> Eyes
  o Blindness
  o Diplopia (3.5)

> Jaw
  o Jaw claudication(4.3)

> Sometimes proximal muscle tenderness

> General
  o Malaise
  o Fever
  o Appears 'depressed'

> Muscle
  o Beaded temporal artery (4.6)
  o Prominent or enlarged temporal artery (4.3)
  o Absent temporal artery pulse (2.7)
  o Tender temporal artery (2.6)
  o Any temporal artery abnormal (2.0)

*Note: the numbers show in brackets represent the values of the positive likelihood ratios (PLR). Note that valve of the PLR is ≤ 2 for scalp tenderness, optic atrophy, ischemic neuropathy, signs of anemia, or any valve of ↑ ESR.

Adapted from: Davey P. *Wiley-Blackwell* 2006, page 412; Simel DL, et al. *JAMA* 2009, Table 49-5, 49-7, page 654 and 649.

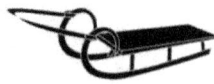

Other Headache Patterns

- Brain tumour (space occupying lesion)
  - Presents on wakening and improves during the day
  - Symptoms due to increased intracranial pressure
  - Generalized, may be more severe in occipital region, worse when lying down or with a Valsalva maneuver
  - May be associated with nausea/vomiting, blurring of vision, papilloedema, transient visual obscuration
  - Recent onset (< 5 months)
  - Worse on lying, coughing, bending early morning
  - Better on sitting, standing
  - Other neurological symptoms, signs
  - ± malignancy unwell, weight loss, fever

- Meningitis
  - Generalized headache, neck stiffness, photophobia, fever
  - Gradual onset (< 24 h)
  - Fever +/- rash
  - ± ↓ BP (systemic blood pressure)

- Increased ICP
  - Generalized headache, worse in the morning, with vomiting and drowsiness

- Cervical spondylosis
  - Occipital headache, neck stiffness

- Temporal arteritis
  - Unilateral headache, blurred vision, tenderness over temporal artery
  - ↑ ESR

- Sinusitis
  - Generalized headache, pressure/fullness behind the eyes/cheek/forehead

Adapted from: Filate W, et al. *The Medical Society, Faculty of Medicine, University of Toronto* 2005, page 172.

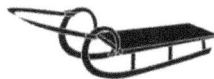

- Give the serious causes of headache in which neuroimaging findings may be normal.

  o Trigeminal or glossopharyngeal neuralgia

  o Giant cell/temporal arteritis

  o Sentinel bleed of aneurysm (warning leak)

  o Inflammation, infection, or neoplastic invasion of leptomeninges

  o Glaucoma

  o Lesions around sella turcica

  o Cervical spondylosis

  o Pseudotumour cerebri

  o Low intracranial pressure syndromes

Source: Ghosh AK. *Mayo Clinic Scientific Press* 2008, Table 19-10, page 759.

- Give the meaning of the **"medial" medullary syndrome**.

  o It is caused by the occlusion of the lower basilar artery or vertebral artery

  o Ipsilateral lesions result in paralysis and wasting of the tongue

  o Contralateral lesions result in hemiplegia and loss of vibration and joint position sense

"Play a crucial role in finding your own humility and humanity."

Grandad

HYPOTHALAMUS

➢ Anatomy (structure)

  o That part of the brain situated in the interpeduncular space

  o Forms the floor of the third ventricle

  o Consists of tuber cinereum and mammilary bodies

  o Tuber cinereum is a sheet of grey matter which stretches from the mammary bodies to the optic chiasm

  o The tuber cinereum is also attatched to the infundibulum (posterior part) of the pituitary.

  o Receives afferents from
    - Olfactory tract
    - Frontal cortex
    - Thalamus
    - pituitary

  o Contains ganglia of sympathetic nervous system

  o Consists of tuber cinereum and mammilary bodies

  o Tuber cinereum is a sheet of grey matter stretching from the optic chiasm to the mammary bodies, attached to which is the infundibulum of the pituitary

➢ Function

  o Coordinates sympathetic and parasympathetic functions

  o Receives afferents from the olfactory tract, frontal cortex, and thalamus

  o The posterior pituitary is traversed by fibres arising in the hypothalamus.

➢ Clinical

• Take a directed history for hypothalamic disease.

  o Truncal obesity

  o Hypogonadism

  o Diabetes insipidus

  o Narcolepsy-irreversible urge to sleep

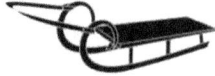

- o Cataplexy-sudden brief loss of power of limbs-eyelids drop, jaw drops, limbs sag, patient falls to the ground but does not loose consciousness

- o Increased sweating, salivation, fever, peptic ulceration, increased gut motility, disturbed appetite, sleep

- o Causes (please see below)

- Perform a focused physical examination of hypothalamic disease.
    - o CNS
        - – Narcolepsy
        - – Cataplexy

    - o Endocrine
        - – Truncal obesity
        - – Hypogonadism
        - – Diabetes insipidus

    - o GI
        - – Salvation
        - – Peptic ulcer
        - – Diarrhea

    - o Skin
        - – Sweating

    - o General
        - – Fever

➢ Causes/associations
    - o Neoplasm
        - – III ventricle
        - – Suprasellar
        - - Chromophobe adenoma

    - o Infection
        - – TB
        - – Syphilis
        - – Encephalitis lethargica

    - o Trauma
        - – Base of skull fracture

    - o Ideopathic

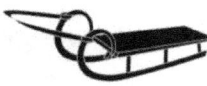

CEREBELLUM, GAIT POSTURE AND MOVEMENT DISORDERS

- ➤ Terminology (movement disorders)
  - ○ Astereognosis
    - – Inability to appreciate size or shape of objects held in his hand.
  - ○ Athetoid movements
    - – Slow, writhing, sinuous movements of periphery
    - – ↑ by emotion and movement.
    - – Due to disease of the extrapyramidal system
  - ○ Choreiform movements
    - – Sudden, brief, involuntary, jerky movements
    - – The same movement is never repeated in succession
    - – Due to disease of the extrapyramidal system
  - ○ Involuntary movements
    - – Tremor, choreiform, athetoid, tic, myoclonic movements
  - ○ Myoclonus
    - – Sudden contraction of large muscle or muscle group
    - – Such as occurs with epilepsy or hiccup (singultus)
  - ○ Tic
    - – Explosive repetition of the same movement, especially of facial muscles
    - – Commonly seen with psychiatric disturbance.
  - ○ Tremor
    - – Extrapyramidal-tremor at rest
    - – Tremor occurring in a body part that is not voluntarily activated and when it is supported completely against gravity.
      - ▪ Disappears with sleep
      - ▪ ↑ by emotion and fine movements
      - ▪ ↓ by strong movements
      - ▪ Intention tremor whose amplitude increases during visually guided movements (eg finger to nose test)
    - – Cerebellar-intention ("action") tremor
      - ▪ absent at rest
      - ▪ ↑ by any voluntary movement
    - – GPI trombone-like tremor of the tongue
      - ▪ Present both at rest and on attempted protrusion
    - – Fine tremors- caused by fatigue, anxiety, emotion, thyrotoxicosis, as well as poisoning with alcohol, tobacco, cocaine, mercury

Adapted from: Simel DL, et al. *JAMA* 2009, Box 38-1, page 506.

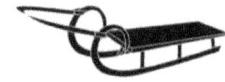

➢ Physiology

● Give the physiological components of gait.

- o Structures Involved in walking
  - – Basal ganglia
    - ▪ Anatomic movements which accompany walking
    - ▪ Initiate walking

  - – Midbrain, locomotor region
    - ▪ Anti-gravity reflexes

  - – Cerebellum
    - ▪ Maintains posture, balance, characteristic of movement (trajectory, velocity, acceleration)

  - – Spinal cord
    - ▪ Sense and proprioception
    - ▪ Anti-gravity reflexes

- o Antigravity support
  - – Provided by reflexes located in the spinal cord and brainstem.
  - – Anti-gravity reflexes are responsible for maintaining full extension of hips, knees, and neck.
- o Stepping
  - – Basic part of movement based on sensory input from soles and body (including inclination forward and from side to side) and integrated at the midbrain level.
- o Equillibrium
  - – Responsible for maiantaining balance and centre and gravity during shifting of weight from one foot to the other.
- o Propulsion
  - – Involves leaning forward and slightly to one side, permitting the body to fall a certain distance before being checked by leg support.

Source: Mangione S. *Hanley & Belfus*, 2000, page 12.

➢ Anatomy
- o "The head ganglion of the proprioceptive system"
- o The cerebellum
  - – not primarily a motor organ
  - – developed phylogenetically from a primary vestibular area and is involved in modulation of motor activity

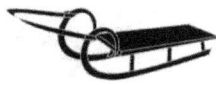

Mastering the Boards: Neurology   A.B.R. Thomson

- receives afferents from the vestibular nuclei, spinal cord and cerebral cortex via the pontine nuclei.
  - o Superior cerebellar peduncle
    - Afferent (sensory) ventral spinothalamic tract
    - Efferent (motor) to midbrain
      - In midbrain associated with cranial nerves III and IV, as well as extrapyramidal tracts

  - o Middle cerebellar peduncle
    - Afferent ← cerebral cortex
    - Efferent → pons

  - o Inferior cerebellar peduncle
    - Afferent ← dorsal spinocerebellar tract
      - Vestibular nuclei
      - Nucleus gracilis
    - Efferent → medulla

➢ Causes/associations

• Give the causes of cerebellar disorders which cause disturbances in the gut.

  - o Congenital/hereditary
    - Friedreich ataxia and other hereditary ataxias
    - Congenital malformations at the level of the foramen magnum
  - o Drugs/ toxins
    - Phenytoin toxicity
    - Alcoholic cerebellar degeneration (there is atrophy of the anterior vermis of the cerebellum)
  - o Tumour
    - Space-occupying lesion in the posterior fossa including cerebellopontine angle tumour
    - Paraneoplastic manifestation of bronchogenic carcinoma
  - o Vascular
    - Brainstem vascular lesion
  - o Demyelination
    - Multiple sclerosis
  - o Common
    - Infectious
      - Viral infections
      - Prion disease (Creutzfeldt-Jakob disease)

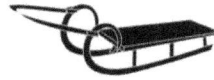

- Metabolic
  - Hepatic encephalopathy
  - Hypothyroidism
  - B12 deficiency
  - Thiamine deficiency
  - Hyperthermia
- Cardiovascular
  - Anoxia
  - Infarction
  - Hemorrhage
- Inherited
  - Friedreich ataxia
  - Ataxia telangiectasia
  - Ramsay- Hunt disease

➢ Types

- o Acute
  - Cerebellar hemorrhage or infarction
  - Trauma
  - Intoxication
  - Migraine

- o Chronic
  - Alcoholic cerebellar degeneration
  - Hypothyroidism
  - Hydrocephalus
  - Chronic infection (panencephalitis, rubella, prion disease)
  - Vitamin E deficiency
  - Paraneoplastic syndrome

"There are three constants in life... change, choice and principles."

Stephen Covey

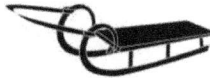

- Give the causes of **spastic and ataxic paraparesis** (upper motor neuron [UMN] and cerebellar signs combined).

  - ○ Congenital   – Arnold-Chiari malformation, or other lesion at the craniospinal junction

  - ○ Infection   – Syphilitic meningomyelitis

  - ○ Infiltration   – Lesion at the craniospinal junction e.g., meningioma

  - ○ Ischemic   – Syringomyelia
    - – Infarction (in upper pons or internal capsule on one side – 'ataxic hemiparesis')

  - ○ Degeneration   – Spinocerebellar degeneration e.g., Marie spastic ataxia
    - – Multiple sclerosis
    - – Spinocerebellar degeneration

Note: Unrelated diseases that are relatively common (e.g., cervical spondylosis and cerebellar degeneration from alcohol) may cause a similar clinical picture.

Adapted from: Talley NJ, et al. *Maclennan & Petty Pty Limited* 2003, page 434.

Alcoholic Cerebellar Degeneration

➢ Defining points

  - ○ An ataxia that affects the trunk and gait (upper body ataxia and dysarthria are less frequent).

  - ○ Atrophy of anterior vermis in cerebellum

  - ○ Gait is broad-based and is progressive, but partially reversible with abstinence

  - ○ May present as a complex called Wernicke encephalopathy (confusion, ataxia, ophthalmoplegia of CN VI)

Adapted rom: Jugovic PJ, et al. *Saunders/ Elsevier* 2004, page 166; Talley NJ, et al. *Maclennan & Petty Pty Limited* 2003, Table 10.32, page 433.

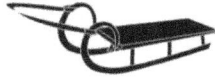

➢ Clinical (all cerebellar signs are ipsilateral)

• Perform a focused physical examination for the cerebellum.

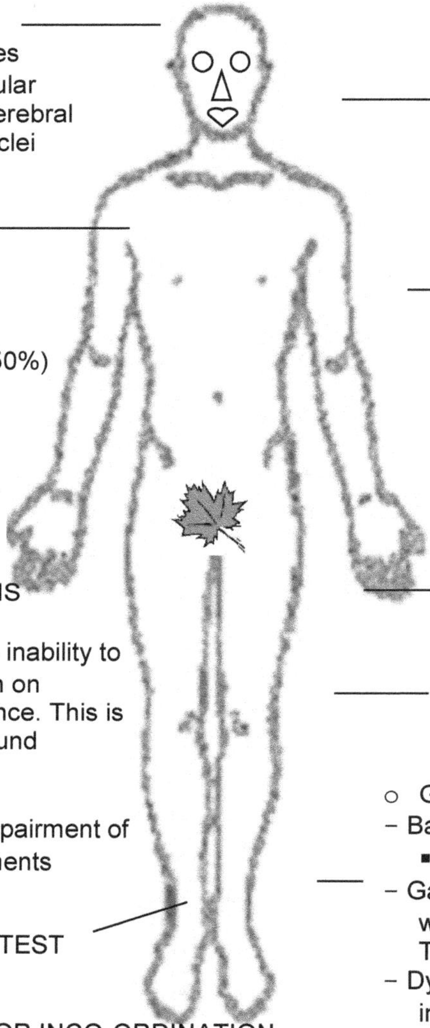

o NYSTAGMUS (75%) ──────
  −The celebrellum receives
  afferents from the vestibular
  nuclei, spinal cord and cerebral
  cortex via the pontine nuclei

o LIMB ATAXIA ──────────
  − Dysmetria (~ 75%)
  − Intention tremor (29%)
  − Hypotonia
  − Dysdiadochokinesia (~ 50%)
  − Arm drift (~ 50%)
  − Rebound

➢ FINGER – NOSE TEST

o DYSDIADOCHOKINESIS
  REBOUND (50%)
  − Rebound phenomenon – inability to
  arrest strong contraction on
  sudden removal resistance. This is
  known as Holmes' rebound
  phenomenon
  − Intention tremor
  − Dysdiadochokinesia – impairment of
  rapid alternating movements
  (clumsy)

      o HEEL – SHIN TEST

o GROSS AND FINE MOTOR INCO-ORDINATION
  −Lack of finger – nose coordination (past-pointing):
  movement is imprecise in force, direction and distance –
  dysmetria

o SPEECH
  − Dysarthria (say "British
  Constitution")
  − Scanning dysarthria: a
  halting, jerking
  dysarthria which is
  usually a feature of
  bilateral lesions

──────o INTENTION
       TREMOR (29%)

                    oLEG
                    - Tone

oKNEE JERKS
  − Pendular
  − Reduced / absent

o GAIT & BALANCE (90%)
  − Balance
    ▪Rhomberg test, Pull test
  − Gait ▪ Normal gait, Toe
    walking, Heel walking,
    Tandem gait, Ataxia
  − Dyssynergia, movements
    involving more than one joint
    are broken into parts
  − Lack of co-ordination of gait
    ▪patient tends to fall towards
    the side of the lesion

Adapted from: Jugovic PJ, et al. *Saunders/ Elsevier* 2004, page 165; Talley NJ,
et al. *Maclennan & Petty Pty Limited* 2003, page 431; McGee SR.
Saunders/Elsevier 2007, page 198; Baliga RR. *Saunders/Elsevier* 2007, pages
143 and 124.

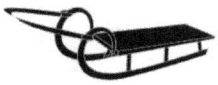

- o The classical clinical triad of cerebellar diseases is ataxia, atonia, asthenia.
- o Note that disorders of movement:
  - Nystagmus: coarse horizontal nystagmus with lateral cerebellar lesions; its direction is towards the side of the lesion.
  - Scanning dysarthria: a halting, jerking dysarthria which is usually a feature of bilateral lesions.
  - Lack of finger-nose co-ordination (past-pointing): movement is imprecise in force, direction and distance – dysmetria.
  - Rebound phenomenon – inability to arrest strong contraction on sudden removal of resistance. This is known as Holmes' rebound phenomenon.
  - Intention tremor.
  - Dysdiadochokinesia – impairment of rapid alternating movements (clumsy).
  - Dyssynergia – movements involving more than one joint are broken into parts.
  - Hypotonia.
  - Absent reflexes or pendular reflexes.
  - Lack of co-ordination of gait – patient tends to fall towards the side of the lesion.
- o Localization
  - Gait ataxia (inability to do tandem walking): anterior lobe (palaeocerebellum).
  - Truncal ataxia (drunken gait, titubation): flocculonodular or posterior lobe (archicerebellum).
  - Limb ataxia, especially upper limbs and hypotonia: lateral lobes (neocerebellum).
- o Eyes
  - Phasic nystagmus
- o Voice
  - Dysarthria
- o Balance
  - Ataxia

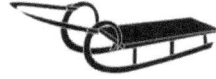

- o Muscle
  - – Intention tremor
  - – Hypotonicity
  - – Dystonicity
  - – Dysdiadis kinesia
- o Reflexes
  - – Pendular
- o Gait
  - – Walk with legs wide apart
  - – Cannot "walk with tight rope" (poor tandem walking)
  - – Poor balance and co-ordination

➤ Special tests

- o Upper extremities
  - – Finger-nose-finger test
    - ▪ Dysmetria (overshooting the target)
    - ▪ Hypermetria (stopping before reaching the clinician's finger)
    - ▪ The patient's finger also may deviate from a smooth course (especially if the clinician shifts the target during the test)
    - ▪ Intention tremor (as the patient's finger approaches the target, an increasing side-to-side tremor may appear)
- o Lower extremities
  - – Rapid Alternating Movements
    - ▪ Dysdiadochokinesia (difficulty with rapid alternating movements)
    - ▪ Rapid pronation and supination of the foream, clapping hands, tapping a table, or stamping the foot.
    - ▪ The movements of patients with cerebellar disease are slower and more irregular in rhythm, range and accuracy.
  - – Heel-Knee-Shin Test
    - ▪ Place the heel of one leg on opposite knee and then slide it down the shin.
    - ▪ A positive response may reveal any combination of ataxia, dysmetria, and intention tremor.

Adapted from: McGee SR. *Saunders/Elsevier* 2007, page 794.

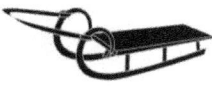

- Give the differences between sensory ataxia and cerebellar ataxia.

Clinical	Cerebellar ataxia	Sensory ataxia
o Site of lesion	– Cerebellum	▪ Posterior column or peripheral nerves
o Deep tendon reflexes	– Unchanged or pendular reflexes	▪ Lost or diminished
o Deep sensation	– Normal	▪ Decreased or lost
o Sphincter disturbances	– None	▪ Decreased when posterior column involved, causing overflow incontinence

Source: Baliga RR. *Saunders/Elsevier* 2007, page 145.

SO YOU WANT TO BE A NEUROLOGIST!

- Give the meaning of **Benedikt syndrome.**

  - o Cerebellar signs on the side opposite the third nerve palsy (which is produced by damage to the nucleus itself or to the nerve fascicle).

  - o Due to a midbrain vascular lesion causing damage to the red nucleus, interrupting the dentatorubrothalamic tract from the opposite cerebellum.

- Give the parts of the cerebellum, and perform a focused physical examination to distinguish which part is causing ataxia.

  - o Paleocerebellum – Gait ataxia (inability to do tandem walking): anterior lobe

  - o Aerchicerebellum – Truncal ataxia (drunken gait, titubation): flocculonodular or posterior lobe

  - o Neocerebellum – Limb ataxia, especially upper limbs and hyponia: lateral lobes

Source: Baliga RR. *Saunders/Elsevier* 2007, page 145.

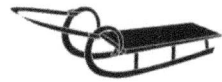

- Perform a focused physical examination for a unilateral cerebellar lesion.

Physical Finding	Frequency (%)
o Ataxia	
– Gait ataxia	80-93
– Limb ataxia	
▪ Dysmetria	71-86
▪ Intention tremor	29
▪ Dysdiadochokinesia	47-69
o Nystagmus	54-84
o Hypotonia	76
– Pendular knee jerks	37
o Dysarthria	10-25

Source: McGee SR. *Saunders/Elsevier* 2007, Table 61-1, page 798

➤ Terminology

- Give four terms to describe the different abnormalities of movement.
    - Tremor
    - Choreiform movements
    - Athetoid movements
    - TIC
    - Myoclonic movements

➤ **Types of Gaits**

- **Anserime** gait
    - Clinical
        - Standing
            - legs spread wide, shoulder sloped forward
            - lumber lordosis, protruding abdomen
        - Walking
            - Getting up from chair: Gower's maneuver – bend forward, hands on knees, slide hands up the thighs and pushing up to standing
            - Short steps, waddling from side-to-side (duck-like waddling)
        - Differentiate from with high stepped gait
    - Causes
        - Dystrophy of girdle muscles
        - Progressive muscular atrophy

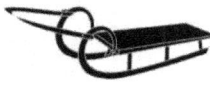

Mastering the Boards: Neurology   A.B.R. Thomson

- **Apraxic** "magnetic gait"
  - Clinical
    - Standing – feet wide apart
    - Walking
      - flexion of upper trunk, arems, knees
      - decreased automatic arm swing
      - shuffling gait
    - Normal sensation and reflexes; Babinski plantar reflex may be up-going (abnormal)
  - Causes/associations
    - Frontal lobe disease
    - Normopressure hydrocephalus
    - Aging

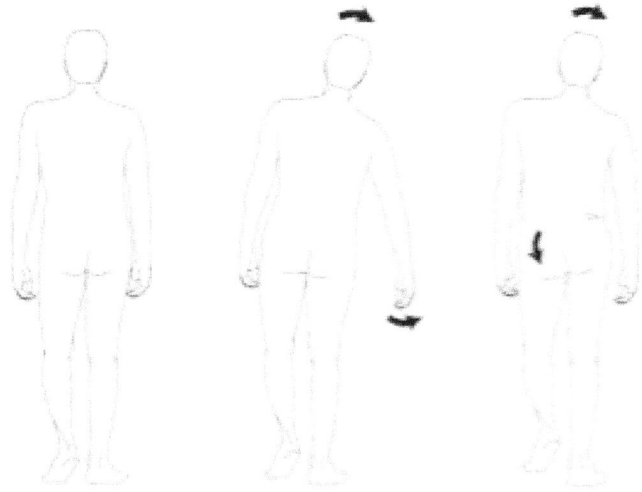

Normal gait   Coxalgic gait   Tendelenburg gait

- **Charcot Marie-Tooth** (CMT) Gait
  - Clinical
    - High steppage gait (even with high elevation of knees)
    - Pes cavus (equinovarus deformity)
    - Plantar flexion
    - Inversion and adduction of foot
    - Calluses/foot ulcers
    - Impaired touch, pain, proprioception sensation
    - Absent deep tender reflex

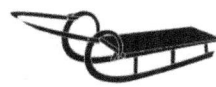

- o Causes
  - – Progressive, hereditary degeneration of peripheral nerves and nerve roots (peroneal nerve paralysis)
  - – Slow, progressive wasting of muscles of feet/legs ("stork legs") and then hands/arms

- **Cerebellar Ataxia** Gait
  - o Clinical
    - – Irregular rate, range, direction of gait
    - – Tendency to fall in any direction
    - – Wide-base gait
    - – Standing – titubation, may lead to falls, worse when feet together, unaffected by opening or closing eyes
    - – Steps- vary in length, swaying (looks like drunken swagger)
    - – Other cerebellar signs present – limbs ataxia, nystagmus

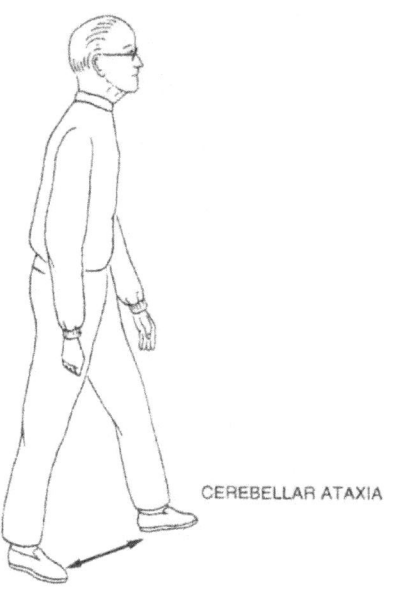

CEREBELLAR ATAXIA

  - o Cause
    - – Cerebellar disease
    - – Chronic alcoholism
    - – Demyelination
    - – Infection
    - – Inherited

- **Coalgic** gait
  - o In both abnormal gaits, the trunk may lean over the abnormal leg during stance (arrow).
  - o In patients with hip pain and coxalgic gait, the trunk lean and accompanying ipsilateral arm movement (arrow) is more dramatic ('lateral lurch"), and the opposite pelvis does not fall excessively.

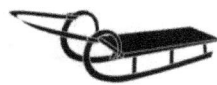

- **High stepped** gait ("foot drop")

  o Clinical
    - No dorsiflexion of ankle while walking: foot is raised high and then brought down quickly, in a flopping manner
    - Asymmetrical wear on soles of shoes
    - Waddling gait if proximal girdle muscles are also affected (eg. motor neuron disease, progressive muscular atrophy); known as the anserine (duct-like waddling) gait.

  o Cause
    - Motor neuron disease
    - Peripheral neuropathy
    - Peroneal neuropathy
    - Spinal muscle atrophy (Charcot Marie Tooth gait)

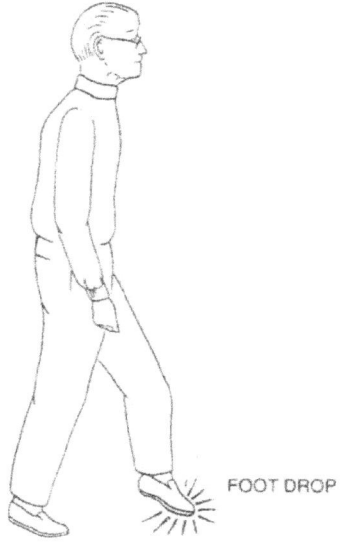

FOOT DROP

- **High-stepping** gait
  o Usually unilateral, and results from foot-drop.
  o Causes
    - Lateral popliteal nerve palsy
    - Poliomyelitis
    - Charcot-Marie-Tooth disease
    - Lead or arsenic poisoning

- **Parkinsonian** Gait
  o Clinical
    - Slow standing up and starting to walk
    - Standing head and chest bent forward, flexed arms at elbows and knees flexed hips
    - Slow small steps with no arm swinging (automatic movement)
    - Festination – accelerating of walking, once walking started
    - Propulsion – tendency to fall forward, calling festination
    - Walking – further forward bending to chest, non-swinging arms, legs bent at ankles, knees, hips
    - Poor balance, poor compensation of flexion/extension, resulting in frequent falls
    - Toes not always on ground

PARKINSON'S DISEASE

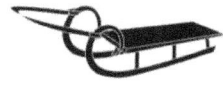

- **Psychogenic** Gait

  - "…… inconsistent , incongruous, and elaborate, often with expressors of great effect, unconvincing develop of weakness or impairment, sudden genuflections, extreme turding, without falling'. (Source: MKSAP 16 2012, Neurology, page 2012).

- **Scissor** gait
  - Seen in spastic paraplegia
  - The adductor spasm may be so severe as to lead to the legs crossing in front of one another

- **Sensory Ataxia** Gait

  - Clinical
    - Standing wide stance
    - High stepping gait
    - Wide gait, worsen when opening/closing eyes; sway/fall only when eyes closed (difficult walking at night)

  - Cause
    - Impaired sensory and proprioception in lower limbs
    - Peroneal nerve palsy
    - Tertiary syphilis

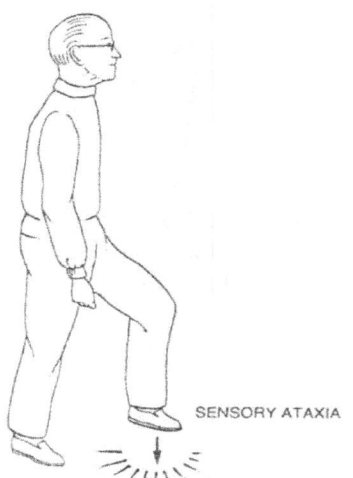

SENSORY ATAXIA

- **Spastic Hemiplegia** (circumduction gait)

  - Clinical
    - Standing: (affected side)
      - Adduction/flexion of fingers, wrist, elbows
      - Extension of ankle, knee, hip
      - Internal rotation of foot
    - Walking (affected side)
      - Upper body tilts to uneffected side
      - Foot/leg of affected side swing in a semi-circle
      - Slow, difficult walk
  - Causes
    - Internal capsule hemisphere CVA

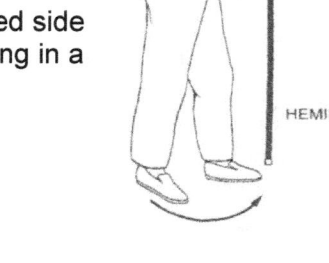

HEMIPLEGIA

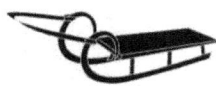

- **Trendelenburg** gait (abnormal gluteus medius and minimus)
  In the Trendelenburg gait (from ineffective or weak hip abductors), the opposite pelvis falls excessively (arrow), and the conspicuous but opposing swings of the upper body and pelvis create the impression of the hinge between the sacral and the lumbar spine.

  - o The patient is bearing weight on the affected right hip, with and ineffective right hip abductors (Trendelenburg gait).
  - o The trunk may lean over the abnormal leg during stance (arrow).

➤ Clinical

  - o During walking, a slight dip of the opposite pelvis is normal during stance phase on one limb.

  - o The finding of excessive drop of the opposite pelvis is the abnormal Trendelenburg gait.

  - o When the abnormality is bilateral, the pelvis waddles like that of a duck.

  - o Like patients with the coxalgic gait ['Colxalgic Gait'], patients with Trendelenburg gait may lean their trunk over the abnormal leg during stance, but the lean lacks the dramatic lurch seen in coalgic gait, and the opposing sways of the ipsilateral shoulder and opposite pelvis make it.

- **Waddling** gait
  - o The legs are held wide apart and the patient shifts weight from one side to the other as he walks.
  - o Lumbar lordosis
  - o Causes
    - – Advanced pregnancy
    - – Proximal weakness (Cushing syndrome, osteomalacia, thyrotoxicosis, polymyositis, diabetes, hereditary muscular dystrophies).

➤ Causes/associations

  - o Occurs when the gluteus medius and menimus do not function properly.

  - o These two muscles abduct the hip, an action that supports the opposite pelvis and prevents it from dropping excessive amounts during the normal single-limb stance.

Adapted from: Burton JL. *Churchill Livingstone* 1971, pages 88 and 89.

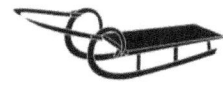

- Take a directed history and perform a focused physical examination of a gait (movement) disorder.

❖ History

  o Worsening of gait disturbance at night (because of darkness)

  o Association with vertigo or light-headedness

  o Association with pain, numbness, or tingling in the limb

  o Presence of muscle weakness

  o Presence of bladder or bowel dysfunction

  o Presence of stiffness in the limbs

  o Problems initiating or terminating walking

❖ Physical

  o Walking: Inspect how the patient

    – Gets up from a chair (useful, for example, in Parkinson disease or limb girgle dydtrophy)

    – Initiates walking

    – Walks at a slow pace

    – Walks at a fast pace

    – Walks on toes (toe-walking cannot be done by patients with Parkinson's disease, sensory ataxia, spastic hemiplegia, or paresis of the soleus or gatrocnemius muscle)

    – Walks on heels (unmasks patients with motor ataxia, spastic paraplegia, or foot drop)

  o Balance

    – Ask the patent to sit in a chair with his/her back straight against the back of the chair.

    – Ask them to keep their arms folded while standing. Can they:

      ▪ Sit without leaning or sliding?

      ▪ Arise from chair in single movement without use of arms (and at end of gait assessment, sit down in a smooth motion without falling)?

      ▪ Stand immediately without need for support?

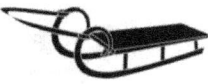

- With the patient standing, ask them to place their feet together (without support). Can they:
  - Stand without support for > 30 seconds?
  - Stand without loss of balance with their eyes closed?
  - Turn their neck to both sides and look upward without loss of balance?
  - Maintain balance despite gentle nudging on sternum (nudge three times)?
  - Stand on 1 leg without loss of balance?
  - Reach up and pick a object off a shelf, then reach down and pick up a object off the floor, without loss of balance (this last maneuver can be done at the end of the patients "walk across the room")?

- Gait
  - Then, ask the patient to walk across room, turn and walk back as quickly as possible. Can they:
    - Initiate gait immediately?
    - Maintain normal step height, clearing the floor with their feet, but by a maximum of 5 cm (greater than this is "high stepping")
    - Maintain a step length between stance toe and swinging heel that is at least the length of the patient's foot?
    - Maintain step symmetry and continuity (raises heel of one foot as other foot touches down)?
    - Maintain a straight path and normal truncal stability (no swaying back, knee flexion, or arm abduction)?
    - Maintain a normal walk stance with feet almost touching as they pass each other (observe from behind)?
    - Turn without discontinuity of steps or motion?

"Is there anyone so wise as to learn by the experience of others?"

Voltaire

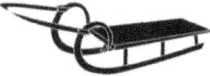

Mastering the Boards: Neurology   A.B.R. Thomson

o The shading indicates the limb with the weak muscle and the black arrows indicate the diagnostic movements.

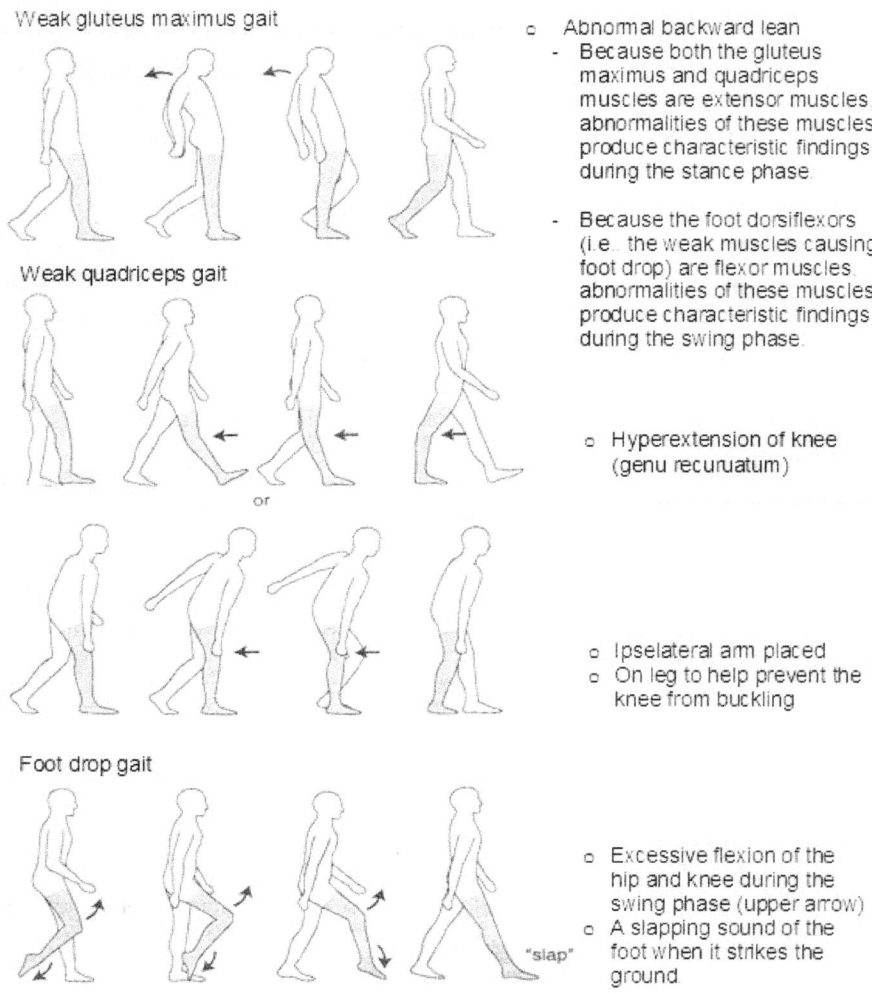

Weak gluteus maximus gait

o Abnormal backward lean
- Because both the gluteus maximus and quadriceps muscles are extensor muscles, abnormalities of these muscles produce characteristic findings during the stance phase.

- Because the foot dorsiflexors (i.e. the weak muscles causing foot drop) are flexor muscles, abnormalities of these muscles produce characteristic findings during the swing phase.

Weak quadriceps gait

or

o Hyperextension of knee (genu recurvatum)

o Ipselateral arm placed
o On leg to help prevent the knee from buckling

Foot drop gait

o Excessive flexion of the hip and knee during the swing phase (upper arrow)
o A slapping sound of the foot when it strikes the ground

"slap"

Adapted from: McGee SR. *Saunders/Elsevier* 2007, pages 12, 13, 60, 61, 64 and 65; Filate W, et al. *The Medical Society, Faculty of Medicine, University of Toronto* 2005, Table 17, page 169; Mangione S. *Hanley & Belfus* 2000, pages 12 to 15; Talley NJ, et al. *Maclennan & Petty Pty Limited* 2003, page 414, Table 10.21; Common types of gait abnormalities (From Swartz MH. *W. G. Saunders* 1997, with permission); and Reproduced with permission of Dr. B. Fisher, (Uof Alberta).

INVOLUNTARY MOVEMENT DISORDERS

- o To be considered here include
  - – Chorea
  - – Dystonia
  - – Essential tremor
  - – Myoclonus
  - – Parkinson disease and Parkinsonism
  - – Post-hypoxic Myoclonus
  - – Restless legs syndrome
  - – Tardive Dyskinesia
  - – Tourette Syndrome
  - – Wilson disease

- o What do the movement disorders have in common?
  - – Most movement disorders (chorea, dystonia, myoclonus, tic, tremor) arise from neurodegenerative disorders with a defect in the basal ganglia (comprised of caudate, globus pallidus, putamen, substantia nigra, subthalamic nuclei, thalamus), which are part of the extrapyramidal motor system which interconnects the cortex, cerebellum and brainstem.

Chorea

- ➢ Definition
  - o Basal ganglia (caudate nucleus) disease causing focal or generalized random jerks or twitches (choreiform movements)

- ➢ Common causes/associations
  - o Dopamine drugs (e.g., for Parkinson disease)
  - o Huntington disease
    - - Progressive degeneration of caudate nucleus
    - - Psychiatric and personality disorders
    - - Dementia
    - - Choreiform movements
    - - Dysarthria
    - - Parkinson

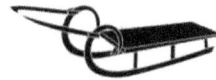

- Take a directed history and perform a focused physical examination for chorea.

  - o Neurological disorder
    - – Post CVA
    - – Huntington's disease (autosomal dominant)

  - o Drugs: e.g., excess levodopa, phenothiazines, the contraceptive pill, phenytoin

  - o Metabolic
    - – Wilson disease
    - – Kernicterus (rare)
    - – Thyrotoxicosis (very rare)
    - – Hypoparathyroidism

  - o Infection
    - – Viral encephalitis (very rare)
    - – Sydenham chorea (rheumatic fever) and other postinfectious states (both rare)

  - o Hematological
    - – Polycythaemia or other hyperviscosity syndromes (very rare)

  - o Vascular and vasculitis

  - o MSK
    - – Lupus

Adapted from: Talley NJ, et al. *Maclennan & Petty Pty Limited* 2003, Table 10.37, page 437; Baliga RR. *Saunders/Elsevier* 2007, page 216.

SO YOU WANT TO BE A NEUROLOGIST!

- Give the name of the characteristic tremor seen in persons with advanced cirrhosis.

  - o Asterixis: Inability of the patient to maintain a voluntary muscle contraction, such as dorsiflexion of wrist. Asterixis consists of a sequence of jerky flexion and extensions.

Source: Mangione S. *Hanley & Belfus* 2000.

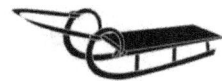

Mastering the Boards: Neurology   A.B.R. Thomson

Clinical Challenge

A 25 yr old woman develops quick muscle jerks with no abnormal facial movements, compatible with chorea. She does not use alcohol, prescription medications, and blood concentrations are normal for sugar, creatinine, calcium and TSH. She is in the third trimester of pregnancy, and she has a family history of a 70 yr old uncle having similar symptoms.

- Give the recommended management.

  o She likely has pregnancy-associated chorea (chorea gravidarum), and needs to be reassured the symptoms will disappear after delivery.

➢ Treatment
  o First-line
    – Propranolol
    – Primidone
  o Second-line
    – Gabapentin
    – Methazolamide
    – Topiramate
  o Deep brain stimulation
    – Ventral intermediate thalamic nucleus

Dystonia

➢ Definition
  o Basal ganglia causing focal or generalized twisting movement and postures.

➢ Clinical
  o Types
    – Eyelids (blepharospasm)
    – Face/jaw (craniofacial dystonia)
    – Neck (spasmatic torticollis)
  o Generalized
    – Anti-cholinergics (high dose)
    – Baclofen

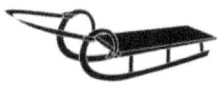

➢ Treatment

- o Focal   – Botulinum toxin
- o Dopamine-responsive dystonia   – Levodopa
- o Non-response to pharmaceuticals   – Bilateral continuous electric stimulation internal nuclei of globus pallidus

---

Clinical Gem

Spastic torticollis is a focal dystonia of the neck, treated with injections of Botulinum toxin.

Hyperkinetic Movement Disorders

➢ Types

- o Tremors
  - – Hyperkinetic rhythmic oscillation of muscles
    - ▪ With activity, no rigidity – essential tremor
    - ▪ With rest, with rigidity – Parkinsonism

- o Dysteria
  - – Contraction of opposing groups of muscles, causing
    - ▪ Repeated movement, or
    - ▪ Abnormal posture

- o Myoclonus
  - – Sudden jerky movement of extremities

- o Chores

Buzzwords in causes of in Hyperkinectic Movement Disorders

- o Essential tremors
  - – Bilateral tremors with activity, decreased with use of alcohol

- o Huntington disease
  - – Hyperkinetic movements, dementia, hallucinations, family history

- o Periodic limb movement disorder
  - – Jerky movements of legs while sleeping →

- o Restless legs syndrome
  - – Decreased by stretc.hing/walking

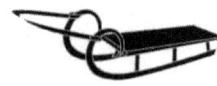

➢ Treatments

  o Cervical dystonia (torticollis)
    – Botulinum toxin injection into dystonic mode, or
    – anticholinergic

  o Drug-induced dystonia
    – Stop offending drug
    – For rapid benefit of severe dystonia
        Benztropine
        Biperidon
        diphenhydramine

  o Essential tremor
    – B-blocker, or primidone

  o PLMD/restless leg
    – Treat associated iron deficiency

  o Syndrome
    – Pramipexole
    – Ropinirole

PRACTICAL PRACTICE

Because periodic limb movement disorder (PLMD) is often associated with restless leg syndrome (RIS), and because RIS is often associated with iron deficiency, it is reasonable to perform appropriate diagnostic blood testing in both of these hyperkinetic movement disorder.

Essential Tremor

➢ Causes/associations

  o Familial (50%)
    – In some families, associated with
        ▪ Anxiety
        ▪ Alcoholism

  o Autosomal dominant inheritance

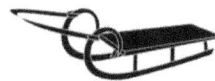

- ➤ Clinical
  - o Shaking when carrying a teacup, putting a glass to the mouth, or trying to eat soup.
  - o May affect handwriting and voice.
  - o Bilateral, usually symmetric postural or kinetic tremor.
  - o Site of tremor
    - – Hands
    - – Left or right (dominant or non-dominant)
    - – Neck
    - – Voice
  - o ↑ with activity
    - – Drugs
      - ▪ β-agonists
      - ▪ Stimulants
      - ▪ Caffeine
      - ▪ SSRIs
      - ▪ Corticosteroids
    - – Anticonvulsants
      - ▪ Lithium
      - ▪ Valproic acid
  - o ↑ by action, postural change, alcohol
  - o Tremor due to neuropathy (postural tremor; arms more than legs)
  - o No rigidity or bradykinesis
  - o Progression
    - – ↑ over time
    - – May become disabling
      - ▪ Ataxia
      - ▪ Dysarthria
      - ▪ Dysmetria
    - – May become at rest as with activity
- ➤ Differential diagnosis
  - o Parkinsonism when essential tremor occurs both hands, occurs at rest, and associated with cerebellar signs
  - o Fragile X tremor ataxia (FXTA) syndrome
    - – Dementia in FXTA, but not in essential tremor
    - – Test for genetic abnormality, especially for family history of mental retardation

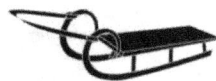

Myoclonus

➢ Definition: "….. single, rapid, shockline muscle jerk … [which] may arise from any level of neuraxis" (Source: MKSAP 16 2012, Neurology, page 54).

➢ Differential diagnosis
  o Physiological
  o Pathological
  – Epilepsy syndromes
  – Encephalopathy
    ▪ Alzheimer disease
    ▪ Hepatic encephalopathy
    ▪ Uremia
    ▪ Post-anoxia/post-trauma

➢ Treatment
  o Anti-myoclonic drugs
  – Valproic drugs
  – Clonazepam

Parkinson Disease and Parkinsonism

➢ Definition:
  o A chronic, progressive, neurogenerative of the substantia niagara in which the diagnosis is made from the clinical features such as tremor, bradykinesia and rigidity.
  o Parkinson disease (PD) is an idiopathic degeneration of the dopaminergic neurons of the substantia nigra of the midbrain causing initially slow progression of asymmetric symptoms and signs
  o Parkinsonism any cause of the symptoms/signs of Parkinson disease, such as
    – Bradykinesia
    – Gait freezing
    – Postural reflex abnormality
    – Resting tremor
    – Rigidity

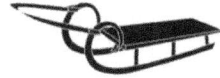

- ➢ Terminology
  - ○ Parkinsonism   – Any cause of the symptoms and signs similar to those associated with Parkinson disease
  - ○ Parkinson disease   – Ideopathic degeneration of dopaminergic neurons of the substantia nigra in the midbrain
    - – Characteristic early asymmetric clinical findings, with slow progression

Note: There is no diagnostic test for Parkinson disease, meaning that the diagnosis is based on clinical findings.

- ➢ Causes/associations
  - ○ Ideopathic
  - ○ Atherosclerosis
  - ○ Post-encephalitis
  - ○ Post-traumatic
  - ○ Tumour (midbrain compression)
  - ○ Syphilis
  - ○ Drugs
  - ○ Hepatolentecular degeneration of Wilson disease
  - ○ Hypoparathyroidism

- ➢ Clinical
  - ○ Early changes noted above
    - – Asymmetric
    - – Slow progression
    - – Responsive to
      - ▪ Levodopa, +/-
      - ▪ Dopamine agonist
  - ○ Late changes
    - – Frequent falls
    - – Ataxia
    - – Autonomic dysfunction
    - – Dementia

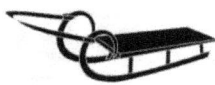

o   Muscle   – Bradykinesia
                              – Rigidity
                              – Tremor (at rest)

o   Reflexes   – Abnormal postural reflex
                              – Autonomic dysfunction
                              – Altered bowel and bladder function

o   Gait   – Freezing of gait
                              – ↑ risk of falls
                              – No ataxia

o   Cognition   – No dementia

Bradykinesia
Tremor   }   Asymmetric onset
Rigidity

o   Resting "cog wheel" rigidity

o   Greasy skin

o   No facial expression = hypomimia

o   Interlectual deterioration

o   On walking
     – No arm swinging
     – Small footsteps with 'shuffling' gait-festinant
     – Difficulty walking and turning-falls
     – Bent posture

o   Non-motor features such as dementia, psychosis and autonomic dysfunction (excessive sweating, bladder frequency/urgency, orthostasis [postural instability]) [and depression] often become the more disabling features as the disease progresses" (Grimes DA, et al. Chapter 23. In: Therapeutic Choices. Grey J, Ed. 6th Edition, *Canadian Pharmacists Association*: Otttawa, ON, 2011, page 282).

o   Early complaints "...... may include fatigue, loss of smell, sleep disroders, general slowness, poor handwriting and a tremulous feeling in one arm, without obvious tremor".

o   "Postural mobility, autonomic dysfunction, dementia, impaired eye movemments, rapid progression and poor response to dopaminergic therapy are not features of early Parkinson disease, and if present suggest a different diagnosis". (Grimes DA, et al. Chapter 23. In: Therapeutic Choices. Grey J, Ed. 6th Edition, *Canadian Pharmacists Association*: Otttawa, ON, 2011, page 282).

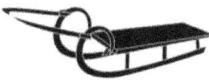

- ➢ Differential
  - o Multiple system atrophy (aka Shy-Drager syndrome)
    - – Ataxia, severe orthoastatic hypotension
  - o Progressive Supranuclear palsy
    - – Parkinsonism, falling backwards, ↓↓ vertical movement of eyes
  - o Lewy body dementia
    - – Parkinsonism, dementia, hallucinations

- ➢ Treatment

  < 65 years
  - o Dopamine agonist
    - – Pramipexole
    - – Ropinirole

          Poor response
            ↓
    - – Levodopa plus carbidopa

  >65 years
  - o levodopa plus carbidopa

- In the context of the patient with Parkinson Disease, give the significance of the development of dyskinesias and worsening of the parkinsonian symptoms/signs.

  - o Each year about 10% of patients > 60 yr who are on levodopa for Parkinson Disease will experience a "weakening off" effect of the levodopa of the initial beneficial

  - o Adding carbidopa to levodopa helps to slow this wearing off effect (blocks conversion of levodopa to dopamine, thereby enhancing/maintaining its benefit)

  - o Patients < 65 develop levodopa "wearing off" faster than in older persons, so are often started on dopamine agonists, rather than with levodopa and carbidopa.

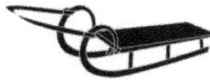

┌───┐

THERAPEUTIC ALERT

- Give the reason why bromocriptine and cabergoline are not used for treatment of parkinsonism symptoms.

  o The use of these older drugs is associated with the development of valvular heart disease.

└───┘

True Parkinsonism

➢ Causes/associations

- o Idiopathic (due to degeneration of the substantia nigra, aka Parkinson disease or "paralysis agitans")
- o Familial
- o Drug/toxins
  - Antagonist of D_2 receptors
    - Neuroleptics (haloperidol, risperidone, resperine, etc.)
    - Anti-emetics (metaclopramide, prochloperazine)
  - Other psychiatric drugs
    - Selective serotonin reuptake inhibitors
    - Tricyclics
    - Lithium
  - Cardiovascular drugs
    - Amiodarone
    - Calcium channel blockers (flunarizine)
    - Atorvastatin
  - Anticonvulsants
    - Valproate
  - Others
    - Cyclosporine
    - Metrodinazole
    - Caffeine & other methylxanthines
    - β-Adrenergic agonists
    - Thyroine
    - Prednisone

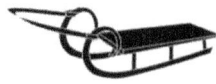

- o Brain damage (e.g cardiac arrest, exposure to manganese or carbon monoide)
- o Postencephalitic – as a result of encephalitis lethargic or von Economo's disease
- o Multiple system atrophy
- o Progressive supranuclear atrophy
- o Post encephalitic
- o Syphilis
- o Midbrain compression
- o Post traumatic
- o Wilson disease (Hepato-lenticular degeneration)
- o Hypoparathyroidism
- o Kernicterus
- o Neurologic
    - Brain tumour
    - Spinal cord trauma
    - Sleep apnea
    - Porphyria
    - Progressive supranuclear palsy
    - Shy-Drager syndrome

PseudoParkinsonism

- o Essential tremor

HemiParkinsonism (presenting feature of a progressive space-occupying lesion)

➤ Pathology

- o Disease process in nigrostriatai pathway
- o Depigmentation
- o Zona compacta neuronal
    - Degeneration
        - Melanin-containing neurons
        - Dopamine-containing neurons
    - Lewy bodies

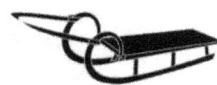

- o Parkinson-plus syndrome
  - – Deposits of neurofibrillary
    - ▪ Basal ganglia
    - ▪ Midbrain
    - ▪ Brainstem
    - ▪ Cerebellum

- ➢ Clinical

- • Give the major clinical features of Parkinsonism.
  - o Motor features
    - – Bradykinesia
      - ▪ ↓ spontaneous movement
      - ▪ Facial masking
      - ▪ ↓ fine/whole-body movement
      - ▪ ↓ arm swinging
      - ▪ Drooling
      - ▪ Monotonous speech
    - – Rigidity
      - ▪ Asymmetric
      - ▪ Arm/hand, axial
      - ▪ Cogwheel
      - ▪ Painful dystonia
    - – ↓ postural reflexes
      - ▪ Instability
        - - Falls
        - - Fractures
      - ▪ Flexion of neck and trunk
    - – Gait
      - ▪ Freezing
      - ▪ Flexion posture
      - ▪ Shuffling (short steps)
      - ▪ Narrowing based
      - ▪ Enbloc turning (rigidity of axial core)
      - ▪ Falls
  - o CNS / psyche
    - – Dementia
      - ▪ Apathy
      - ▪ Central pain
      - ▪ Compulsive/addictive behaviour
      - ▪ Confusion
      - ▪ Dementia
        - - Diffuse Lewy disease
      - ▪ Depression/anxiety
      - ▪ Hallucination
      - ▪ Hypersexuality
      - ▪ Psychosis
      - ▪ Sleep fragmentation

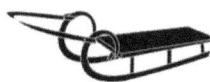

- o Autonomic
  - – Bladder/sexual dysfunction
  - – Dysfunction
  - – Postural hypotension
  - – Salivation
  - – Sweating
- o Parkinson-plus syndrome

- Perform a directed physical examination for Parkinson disease.
  - o The most typical pathological hallmarks of Parkinson disease are:
    - – Neuronal loss with depigmentation of the substantia nigra
    - – Lewy bodies, which are eosinophillic cytoplasmic inclusions in neurons consisting of aggregates of normal filaments

➤ Differential: Types of Parkinsonian syndrome

If:	If:	If:	If:	If:
Sudden onset + stuttering	Symtometrical disease	Marked postural hypotension 5 BP ≥ 30 mmHg fall	Early progressive dementia	Axial rigidity
Progression +minimal tremor +lower limbs much more affected than upper limb	Younger patient Taking dopamine Antagonists or lithium	Sphincter disturbance (impotence or urinary symptoms) Cerebellar signs	Noctural wandering +/- confusion	Failure of vertical gaze ↓ Consider **progressive Supranuclear palsy**
↓ Consider **vascular** Parkinsonism:	↓ Consider **drug- induced** Parkinsonism	↓ Consider **multisystem atrophy**	↓ Consider **dementia with lewy bodies**	

Adapted from: Davey P. *Wiley-Blackwell* 2006, page 386.

- o Diagnosing Parkinson disease
  - – Prominent rigidity on initial examination, tremor, tremor as initial symptom, tremor-dominant disease, signs are asymmetric
  - – Bradykinesia; a combination of tremor, bradykinesia, rigidity; paralysis or weakness, impaired consciousness, asymmetric disease, brady kinesia (akinetic/rigid disease)
  - – Good response to levodopa have a positive predictive ratio (PLR) < 2 for diagnosing Parkinson disease

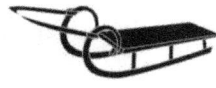

- o Face
  - – Mask-like facies
  - – Absent blinking
  - – Titubation (tremor of head)
  - – Dribbling
  - – Sialorrhea
  - – Facial seborrhoea, depressed, tendency to protrude tongue/ tongue tremor (mask-like face)
- o Speech
  - – Soft, faint, monotones (monotonous)
  - – Repetition of the end of a word (phalilalia)

- o Co-ordination test
  - – Coarse motor control
    - ▪ Heel from knee to ankle test
    - ▪ Finger to nose test
  - – Fine motor control
    - ▪ Rapid alternating movements – tapping feet
    - ▪ Rapid alternating movements – Thumb-finger opposition
    - ▪ Rapid alternating movements – Pronate-supinate hands
  - – Posture and gait
    - ▪ Regular, toe, heel, and tandem gait assessments (start hesitation, shuffling steps, loss of arm swing)
    - ▪ Examines rising from chair, and walking and turning
    - ▪ Looks for festinant gait, foot shuffling, loss of arm swing, postural instability (stooped), flexed posture, pro/retropulsion (attempt provocation with push), slow (en bloc) turning
    - ▪ Heel from knee to ankle test, finger to nose test
    - ▪ Looks for loss of spontaneous movements
    - ▪ Blank facies
    - ▪ Stare with decreased blinking and widened palpebral fissures
    - ▪ Writing test for micrographia
- o Limbs
  - – Bradykinesia
  - – Kinesia paradoxical- ability to perform rapid but not slow movements Resting tremor (may be accentuated by person concurrently performing subtraction of "serial 7's")
  - – Cogwheel rigidity
  - – Chorea jerky, abrupt, involuntary movements

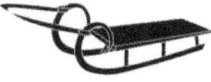

- o Motor examination
  - – Inspection
    - Muscle bulk
    - Fasciculation
    - Muscle tone
  - – Tone (palpation)
    - Upper extremities
    - Lower extremities
    - Asymmetry
    - Graded
    - Checks for rigidity with cogwheeling (intensified wtih clenching other hand into fist) (upper and lower extremities)
      - - Tests by flexion-extension of elbow or supination-pronation of wrist

Special tests for bradykinesia
- o Tapping the fingers
- o "Twiddling"

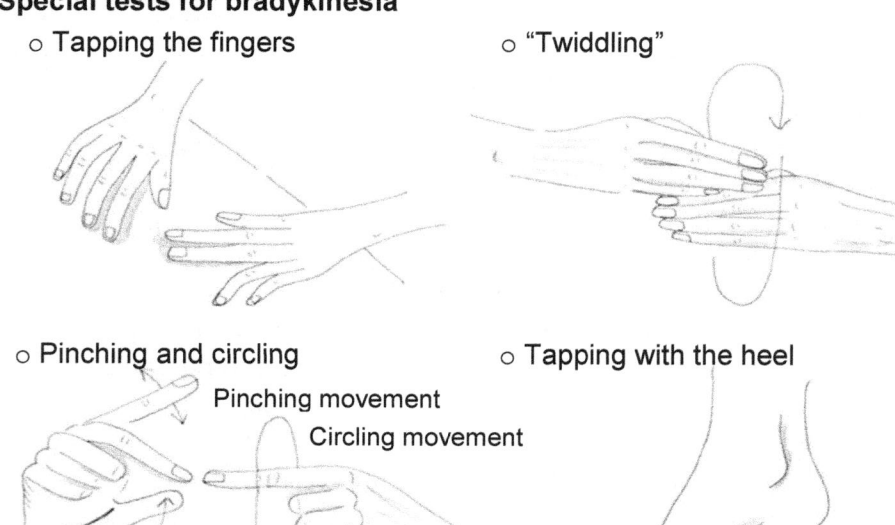

- o Pinching and circling
  - Pinching movement
  - Circling movement
- o Tapping with the heel

Adapted from: Simel DL, et al. *McGraw-Hill Medical* 2009, Figure 38-1, page 507.

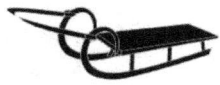

Mastering the Boards: Neurology   A.B.R. Thomson

Glabella Tap Test

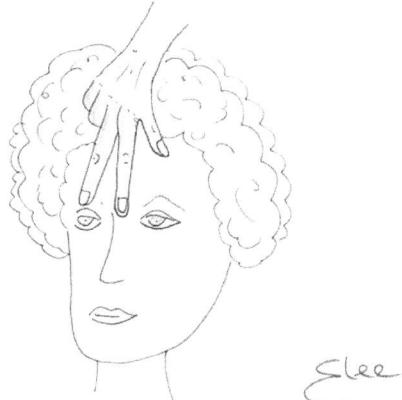

Adapted from:, Simel DL, et al. *McGraw-Hill Medical* 2009, Figure 38-2, page 508 and Filate W, et al. *The Medical Society, Faculty of Medicine, University of Toronto* 2005, Figure 38-1, page 507.

SO YOU WANT TO BE A NEUROLOGIST!

A patient is thought to possibly have Parkinsonism, but striatonigral degeneration, Shy-Drager syndrome, and olivopontocerebellar atrophy needs to be excluded.

- Perform a focused physical examination to diagnose the patient's type of multisystem atrophy.

  o Striatonigral degeneration
    - Resembles Parkinson's disease, but without tremor
    - Does not respond to anti-Parkinson medications

  o Shy- Drager syndrome:
    - Parkinson disease plus autonomic neuropathy (especially postural hypertension)
    - Impotence
    - Bladder disturbances

  o Olivopontocerebellar atrophy
    - Extrapyramidal signs plus cerebellar ataxia
    - Autonomic neuropathy plus anterior horn call degeneration

Adapted from: Baliga RR. *Saunders/Elsevier* 2007, page 245.

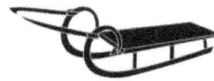

Mastering the Boards: Neurology   A.B.R. Thomson

- Give "the best" clinical test for the presence of Parkinson disease.
  - o The presence of all three of
    - − tremor
    - − bradykinesia
    - − rigidity
  - o Also useful are the presence of
    - − positive glabella tap
    - − soft voice
    - − difficulty or inablilty to walk heel-to-toe.

➤ Clinical

- Perform a focused physical examination for Parkinsonism.
  - o Tone
    - − Increased
    - − Cog-wheel or lead-pipe rigidity
    - − Featureless face
    - − Flexed posture
    - − Festination
      - ▪ Increasing speed of gait on walking
      - ▪ When patient is gently pushed, festination increases
  - o Upper body dyskinesia
    This must be present – it is a symptom complex containing many of the following features:
    - − Slowness of movement (bradykinesia)
    - − Poverty of movement (mask-like facies, diminished arm swing)
    - − Difficulty in intiating movement
    - − Diminished amplitude of repetitive alternative movement
    - − Inordinate difficulty in accomplishing some simultaneous or sequential motor acts
  - o Rigidity
    This is usually but not always present:
    - − Leadpipe rigidity, where the increase in tone is equal in fleors and etensors of all four limbs but slightly more in fleors, resulting in a part fleed 'simian' posture
    - − Cog-wheel rigidity is due to superimposed or underlying tremor

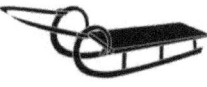

- o Postural instability; usually a late feature; may cause frequent falls
  - – Gait
  - – Festinant gait, in a posture of slight flexion

- o Tremor
  Absent in about one third of patients with Parkinson's disease at presentation and throughout its course in some
  - – Resting, pill, pronation and supination rolling tremor of the upper limb
  - – Intermittent
  - – Intensified by emotion or stress, and disappears during sleep
  - – The legs, head and jaw may shake as well distressing; the teeth may pound together until they become unbearably painful
  - – Tremor
    - ▪ Athetoid
    - ▪ Choreiform
    - ▪ Hemiballismus

- o Speech
  - – Monotonous

- o Writing
  - – Micrographia

- o Reflexes – positive globellar tap

- o Sleep disorders

- o Autonomic involvement

- o Neuropsychiatric
  - – Hallucinations
    - ▪ Medication effect (exclude RBD)
  - – Depression
    - ▪ Loss of serotonergic neurons
  - – Cognitive impairment
    - ▪ Badyphrenia
    - ▪ Dementia (consider DLB)
  - – Sensory symptoms
  - – Abnormal behaviour

- o Anxiety
  - – Akathisia
  - – Stressors

- o Sleep disorders

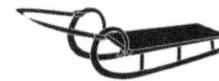

- o Autonomic involvement
- o Sensory symptoms
- o Abnormal behaviour
- o Other manifestations in Parkinson disease

Manifestation	Cause
– Pain	▪ Early morning dystonia ▪ Motor fluctuations ▪ Mechanical
– Arm paresthesia	▪ May reflect insufficient levodopa treatment
– Fatigue	▪ Multifactorial
– Diplopia	▪ Medication effect ▪ Poor convergence
– Pathologic gambling	▪ Activation of D3 receptors in limbic striatum
– Hypersexuality	

Abbreviation: DLB, dementia with Lewy bodies; MAO, monoamine oxidase; RBD, rapid eye movement sleep behaviour disorder; SSRI, selective serotonin reuptake inhibitor

Adapted from: Talley NJ, et al. *Maclennan & Petty Pty Limited* 2003, page 436,437; Hauser SC, et al. *Mayo Clinic Gastroenterology and Hepatology Board Review, 3rd Review*, page 778 and 779.

- • Give the performance characteristics (likelihood ratios) of clinical findings for Parkinson disease.

Symptoms	PLR	NLR
o Shuffling gait	3.3-15	0.32-0.50
o Bradykinesia (difficultly rising from a chair)	1.9-5.2	0.39-0.58
o Loss of balance	1.6-6.6	0.29-0.35
o Tremor	1.4-11	0.24-0.60
o Rigidity	1.3-4.5	0.12-0.93

Abbreviations: PLR, positive likelihood ratio; NLR, negative likelihood ratio
Source: Simel DL, et al. *JAMA* 2009, Table 38-4

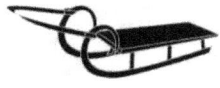

Finding	PLR	NLR
o Diagnosing Multiple System Atrophy		
– Rapid progression	2.5	0.6
– Speech and/or bulbar signs	4.1	0.2
– Autonomic dysfunction	4.3	0.3
– Cerebellar signs	9.5	0.7
– Pyramidal tract signs	4.0	Ns
– Downgaze palsy and postural instability within first year of symptoms	60.0	0.5
o Tremor		
– Arms or leg shake	1.4 -17	0.24- 0.25
– Tremor of head or limbs	11	0.26
o Rigidity		
– Rigidity and bradykinesia	4.5	0.12
– Muscle stiffness	2.3	0.73
o Facies and general symptoms or historical findings		
– Feet freeze	3.7	0.55
– Face less expressive	2.1	0.54
o Bradykinesia		
– Difficulty rising from chair	1.9- 5.2	0.39- 0.58
o Posture and motor tasks		
– Loss of balance	1.6 –6.6	0.29- 0.35
– Shuffling gait	3.3- 15	0.32 – 0.50
– Trouble turning in bed	13	0.56 (0.41-0.76)
– Trouble opening jars	6.1	0.26 (0.14-0.48)
– Trouble buttoning	3.0	0.33 (0.19-0.60)
– Uncontrolled limbs	1.3 (0.53-3.1)	0.93 (0.72-1.2)
– Micrographia (fine motor)	2.8 –5.9	0.30- 0.44
o Tremor		
– Tremor	1.5	0.47
– Tremor with rigidity and bradykinesia	2.2	0.50
o Rigidity		
– Rigidity	2.8	0.38
– Rigidity with bradykinesia	4.5	0.12

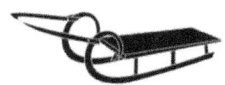

Finding	PLR	NLR
○ General findings		
– Glabella tap	4.5	0.13
– Voice softer	3.7	0.25
– Change in speech	2.6	0.73
– Asymmetric disease	1.8	0.61
– Levodopa response	1.2	0.63
○ Bradykinesia	-	-
○ Posture and motor tasks		
– Difficulty or inability to walk heel to toe	2.9	0.32

Abbreviation: NLR, negative likelihood ratio; PLR, positive likelihood ratio

---

SO YOU WANT TO BE A NEUROLOGY RESIDENT!

- Describe the abnormal reflexes which occur in Parkinsonism!
  - ○ That was a terrible trick: the deep tendon reflexes are normal.

Probability

Decrease ← → Increase

-45%	-30%	-15%		+15%	+30%	+45%

NLR | 0.1 0.2 0.5 1 2 5 10 | PLR

Sen N out – <u>Sen</u>sitive test; when negative, rules <u>out</u> disease

Sp P in – <u>Sp</u>ecific test; when positive, rules <u>in</u> disease

Adapted from: McGee SR. *Saunders/Elsevier* 2007, Box 57-2, page 729; Simel DL, et al. *JAMA* 2009, Table 38-2 and Table 38-3, pages 509 and 510.

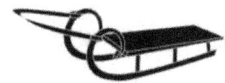

- Take a directed history and perform a focused physical examination to distinguish between Parkinson disease and atherosclerotic Parkinsonism.

	Parkinson disease[1]	Artherosclerotic Parkinsonism[2]
o Dementia	No	Yes
o Bilateral UMN signs	No	Yes
o Reflexes increased	No	Yes
o Extensor plantar responses	No	Yes
o Increased deep tendon reflexes	No	Yes
o Pseudobulbar palsy	No	Yes
o Epilepsy	No	Yes

[1] idiopathic destruction of basal ganglia
[2] atherosclerotic ischemia

- Parkinsonism may be caused by a number of conditions. Give the typical features which distinguish progressive supranuclear palsy, Lewy body dementia, and medication-associated disorder from Parkinson disease.

  - Progressive supranuclear palsy
    - ↓ vertical movement of eyes
    - Backward falls
  - Dementia with Lewy bodies
    - Dementia
    - Hallucinations
  - Medication-associated Parkinsonism
    - History of drug intake
      - Prokinetics
      - Anti-psychotics
      - Reserpine
      - Methydopa
      - Lithium

➢ Pathogenesis

  - About 10% of Parkinson disease patients have a family history. Give the molecular basis.

  - Mutation in LRRK2 gene → abnormal proteolysis of ubiquitin → formation of abnormal protein, α-synuclein → formation of Lewy bodies → destruction of dopaminergic cells

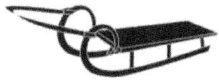

~~~
DO YOU STILL WANT TO BE A NEUROLOGIST AND HAVEN'T GIVEN
UP YET?

Some persons with Parkinson disease have other neurological deficits. These
are called "Parkinson plus syndromes".
• Give examples of Parkinson-plus-syndromes.

    o Steele – Richardson – Olszewski (SRO) disease (akinesia, aial
      rigidity of the neck, bradyphrenia, supranuclear palsy)

    o Multiple system atrophy (MSA)
        – Olivopontocerebellar degeneration
        – Strionigral degeneration
        – Progressive autonomic failure (Shy – Drager syndrome)

    o Basal ganglia calcification

Source: Baliga RR. *Saunders/Elsevier* 2007, page 142.
~~~

~~~
DO YOU STILL WANT TO BE A NEUROLOGIST?

•   In the content of mild Parkinsonism, what other neurological or
    endocrine conditions may demonstrate a slightly abnormal facies.

    o Neurological      – Mild pseudobulbar palsy
    o Endocrine         – Hypothyroidism
                        – Acromegaly
                        – Paget's disease

Source: Davies IJT. *Lloyd-Luke (medical books) LTD* 1972, page 290.
~~~

• Give the difference between rigidity, spascity, gegenhalten, tardive
  dyskinesia and the wheelchair sign.

    o Rigidity
        – ↑ tone affecting opposing muscle groups equal
        – Is present throughout the range of passive movement
        – When smooth it is called 'leadpipe' rigidity
        – When intermittent is termed 'cog-wheel' rigidity
        – Common in extrapyrimidal syndromes
            ▪ Wilson disease
            ▪ Creutzfeldt-Jakob disease.

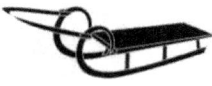

Mastering the Boards: Neurology   A.B.R. Thomson

- o Spasticity (the clasp-knife type) is characterized by
  - ↑ tone which is maximal at the beginning of movement and suddenly decreases as passive movement is continued
  - Occurs chiefly in flexors of the upper limb, and etensors of the lower limb (antigravity muscle)
- o Gehenhalten, or paratonia
  - ↑ muscle tone varies and becomes worse the more the patient tries to relax
- o Tardive dyskinesia
  - Seen in patients taking neuroleptics
  - Orofacial dyskinesia such as
    - Smacking
    - Chewing lip movements
    - Discrete dystonia
    - Choreiform movements and, rarely, rocking movements
- o Withdrawal of the "Wheelchair sign" in Parkinson patients with advanced disease and "on-off" motor fluctuations require a wheelchair when "off" and when "on" are seen to walk about (sometimes pushing the chair!).
  - These patients are rarely permanently wheelchair-bound
  - In contrast, those who never leave their wheelchair usually do not have Parkinson's disease.

Adapted from: Baliga RR. *Saunders/Elsevier* 2007, page 139; McGee SR. *Saunders/Elsevier* 2007, pages 139 and 140.

➢ Treatment
  - o Manage patient's overall needs, expectations activity, sleep, complications
  - o Classes of drugs
    - Dopamine agonists
      - Pramipexole
      - Ropinirole
      - AEs
        - Sedation
      - Compulsive behaviours
    - Levodopa plus carbidopa
      - ↓ effect over time
      - AE dyskinesia
    - Dopamine precursors plus decarboxylase inhibitor levodopa plus carbidopa

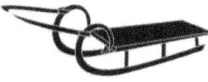

- Catechol-o-methyltransferase inhibitors
- Dopamine/anti-cholinergic/glutamine inhibitor
- Monoamine oxidase type B inhibitor
  - Wearing-off
    - Motor fluctuations → return of parkinsonian symptoms
    - Dyskinesias (twisting, writhing movements occurring 5 yrs within in 50%)
    - Amantadine, a dopaminergic/anti-cholinergic/glutamine antagonist may be of some benefit for the wear-off dyskinesia
    - Depp-brain stimulation of
      - Subthalamic nucleus
      - Globus pallidus interna
  - Tremor refractory to medication
    - Deep-brain stimulation of ventral intermediate thalamus
  - Deep-brain stimulation (subthalamic)

- Give the likely diagnosis and recommended diagnostic imaging.

  - MRI of the cervical spine is necessary to exclude traumatic compression of the spinal cord, but the diagnosis is clinical.

SO YOU WANT TO BE A NEUROLOGIST!

- Give the rationale for combining levodopa with carbidopa.

  - Levodopa is metabolized to dopamine

  - Dopamine may cause adverse effects (AEs)

  - ↓ AEs with levodopa by adding carbidopa to ↓ conversion of the levodopa to dopamine

  - Theoretically bromocriptine and cabergoline might be useful for Parkinson disease

- Give the major AE which explains the non-use of these drugs.

  - ↑ risk of developing valvular heart disease.

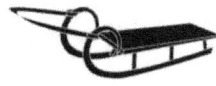

After years of effective treatment of their Parkinson disease, some patients develop **incapacitating symptoms**.

- o Motor fluctuations
    - – Tremor
    - – Slowness
    - – Gait impairment

- o Dyskinesia
    - – Involuntary twisting/writhing movement shortly after taking their medication
    - – Ballistic movements

- • Give the likely diagnosis and recommended treatment for these in capacitating symptoms.

    - o About ½ of patients treated for < 5 yr with a dopamine agonist or levodopa will develop motor fluctuations and dyskinesia.
    - o Recommended treatment is deep brain stimulation of
        - – Globus pallidus internam or
        - – Subthalamic nucleus

A patient with Parkinson disease falls, and immediately afterwards notes weakness of her legs and sufficient that she cannot walk. There is no neck pain, signs of an UML lesion, no sensory loss or incontinence of urine or stool.

- • In the patient with suspected Parkinson disease, give the significance of a lack of response to levodopa, in terms of the diagnosis and the likely pathology.

    - o Diagnosis
        - – A lack of sustained responsiveness to levodopa suggests
        - – Atypical Parkinsonism, rather than Parkinson disease
        - – The disease process has likely extended beyond to nigrostraital pathway, and the patient has atypical Parkinsonism

    - o Pathology
        - – In Parkinson disease the disease process is in the nigrostriatal pathway
        - – When there is an atypical response to levodopa

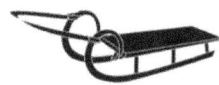

CLINICAL CHALLENGES

- An elderly patient is diagnosed with Parkinson disease. He progresses to develop visual hallucinations despite being on a dopaminergic drug. Give the rational for a study for a possible sleep disorder, and recommended changes in his pharmaceutical management.
  - For Lewy body disease, dopamine agonists are contraindicated.
  - Place on levodopa for symptoms management

- Parkinson disease as well as vascular parkinsonism may affect the lower body, and reduce leg function in the supine and sitting positions. Parkinson disease may cause gain disturbance, gait abnormalities, and dysfunction of the bowel and bladder (Parkinson-plus Shy-Drager syndrome).

In such a patient, the leg function in the supine and sitting position was curiously normal. Give the name of the treatable condition that needs to be considered, how is it diagnosed and treated.

- NPH (normal pressure hydrocephalis) causes
  - ↓ cognition
  - Abnormal gait
  - Urinary urgency / incontinence
- Diagnosis
  - ↑ CSF pressure > 150 mm H_2O
  - MRI brain
    - Enlarged ventricles
    - No salcal atropy or obstruction
- Treatment surgically placed, with externally controlled programmable value

SO YOU WANT TO BE A NEUROLOGIST!

- Give how do you distinguish clinically rigidity from spasticity.
  - Rigidity
    - Increased muscle tone through all parts of the movement of the joint
    - Usually seen in degenerative neurological conditions e.g. Parkinsonism
  - Spasticity
    - Increasing muscle tone as muscle is stretc.hed more and more, followed by a giveaway phenomenon of protectone relaxation, leading to a jack-knife loss of tone
    - Usually due to damage to the pyramidal (corticspinal) tract

Adapted from: Mangione S. *Hanley & Belfus* 2000, page 414.

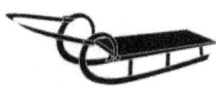

➢ Differential diagnosis for Parkinson disease
  o Ideopathic (degeneration of substantia nigra)
    – Drugs
      ▪ Neuroleptics
      ▪ Metoclorpimide
    – Toxins
      ▪ MPTP (drug abusers), manganese, carbon disulfide, CO

Abbreviations: CO, carbon monoxide

➢ Differential diagnosis of **Parkinson – plus syndromes**

Manifestation	Suspect
o Poor response to levodopa	– Any parkinson-plus syndrome (MSA & PSP may respond)
o Early falls	– PSP & MSA
o Severe OH & urologic Sx	– MSA
o Cerebellar signs	– MSA or spinocerebellar degeneration
o Vertical gaze	– PSP
o Asymmetric apraxia	– Corticobasal degeneration
o Early dementia	– Dementia with Lewy bodies of Creutzfeldt-Jakob disease

Abbreviations: MSA, multiple system atrophy; OH, orthostatic hypotension; PSP, progressive supranuclear palsy; S, symptoms

Source: Hauser SC, et al. *Mayo Clinic Gastroenterology and Hepatology Board Review*. 3rd Review, page 78.

• Give the typical changes on pathology which suggest a Parkinson-plus syndrome.

  o Diagnostic imaging
    – Atrophy of
      ▪ Brainstem
      ▪ Midbrain

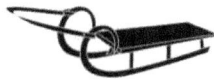

SO YOU WANT TO BE A NEUROLOGIST!

- In the context of a gait disturbance, give what you understand by the term 'astasia abasia'.
    - Seen in psychogenic disturbances in which the patient is unable to walk or cannot stand.
    - The patient falls far to the side on walking, but usually regains balance before hitting the ground.
    - The legs may be thrown out wildly, or the patient may kneel with each step.

- Give what you understand by the term 'marche a petits pas'.
    - A gait in which the movement is slow and the patient walks with very short, shuffling and irregular steps, with loss of associated movements.
    - Seen in normal-pressure hydrocephalus.
    - This gait bears some resemblance to that seen in Parkinson disease.

Source: Baliga RR. *Saunders/Elsevier* 2007, Case 61, page 181.

- Give the simple maneuver performed during the physical examination will help to distinguish cerebellar ataxia from sensory ataxia.
    - Ataxia (clumsiness) due to cerebellar lesions persists when the eyes are closed
    - Sensory ataxia improves when the eyes are open

- Give the hematological abnormalities may be associated with chorea.
    - Polycythemia vera
    - Neuroacanthocytosis (chorea – acanthocystosis)

- Give the meaning of Hemiballismus.
    - Sudden onset of unilateral, involuntary, flinging movements of the proximal upper limbs

    - Cardiovascular disease (source of emboli)
        - Atrial fibrillation
        - Valvular heart disease
        - Severe left ventricular dysfunction, travelling to the ipsilateral subthalamic nucleus of lungs and causing an infarction

    - Unilateral, involuntary, flinging movement of the proimal upper limbs

Source: Baliga RR. *Saunders/Elsevier* 2007, page 218.

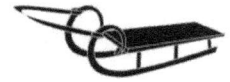

In addition to Friedreich's ataxia, give the other syndromes associated with spinocerebellar degeneration.

- Roussy-Levy disease: hereditary spinocerebellar degeneration with atrophy of lower limb muscles and loss of deep tendon reflexes.
- Refsum disease
- Machado-Joseph disease – dominant inheritance (first described in families of Portuguese origin)
  - Progressive ataxia, ophthalmoparesis, spasticity, dystonia, amyotrophy and Parkinsonism
- Dentatorubral pallidoluysian atrophy, similar to Machado-Joseph disease but maps on the short arm of chromosome 12 rather than 14.

Source: Baliga RR. *Saunders/Elsevier* 2007, page 193.

Post-Hypoxic Myoclonus

➢ Types
  - Cardiac arrest or delayed cardiopulmonary resuscitation may lead to post-hypoxic myoclonus
  - Hypoxia of the cortex leaves the cortex hyperexcitable

➢ Clinical
  - Muscle jerks which are increased by exercise or muscle stimulation
  - "Negative" myclonus – sudden ↓ of a sustained posture (asterixis)

Restless Legs Syndrome (RLS)

➢ Definition
  - Abnormality in central dopamine pathways, often familial or autosomal dominant inheritance.
  - Is a neurologic disorder characterized by an unpleasant sensation in the legs accompanied by an urge to move the legs, especially at bedtime.
  - These symptoms occur when the limbs are at rest, and are relieved by movement.
  - In severe cases, symptoms may extend to the arms and trunk.
  - Symptoms are commonly bilateral and symmetrical, but on occasion can be unilateral.

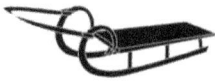

➢ Terminology

- o *Intermittent* RLS is defined as symptoms that are troublesome enough to require treatment but not frequent enough to require daily therapy
- o *Daily* RLS involves symptoms that are frequent and bothersome enough to require daily therapy
- o Patients with *refractory* RLS are those who experience inadequate response and/or intolerable side effects and/or "augmentation"

Reproduced with permission: Therapeutics Choices. Sixth Edition. Ottawa, Canada: *Canadian Pharmacist Association* 2012, page 274.

➢ Causes /associations
- o CNS   – Peripheral neuropathy

- o MSK   – Rheumatoid arthritis
  - – Fibromyalgia

- o Kidney   – Chronic renal disease

- o Blood   – Iron deficiency

- o Endocrine   – Diabetes
  - – Pregnancy

➢ Clinical
- o Motor   – Tonic flexor spasm of the leg (periodic limb movements)
- o Sensory   – Intolerable tingling (dysesthesias)
- o Onset   – When drowsy or sleepy
- o Off-set   – Symptoms retrieval with activity

➢ Diagnosis

All of the following 4 criteria are required for a diagnosis of RLS:
- o An urge to move the legs, usually accompanied or causes by unpleasant sensations in the legs.
- o Symptoms begin or worsen during periods of rest or inactivity such as lying or sitting.
- o Symptoms are partially or totally relieved by movement, such as walking or stretching, for at least as long as the activity continues.
- o Symptoms are worse in the evening or at night than during the day, or occur only in the evening or at night.

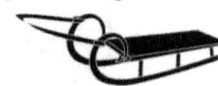

- o Supportive clinical features include
  - – A positive family history
  - – Response to dopaminergic therapy
  - – Periodic limb movements during wakefulness or during sleep

➢ Treatment
  - o Treat associated conditions (e.g., iron deficiency)
  - o Optimize sleep habits
  - o Pharmaceutics
    - – Dopaminergics
    - – Opioid codeine
    - – Benzodiazepine

Cautionary note

- o Persons with restless leg syndrome treated with levodopa may develop adverse effects of
  - – Dependence
  - – Rebound

Tardive Dyskinesia

➢ Definition

- o Movement disorders associated with the dopamine antagonists (D2-receptor agents)

➢ Types

o Acute dystonia	–	Sudden dystonic spasm of head, face, neck, throat or eye (oculogyric crisis)
o Acute akathisia	–	Sudden onset of restlessness and a need to move around
o Tardive Dyskinesia	–	Late-appearing, persisting and
	–	Repetitive choreiform movements of head and neck
o Dystonia	–	Spasms of muscles of head and neck, arms and trunks
o Akathisia	–	Sensation of restlessness and need to move around
o Parkinsonism-like presentation	–	Induced by drugs
	–	Resolves when dopamine-antagonists

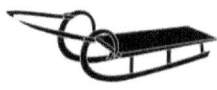

Tourette Syndrome

- ➤ Definition
  - o Tourette syndrome is a disorder which causes ".... repetitive, stereotyped, purposeless brief movements from a background of normal motor activity"
    - – Movements and sounds .... that emerge suddenly (Source: MKSAP 16 2012, Neurology, page 55)

- ➤ Clinical
  - o Movements and sounds, as noted above
  - o Psychiatric symptoms
    - – OCD (obsessive-compulsive disorder)
    - – Attention-deficit +/- hyperactivity
    - – Generalized
      - ▪ Anxiety
      - ▪ Panic
      - ▪ Phobia
      - ▪ Mood disorder

- ➤ Treatment
  - o 1st line
    - – α-agonists
      - ▪ Clonidine
      - ▪ Guanfacine
      - ▪ Clonazepam

  - o 2nd line
    - – Anti-dopaminergic agents
    - – Catecholamine-depleting agents
      - ▪ Reserpine
      - ▪ Tetrabenazine
    - – Neuroleptic drugs

  - o Focal tics
    - – Botulinum toxin

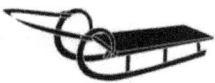

Wilson Disease

➤ Definition

 o "…. an autosomal recessive inborn error of metabolism caused by a mutation of the copper P-type adenosine triphosphate encoded on chromosome 13q14.3, [which] leads to a failure of copper excretion in bile, which results in copper accumulation in the liver and brain (Source: MKSAP 16 2012, Neurology, page 55).

➤ Clinical

• Give the neurologic presentations of Wilson disease.

 o Eye — Kayser Fleischer ring
   ▪ Copper deposited in Descemet membrane of cornea

 o Basal ganglia — Dystonia
   — Ataxia

 o Cerebellum — Tremors
   Large-amplitude (wing-beating) tremor
   — Dysmetria

➤ Treatment

• Give the name of the drug used as maintenance therapy in Wlson disease which is **not** to be used in pregnancy (FDA category D).

 o Desferoximine

 Note:
   — Use zinc or triampterine
   — Do not suddenly stop copper
   — Lowering medication

• Give the name of the only life-saving treatment for Wilson disease in a person presenting with acute liver failure (hepatic encephalopathy and coagulopathy).

 o Liver transplant
   — To do so might precipidate life-threatening acute liver failure (ALF)

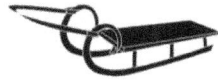

TREMOR

➤ Definition
  o Tremors are involuntary movements that result from alternating contraction and relaxation of the group of muscles.
  o Rhythmic oscillations about a joint or a goup of joints.

➤ Terminology
  o Athetoid movements
    – Slow
    – Writhing
    – Sinuous
    – Movements of periphery
    – By emotion, voluntary movement
    – Cause – disease of extrapyramidal system

  o Choreiform movements
    – Sudden
    – Brief
    – Jerky
    – Involuntary
    – By emotion, voluntary movement
    – Same movement never repeated in succession
    – Cause – disease of extrapyramidal system

  o Myoclonus
    – Sudden contraction of a large muscle or muscle group.
    – Hiccups ("singultus") are an example of myoclonus
    – Epilepsy may be associated with myotonic movements

  o Tremor
    – Extrapyramidal
      • Tremor at rest
      • ↓↓ with sleep, strong movements
      • with emotion, fine movements
      • Course
      • "compound" (affects many joints)
    – Cerebellum
      • Intention tremor
      • ↓↓ at rest
      • as range of movement is increased
    – GPI
      • Tongue: backward and forward trombone – like tremor
      • Tremor present both at rest and with attempted protrusion of the tongue

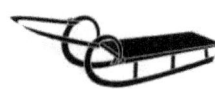

- Fine tremor
  - Cause by
    - Fatigue
    - Anxiety
    - Emotion
    - Thyrotoxicosis
    - Rx: alcohol, tobacco, cocaine, mercury

- o TIC
  - Explosive repetition of the same movement
  - Commonly seen in facial muscles
  - May be associated with psychiatric disturbance

➤ Types of tremors

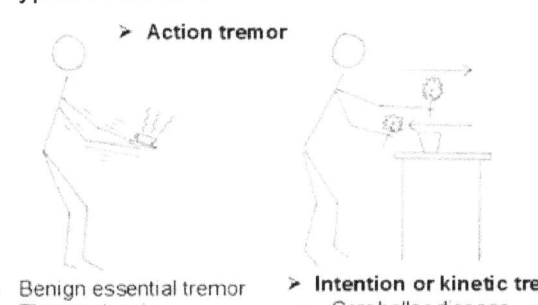

➤ **Action tremor**

- o Benign essential tremor
- o Thyrotoxicosis
- o Anxiety

➤ **Intention or kinetic tremor**
- o Cerebellar disease
- o Severe forms of other tremor

➤ **Resting tremor**

- o Parkinson's
- o Rare causes: Hg poisoning, Wilson's disease, syphilis

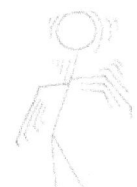

➤ **Chorea**
- o Continuous movements
- o Facial grimacing
- o Teeth grinding
- o Worse with walking
- o 'Fidgety'
- o 'Won't sit still'
- o 'Always crossing and re crossing legs'

- o Drugs (e.g L-dopa, anti psychotics)
- o Huntington's disease
  - SLE
  - Contraceptive pill
  - Thyrotoxicosis
  - Hyperviscosity syndrome
  - Pregnancy

Sustained abnormal tone & posture

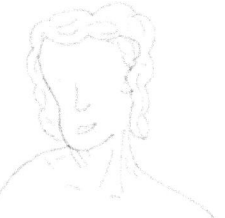

- o 'writer's cramp'
- o Torticollis

➤ **Dystonia**

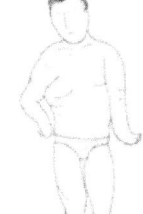

- o Generalized

Adapted from: Simel DL, et al. *JAMA* 2009, Box 38-2, page 508; Davey P. *Wiley-Blackwell* 2006, page 105 and Ghosh AK. *Mayo Clinic Scientific Press* 2008, page 778; Davey P. *Wiley-Blackwell* 2006, page 104.

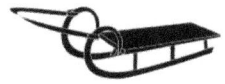

Physiologic Tremor
- o Variable
- o Enhanced form is visible, postural, and has a high frequency (8-12/s)
- o No underlying neurologic disease
- o Cause is usually reversible (e.g., caffeine)

Intention Tremor (Cerebellar)
- ➢ Clinical
  - o Limbs or head tremor
  - o ↑ with alcohol
  - o ↑ by involuntary movement
  - o Contra-axial
  - o Symmetrical
  - o Examples
    - Chorea
    - Athetosis
    - Hemiballismus
    - Fasciculation
    - Torticollis
    - Clonus

Postural and Action (Kinetic) **Tremor**

- ➢ Clinical
  - o Tremor that occurs while voluntarily maintaining a position against gravity (postural)
  - o Kinetic
  - o Tremor occurring during any voluntary movement
  - o Tremor occurring during voluntary movements that are not target directed
  - o Task Specific. Tremor that appears or is exacerbated by specific tasks (e.g., writing)
  - o Fast tremor throughout movement seen best with arms and hands outstretched
  - o Exaggerated physiological tremor

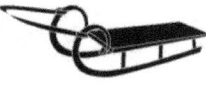

➢ Causes/associations
- o Anxiety
- o Sleep deprivation
- o Fatigue
- o Cold
- o ß-agonist drugs
- o Withdrawal of alcohol, caffeine, or lithium
- o Hyperthyroidism or hypoglycemia
- o Brain damage seen in Wilson's disease, syphilis

Rest Tremor (as seen in Parkinsonism)

➢ Clinical
- o Slow frequency (4-6 / sec) tremor at rest
- o As seen in Parkinsonism
- o The hands have characteristic motion of
  - – Pill rolling
  - – Alternating flexion/extension of fingers or hands
  - – Alternating pronation/supination of forearms
- o Asymmetrical
- o Hands, legs, chin, jaw, but not the head
- o Rigidity, bradykinesia
- o ↓ during movement, sleep
- o ↑ by emotional distress
- o No consistent response to alcohol

- Perform a focused physical examination for different types of abnormal involuntary movements.
  - o Tremor
    - – Rapidly repeated single movement
  - o Athelosis
    - – Slow, writhing, purposeless movements

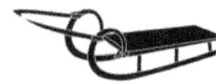

- o Chorea
  - – Semi-purposeful movements eg, repeatedly pulling at bedclothes
- o Myoclonus
  - – Sudden, rapid movement of a muscle group
- o Tic
  - – Repeated complicated movement
- o Tonic – clonic movemnets (convulsion)
- o Jacksonian epilepsy

Adapted from: Davies IJT. *Lloyd-Luke (medical books) LTD* 1972, pages 289 and 302.

The commonest types of involuntary movements are tremor, athetosis and clonus.

- Perform a focused physical examination to determine the cause of each tremor, athetosis, and chorea.
  - o Tremor
    - – Senility
    - – Familial
    - – Basal ganglia Parkinsonism
    - – Alcoholism
    - – Cerebellar disease
    - – Thyroid disease
    - – Thyroid disease-thyrotoxicosis
    - – Psychogenic
  - o Athetosis
    - – Familial
    - – Psychogenic
    - – Basal ganglia disorders
  - o Chorea
    - – Senility
    - – Psychogenic inherited – Huntington's chorea
    - – Rheumatic fever-Sydenham's chorea
    - – Pregnancy ("chorea gravidarum")

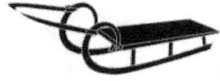

BRAINSTEM

A useful trick:

- o Think of the brainstem as being part of the spinal cord, with the cranial nerves added on.
- o The brainstem is comprised of the midbrain, pons and medulla.
- o There is crossed hemiplegia with disease involvement of the brain stem.

➤ Anatomy
  - o Fibres from the internal capsule of the cortex pass to the cerebral peduncle
  - o Fibres from the cerebral peduncle to the brainstem
  - o The brain stem is comprised of the midbrain, pons and medulla
  - o Fibres from the brain stem pass to the spinal cord
  - o The brain stem receives the motor and sensory fibres of the cranial nerves also contain the nuclei of the cranial nerves, and their interconnections
  - o The motor fibres of the cranial nerves decussate (cross) higher up the brain stem than do the pyramidal fibres
  - o The fibres running from the nuclei of the cranial nerves are lower motor neurons
  - o Because the cranial motor fibres cross higher than the motor fibres from the pyramidal tract, there may be weakness of the crnial muscles on one side, and weakness of the opposite side of the body
  - o Crossed hemiplegia occurs because of damage to a cranial nerve after it crosses, and damage to the pyramidal tract after it crosses

Source: Davies IJT. *Lloyd-Luke (medical books) LTD* 1972, Figure 11, page 243 and 247

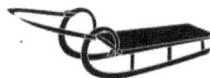

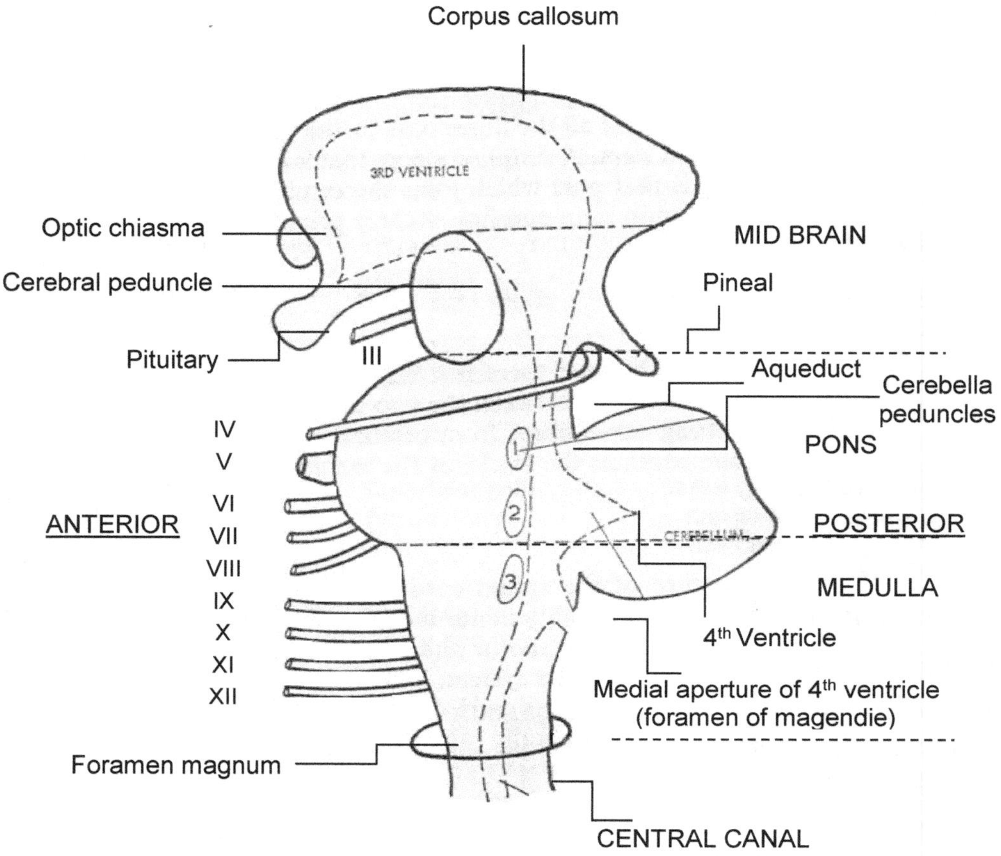

Corpus callosum

3RD VENTRICLE

Optic chiasma

Cerebral peduncle

Pituitary

III

IV
V
VI
ANTERIOR VII
VIII
IX
X
XI
XII

Foramen magnum

MID BRAIN

Pineal

Aqueduct

Cerebella peduncles

PONS

CEREBELLUM

POSTERIOR

MEDULLA

4th Ventricle

Medial aperture of 4th ventricle
(foramen of magendie)

CENTRAL CANAL

The brain stem showing the midbrain, pons and medulla as well as the origin
of the cranial nerves.

Adapted from: Davey P. *Wiley-Blackwell* 2006, page 243.

"Let's change the interactions between alerting,
orienting and executive functions, and control in a
standard curing paradigm."
Grandad

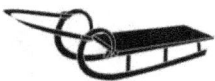

Mastering the Boards: Neurology   A.B.R. Thomson

Anatomy - **Midbrain**

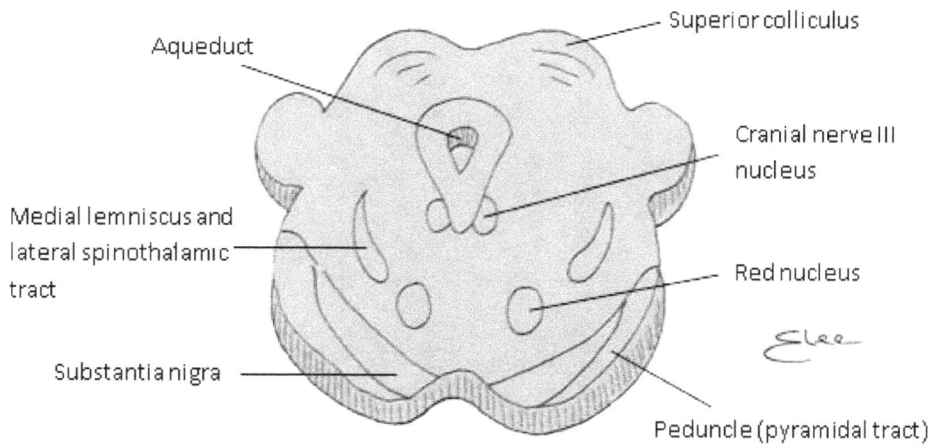

Adapted from: Talley NJ, et al. *Maclennan & Petty Pty Limited* 2003,Figure 10.8, pages 365, 371, 380.

Anatomy - **Medulla**

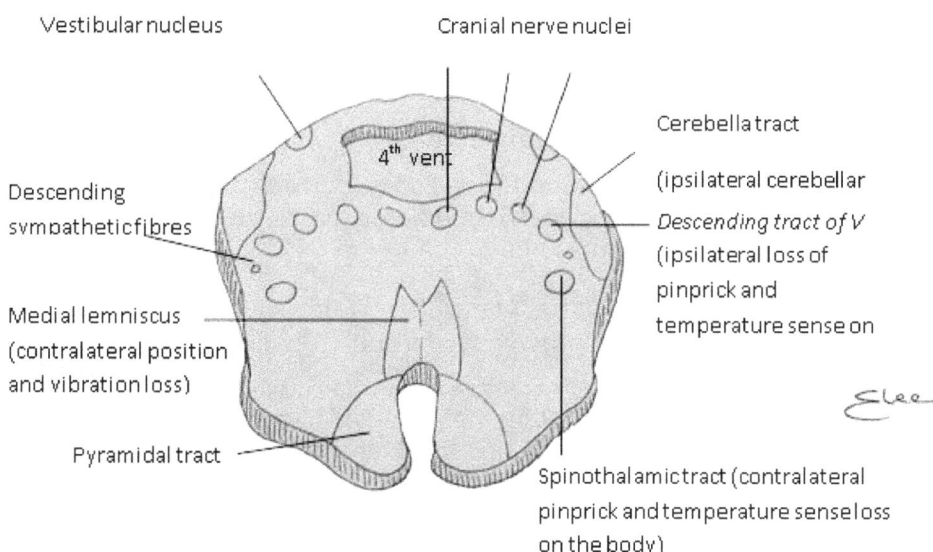

Adapted from: Talley NJ, et al. *Maclennan & Petty Pty Limited* 2003, Figure 10.17, page 380.

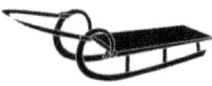

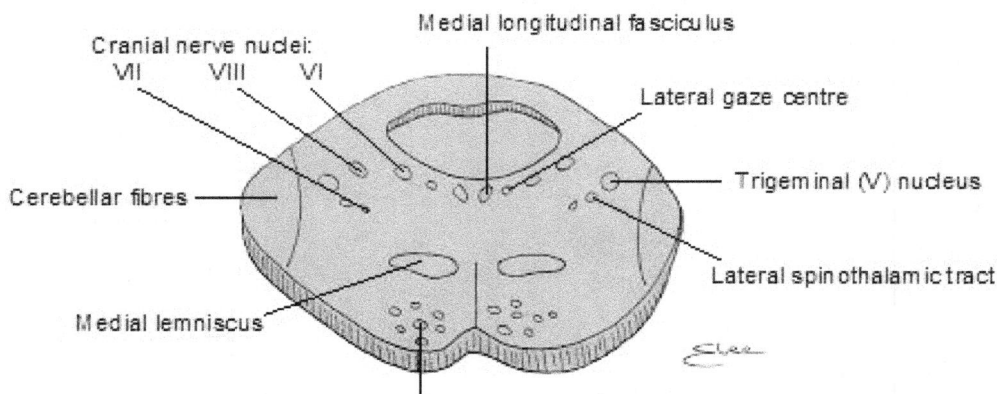

Anatomy - **Pons**

Cranial nerve nuclei:
VII   VIII   VI

Medial longitudinal fasciculus

Lateral gaze centre

Trigeminal (V) nucleus

Cerebellar fibres

Lateral spinothalamic tract

Medial lemniscus

Motor fibres (corticobulbar and corticospinal)

Adapted from: Talley NJ, et al. *Maclennan & Petty Pty Limited* 2003, Figure 10.11, page 371.

➢ Brainstem Neuroanatomy

• Clinically important structures which are seen in the brain stem are:

   o Medial longitudinal bundle

      – Interconnects the nuclei of the cranial nerves, and

      – Is concerned with co-ordination of face and eye movements.

   o Ascending tract of the trigeminal nerve

      – Contains proprioceptive and touch fibres, corresponding to the posterior columns. The fibres immediately cross the midline and join the medial lemniscus.

   o Descending tract of the trigeminal nerve

      – Carries pain and temperature impulses corresponding to the lateral spinothalamic tract.

      – Descends to the level of C.2 on the same side as it enters, and then crosses the midline and joins the lateral spinothalamic tract.

   o Tractus solitaries

      – Contains fibres conveying taste.

   o Corticospinal tracts

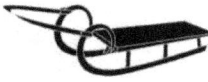

o Nuclei of the cranial nerves.

- The oculomotor nerve emerges from the midbrain close to the cerebral peduncle
  ▪ A lesion in this area gives rise to a lower motor neurone oculomotor palsy on the same side and a hemiplegia on the opposite side (Weber syndrome).

- Pons: abducens, trigeminal, facial and auditory

- Medulla: glossopharyngeal, vagus accessory and hypoglossal nerves

- **Pyramidal system-** internal capsule, midbrain, pons, medulla

  o Pyramidal fibres decussate in medulla to form pyramidal tracts

  o The pyramidal tracts pass down the later columns to enter the grey matter of the anterior horns, where they synapse with the anterior horn cells

  o In the brain stem, the pyramidal tracts give off fibres to the contralateral motor cranial nerve nuclei

  o A few pyramidal fibres do not decussate in the medulla but go down the same side as the anterior cortico-spinal tract

  o The neuroanatomic parts which constitute the pyramidal system

o Internal capsule

o Midbrain ⟶ o Some fibres of the pyramidal tract go to the contralateral motor cranial nerve nuclei

o Pons

A few pyramidal fibres ⟵ Medulla ⟶ Pyramidal fibres decussate do not decussate, but to form pyramidal tracts go down the same side as the anterior cortico-spinal tract

Lateral columns anterior horn cells

Source: Davies IJT. *Lloyd-Luke (medical books) LTD* 1972, Figure 12, page 243.

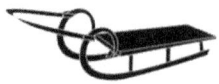

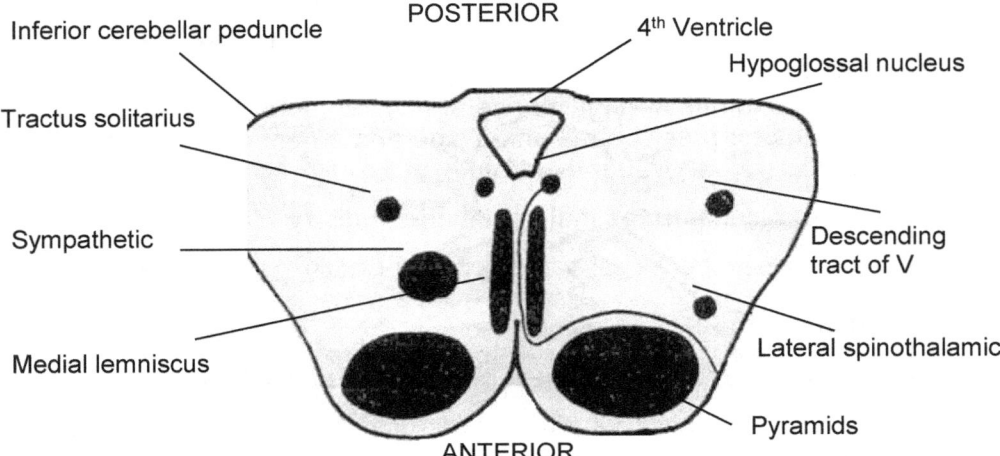

Cross-section of the medulla showing the position of the important tracts.

Adapted from: Davey P. *Wiley-Blackwell* 2006, page 247.

- o The lateral spinothalamic (pain and temperature), which continues through the medulla as the lateral spinothalamic tract and then also joins the medial lemniscus in the pons.

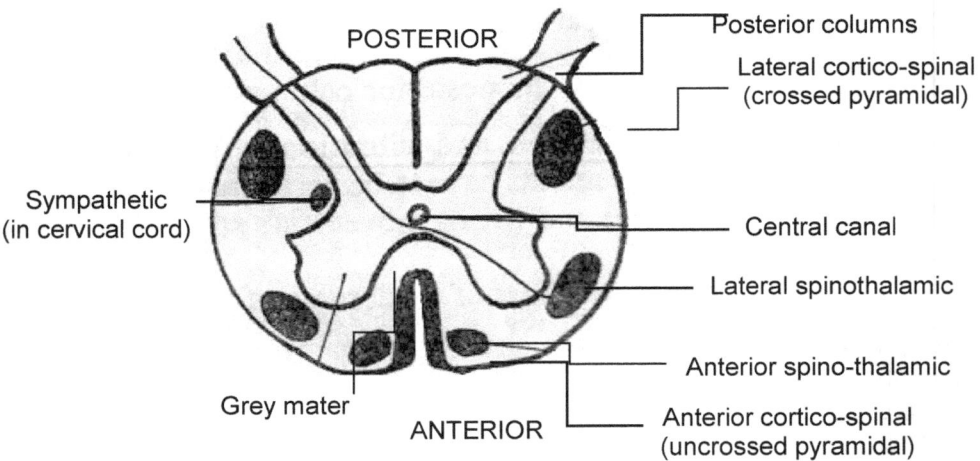

Adapted from: Davey P. *Wiley-Blackwell* 2006, page 243.

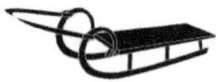

- **Tracts in the Brain Stem**

  - Posterior columns
    - Fibres in the cord
      - uncrossed → medial lemnisci
      - crossed → medulla

  - Anterior spinothalamic
    - Fibres in cord → reticular substance in medulla → medial lemniscus of the pons, crossing several segments above entry → thalamus

  - Lateral spinothalamic
    - Fibres in cord → medulla → medial lemniscus of pons, crossing immediately above entry → thalamus

The sensory tracts which end in the spinal cord at the medulla include fibres from the periphery, as well as the cranial nerves.

Tract	Sensory Impulses	Site of Decussation
o Posterior columns	o Proprioception o Vibration o Deep pain o Some light touch	− In the medulla, after forming medial lemniscus
o Anterior spinothalamic	o Light touch	− In the spinal cord several segments above their entry
o Lateral spinothalamic	o Superficial pain o Temperature o Tickle	− In the spinal cord immediately above entry
o Spinocerebellar	o Concerned with muscle tone and co-ordination	− Probably do not cross

Source: Davey P. *Wiley-Blackwell* 2006, page 245.

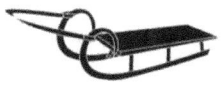

- Translational Neuroanatomy

- Give the sites and causes of a bilateral pyramidal lesion of both lower legs.

  o Sites
    - Lesion of cord
    - Bilateral parasagittal cortical lesion

  o Causes crucial dominance
    - Parasagittal meningioma
    - Sagittal sinus thrombosis
    - Subdural hematoma
    - Thrombosis of both anterior cerebral arteries

- Take a directed history and perform a focused physical examination for disease of the brainstem.

- History (the "D's")
  o Diplopia (CN III, IV or VI)
  o Decreased sensation in the face (CN V)
  o Decreased strength in the face (CN VII)
  o Dizziness and deafness (CN VIII)
  o Dysarthria and dysphagia (CN IX, X, XII)

- Physical
  o Ipsilateral cranial nerve abnormalities, plus contralateral
    - Corticospinal tract changes
      ▪ Ataxia
    - Diplopia
      ▪ Nystagmus
      ▪ ↓ corneal reflexes
      ▪ Facial weakness
      ▪ Facial numbness
      ▪ Deafness
      ▪ Dysarthria
      ▪ Palate paralysed
      ▪ Gag reflex ↓
      ▪ Tongue deviation

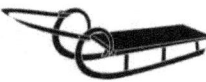

- o Contralateral changes in
  - – Pyramidal tract
    - ▪ Hemiparasis (weakness)
    - ▪ ↑ reflexes
    - ▪ ↑ tone
    - ▪ Babinski sign positive
  - – Spinothalamic tract
    - ▪ Hemianaethesia (numbness: ↓ in all sensory modalities)

Source: Mangione S. *Hanley & Belfus*, 2000; and Ghosh AK. *Mayo Clinic Scientific Press* 2008, page 762.

Babinski sign

- o Dorsiflexion of the big toe when the sole of the foot is stimulated from the lateral to the medial side
- o Dorsiflexion (Babinski sign is positive) indicates an UMN lesion of the pyramidal (aka corticospinal) pathway

Source: Mangione S. *Hanley & Belfus* 2000.

- Perform a focused physical examination for **locked-in state**.

➢ Definition
  - o Localized damage to brainstem, usually between the upper third and lower two-thirds of the brainstem

➢ Clinical
  - o Patient is awake
  - o Only function is CN III and VI (eye moves and can be kept open)
  - o Patient's eyes may follow the MD as he/she moves around ("tracking")
  - o Patient can see and hear, but has no movement or sensation

---

SO YOU WANT TO BE A NEUROLOGIST!

- The plantar response is extensor in the first year of life, in deep coma, and in lesions of the pyramidal tract. Under what clinical circumstances may this response be falsely negative?
  - o Loss of sensation on the sole of the foot
  - o Hallux rigidus
  - o Paralysis of extensor hallicus longus (L4,5)

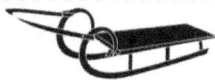

- Perform a focused physical examination for an ischemic event involving the midbrain, pons, as well as the lateral and medial portions of the medulla.

	Site	Clinical
• Midbrain	o Midbrain	
	– Severe	▪ Cerebral pedicles – Quadriplegia ▪ Ipsilateral III, IV – LMN oculomotor and trachear pulses – Impaired conjugate movements of eyes
	– Mild	▪ Crossed hemiplegia (corticospinal tract and CN III involvement)
	o Hemiballismus	– Part of thalamus involved
	o Thalamic syndrome	
	o Akinetic mutism (aka coma vigil)	
	o Peri-pineal area	– Impaired upwards movement of eyes
• Pons	o Unique features – Pin-point pupils – Hyperventilation o Cranial nerves – LMN lesion	▪ IV – abducent – Impaired leteral gaze ▪ V – trigeminal ▪ VII – facial ▪ VIII – auditory

Site		Clinical	
	o Sensation	– Unilateral sensory loss – The anterior and lateral spinothalamic tracts: location of sensory loss depends on whether the medial lemniscus is involved before or after entry of fibres	
	o Motor	– Corticospinal tracts	▪ Contralateral hemiplagia
	o Sympathetic system	– Horner's syndrome	
	o Cerebellar tracts	– Cerebellar signs	
• Medulla	o Cranial nerves	– VIII (vestibular branches) – IX (glossopharyngeal – X (vagus)	▪ Dysarthria ▪ Dysphagia ▪ Vocal cord paralysis
	o Sensation	– Medial lemniscus	▪ Contralateral loss of position and vibration
	o Motor	– Corticospinal tract	▪ Contralateral hemiplegia
	o Cerebellum	– Cerebellar peduncle	▪ Unilateral cerebellar signs
• Lateral medulla*	o Cranial nerve	– CN V	▪ Ipsilateral loss of sensation of face
	o Sensory	– Lateral spinothalamic	▪ Contralateral loss of pain and temperature
	o Sympathetic	– Ipsilateral Horner's syndrome	

*lateral medullary syndrome

• Medial medulla	o Cranial nerve XII	– Unilateral atrophy of the tongue	
	o Sensation	– Medial lemniscus	

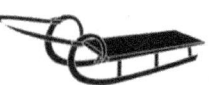

Mastering the Boards: Neurology   A.B.R. Thomson

- Take a directed history and perform a focused physical examination to distinguish between bulbar versus pseudobulbar palsy, and their cause.
  - o Bulbar palsy
    - Clinical
      - CN VII, IX, X, XII
      - Labio-glosso-palato-pharyngeal bilateral LMN lesion
    - Causes
      - Inflammation
        - Poliomyelitis
        - Acute ascending peripheral neuritis
        - Encephalitis lethargic
        - Bolulism
        - Syphilis
  - o Pseudobulbar palsy
    - Clinical
      - Tongue – spastic
      - Palate – paralysed
      - Jaw jerk positive
      - Face fixed, emotionless
      - Pyramidal signs
      - Emotions disturbed
    - Causes/associations
      - Bilateral cerebral thrombosis
      - Motor neuron disease
      - Multiple sclerosis

SO YOU WANT TO BE A NEUROLOGIST!

- Give examples of neurological conditions which undergo **remission and relapses**.

  - o Multiple sclerosis (MS)
  - o Infections (of CNS)
  - o Myasthenia gravis (MG)

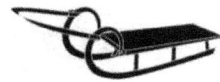

- Take a directed history and perform a focused physical examination to distinguish between pseudobalbar and bulbar palsy.

	Pseudobulbar Palsy (UMN)	Bulbar Palsy (LMN)
o Prevalence	– Common	▪ Rare
o Type of lesion	– UMN	▪ LMN, muscle
o Site of lesion	– Bilateral, usually in the internal capsule	▪ Medulla oblongata
o Tongue	– Small, stiff and spastic	▪ Flaccid, fasciculations
o Speech	– Slow, thick and indistinct	▪ Nasal "twang"
o Nasal regurgitation	– Not prominent	▪ Prominent
o Jaw jerk	– Brisk	▪ Normal or absent
o Other findings	– UMN lesions of the limbs	▪ LMN lesions of the limbs
o Affect	– Emotionally labile	▪ Normal affect
o Causes	– Strokes – Multiple sclerosis – Motor neuron disease – Creutzfeld-Jakob disease	▪ Motor neuron disease ▪ Poliomyelitis ▪ Guillain-Barre syndrome ▪ Myasthenia gravis ▪ Myopathy

Adapted from: Baliga RR. *Saunders/Elsevier*, 2007, page 227; Talley NJ, et al. *Maclennan & Petty Pty Limited* 2003, Table 10.6, page 384.

Clinical Tips

- o Hemiplegia may be
    - – UMN (upper motor neuron) disease
    - – Extrapyramidal disease
    - – Hysterical disorder

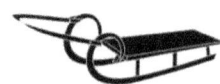

INCREASED INTRACELLULAR PRESSURE (ICP)

Normal Pressure Hydrocephalus (NPH)

➢ Definition
  o Cognition decline
    − ↓ memory
    − Executive function
  o Gait abnormal
    − Shuffling
    − Wide base
    − Retropulsion
    − Pull test abnormal
    − Freezing
      ▪ Turning
      ▪ Starting to stop
  o Urinary frequency/incontinence
  o CSF (cerebrospinal pressure) 150 mm Hg

➢ Associations
  o ↓ absorption of CSF from previous
    − Meningitis
    − SAH (subarachnoid hemorrhage)

SO YOU WANT TO BE A NEUROLOGIST!

• Give the difference in the physical examination of the abnormal gait which help to distinguish NPH (normal pressure hydrocephalus) from Parkinson disease, or parkinsonism-like disorders with lower-body parkinsonism.

  o In NPH, leg function in the supine and sitting positions is normal or almost normal

---

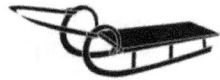

Mastering the Boards: Neurology   A.B.R. Thomson

Hydrocephalus

➤ Clinical

- Take a directed history to distinguish communicating from obstructive (non-communicating) **hydrocephalus**.
  - o Impaired mental state, gait as well as urinary problems, plus
  - o Obstructive hydrocephalus also shows
    - – Nausea and vomiting
    - – Lethargy
    - – Headache
    - – Visual changes

Source: Mangione S. *Hanley & Belfus* 2000, page 762.

Idiopathic Intracranial Hypertension
  - o IIH (aka pseudotumour cerebri) is often diagnosed in obese females with headache, altered vision with papilledema and CN VI palsy and tinitis.
  - o ↑ CSF pressure on lumbar punature (> 250 mm H_2O)
  - o Ventricles may be narrow, but often MRI is normal

➤ Causes/associations

- Give the causes of **benign intracranial hypertension** (Pseudotumour celebri)

  - o CNS
    - – Addison disease
    - – Head injury
    - – Sagital sinus thrombosis (SST)
    - – Scarring from previous meningitis
  - o CVS.
    - – ↑ RV (right ventricular) pressure
    - – SVC (superior venacava syndrome)
    - – AV malformation and shunt

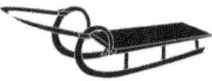

- o Endocrine
  - – Obesity
  - – Pregnancy
  - – Polycystic ovary syndrome
  - – Hypoadrenalism
  - – Hypoparathyroidism

- o Blood
  - – Anemia
  - – Polycythemia

- o Drugs
  - – Tetracycline, chlortetracycline, nalixide acid, oral contraceptive agents
  - – Anabolic drugs
    - ▪ Steroids
    - ▪ Growth hormones
  - – High intake of vitamin A
  - – Change in steroid dosage

- o GU
  - – Pregnancy
  - – Menarche

Adapted from Davies: IJT. *Lloyd-Luke (medical books) LTD* 1972, page 286.

- Perform a focused physical examination for the causes of benign intracranial hypertension (**pseudotumour cerebri**).

  - o Drugs
    - – Change in corticosteroid dosage
    - – Chlortetracycline, nalidixic acid, oral contraceptives

  - o Head
    - – Head injury
    - – Sagittal sinus thrombosis
  - o Female reproductive
    - – Pregnancy
    - – Obesity
    - – Menarche

  - o Hematology
    - – Anemia
    - – Polycythemia

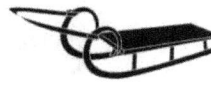

- Metabolic
  - Addison disease
  - Hypoparathyroidism

➢ Treatment
  - Treat underlying cause, if present, including weight reduction
  - Acetazolamide, 250-500 mg po bid, up to 4 g /day (to ↓ CSF production)
    - Multiple LPs
    - Shunting
    - Ophthalmologic procedures in situation of ↑ loss of vision

- Give the clinical effect of **uncus herniation** (temporal lobe).

  - Causes sequential compression of the brainstem
    - Thalamus
    - Midbrain
    - Pons
    - Medulla

- Take a directed history and perform a focused physical examination for **increased intracranial pressure** (↑ ICP).

  - History
    - Headache
    - Vomiting
    - Epilepsy
    - Mental changes
  - Papilledema (blockage of retinal veins)
  - False localising signs
  - Signs of temporal pressure cone

- Perform a focused physical examination for a **temporal pressure cone**.

➢ Translational neuroanatomy
  - With an increase in the intracranial pressure (ICP), the temporal lobes and the midbrain may be forced through the hiatus formed by the two free edges of the tentorium

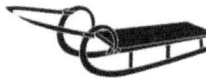

- o This places pressure on
  - – Cerebral peduncles
  - – Midbrain
  - – CN III/VI
  - – Posterior cerebral arteries

- ➢ Physical findings
  - o Contralateral hemiplegia (pressure on cerebral peduncle on side of tumour)
  - o Ipsilateral CN III palsy - fixed dilated pupil
  - o Ipsilateral CN VI – paralysis of ipsilateral rectus muscle
  - o Posterior cerebral artery occlusion – homonymous hemianopia
  - o Midbrain infarction

- ➢ In the context of increased intracranial pressure, perform a focused physical examination for a "**false localizing sign**" for hemiplegia.
  - o Increased intracranial pressure from a tumour will usually place pressure on the same side as the cerebral peduncle, and thereby cause a contralateral hemiplegia
  - o Sometimes a brain tumour will displace the brain to the side, putting pressure on the cerebral peduncle on the side opposite to the Tumour
  - o This causes ipsilateral hemiplegia, so that the paraplegia will appear on the same side as the tumour
  - o The localization of the paraplegia to the same as the tumour, rather than opposite side as would be expected, is known as a "false localising sign"

- • Perform a focused physical examination for a **foramen magnum pressure cone**.

- ➢ Translational neuroanatomy
  - o If the increased intracranial pressure increases in the posterior fossa, the posterior fossa part of the cerebellum is pushed through the foramen magnum, and the medulla is forced downwards with compression exerted on the anterior and posterior parts of the medulla.
  - o When herniation is due to a congenital anomaly, the foramen magnum pressure cone is due to an Arnold-chiare malformation.

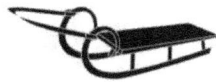

- ➤ Physical findings
  - o Anterior pyramidal tracts
  - o Posterior column nuclei compression of loss of proprioception
  - o Bulbar palsy
  - o Pain in neck
  - o Cerebellar signs
  - o Obstructive hydrocephalus if the forth ventricle is brocked
  - o Associated with syringomyelia, meningocele

Crossed Hemiplegia

- ➤ Anatomy
  - o The fact that the upper motor neurons of the cranial nerves decussate at a higher level than the decussation of the pyramids explains the phenomenon of crossed hemiplegia, i.e., weakness of the opposite side of the body with weakness of the cranial nerve muscles on the same side.
  - o A lesion which damages the cranial nerve after it has decussated, which also damages the pyramidal tract before it has decussated, will cause a crossed hemiplegia.

- ➤ Causes/associations
  - o The best known of crossed hemiplegias are:
    - The posterior columns, which contain uncrossed fibres, form the medial lemnisci which decussate in the medulla.
    - The anterior spinothalamic (light touch) which forms the reticular substance in the medulla, and then joins the medial lemniscus in the pons.

- ➤ Clinical

- • Perform a focused physical examination to distinguish between an intramedullary from an extramedullary cord lesion.

	Intramedullary	Extramedullary
o Root pain	– Rare	▪ Common
o Corticospinal signs	– Late onset	▪ Early onset
o LMN signs	– Extend for several segments	▪ Localized

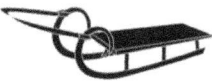

	Intramedullary	Extramedullary
o Sensory loss	– Dissociated sensory loss (pain and temperature) may be present	▪ Brown-Sequard syndrome if lateral cord compression
o Sacral sparing	– May have sacral sparing	▪ No sacral sparing
o CSF fluid	– Normal or minimally altered	▪ Early, marked abnormalities

Abbreviations: CSF, cerebrospinal fluid; LMN; lower motor neuron

Adapted from: Talley NJ, et al. *Maclennan & Petty Pty Limited* 2003, Table 10.28, page 427.

- **Lateral Medullary Syndrome**

➢ Definition
   o The LMS results from infarction of a wedge-shaped area of the lateral aspect of the medulla and inferior surface of the cerebellum, due to occlusion of any of the following five vessels:
     – Posterior inferior cerebellar artery
     – Vertebral artery
     – Superior, middle or inferior lateral medullary arteries

   o The deficits are caused by involvement of one side of the nucleus ambiguous, trigeminal nucleus, vestibular nuclei, cerebellar peduncle, spinothalamic tract and autonomic fibres.

   o Cerebellar signs on the same side (including ipsilateral Horner syndrome).

   o Pain and temperature sensory loss on the opposite side (dissociated sensory loss).

Adapted from: Baliga RR. *Saunders/Elsevier* 2007, page 222.

- **Medial Medullary Syndrome**

- Take a directed history and perform a focused physical examination for Wallenberg syndrome Lateral Medullary Syndrome (LMS).

   o History
     – Severe nausea, vomiting, nystagmus (involvement of the lower vestibular nuclei).
     – Limb ataxia (involvement of the inferior cerebellar peduncle).
     – Intractable hiccups, dysphagia (ninth and tenth cranial nerve involvement).

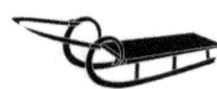

- Physical
  - Ipselateral contralateral loss of pain and temperature sensation
  - Nystagmus
  - Ipsilateral involvement of CN V, VI, VII, VIII
  - Bulbar palsy:
    - Impaired gag
    - Sluggish palatal movements
  - Horner syndrome
  - Ipselateral cerebellar signs on the same side
  - Contralateral pain and temperature sensory loss on the opposite side (dissociated sensory loss).

SO YOU WANT TO BE A NEUROLOGIST!

- Give the **site of the lesion** in the lateral medullary syndrome.

  - Infarction of a wedge-shaped area of the lateral aspect of the medulla and inferior surface of the cerebellum.
  - The deficits are caused by involvement of one side of the nucleus ambiguus, tigeminal nucleus, vestibular nuclei, cerebellar peduncle, spinothalamic tract and autonomic fibres.

- Give the reason why a lesion of the lateral side of the medulla cause ipsilateral loss of sensation of the face, but contralateral loss of sensation (pain and temperature).

  - A lesion of the lateral side of the medulla affects the descending tract of cranial nerve V (trigeminal nerve) before it crosses in the cranial portion of the spinal cord, whereas the fibres of the lateral spinothalamic tract cross after they enter the spinal cord.

- Give the meaning of the medial medullary syndrome.
  - Occlusion of the lower basilar artery of vertebral artery.
  - Ipsilateral lesions result in paralysis and wasting of the tongue.
  - Contralateral lesions result in hemiplegia and loss of vibration and joint position sense.

Source : Baliga RR. *Saunders/Elsevier*, 2007, page 230.

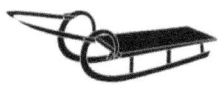

Mastering the Boards: Neurology   A.B.R. Thomson

SPINAL CORD

➢ Anatomy: Spinal cord - Transverse section

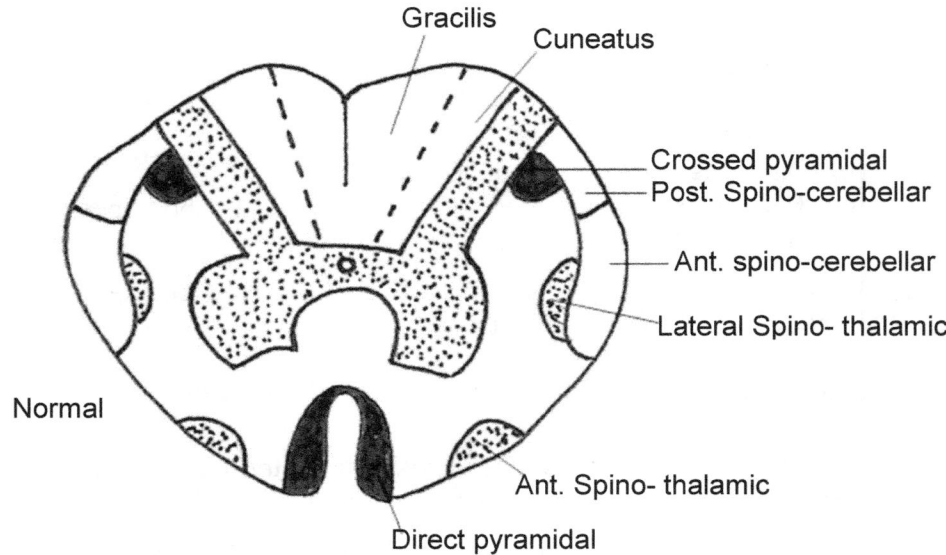

Adapted from: Burton JL. *Churchill Livingstone* 1971, page 83.

- o Spinal pathways
  - – The sensations of pain and vibration enter the posterior nerve tracts, to cells in the posterior horn in the posterior column, and terminate in the nucleus gracilus and cuneatus
  - – From these nuclei are derived the deep arcuate fibres, which cross the midline to form the sensory decussation
  - – In the medulla the sensory decussation is continued upwards as the medial lemniscus, which at this level is not yet split
  - – In the pons the medial lemniscus divides into right and left parts, and is joined by the lateral spinothalamic tract
  - – This continues through the midbrain into the posterior limb of the interval capsule, and terminates mainly in the thalamus

Adapted from: Davies IJT. *Lloyd-Luke (medical books) LTD* 1972, page 244.

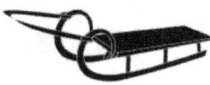

➤ Causes/associations

- Give the causes of spinal cord disorders.
  - Paraplegia or quadriplegia due to complete transverse lesions
  - Effect depends on level (e.g., C1-C3: death from respiratory paralysis)
  - Two stages:
    - Two stages:
      - Loss of all reflex activity below level of lesion
      - Atonic bladder/bowel with overflow incontinence
      - Gastric dilatation
      - Loss of vasomotor control
    - Heightened reflex activity
      - Hyperactive tendon reflex
      - Frequency and urgency of urination, automatic emptying of bladder
      - Hyperactive vasomotor and sweating reactions
  - Central cord syndrome
    - Occurs more often in older people or in patients with cervical spondylosis
    - Weakened hands with impaired pain sensation (most prominent symptom)
  - Relatively little long tract signs

➤ Types of spinal cord disease
  - Anterior cord syndrome
    - Caused by infarction in anterior spinal artery territory or Tumour invasion or inflammatory myelitis in similar region
    - Paraplegia or quadriplegia
    - Bilateral loss of pain and temperature sensation below the lesion
    - Sparing or posterior column (joint position and vibration) sense
  - Conus Medullaris and Cauda Equina syndrome
    - Pain localized to the low back
    - Severe radicular pain in the legs
    - Loss of bladder and bowel control
    - Laxity of the anal sphincter
    - Erectile dysfunction
    - Loss of sensation in sacral segments (saddle parathesia)
    - Often asymmetric leg weakness with upper and lower motor neuron signs

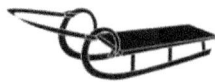

- o Spinal cord syndromes
  - – Motor
    - ▪ Atrophy and areflexia of the arms
    - ▪ UMN lesion of legs
  - – Sensory
    - ▪ Loss of pain and temperature over neck, shoulders and arms
- o Subacute combined degeneration
  - – Motor
    - ▪ UMN signs in both lower limbs
  - – Sensory
    - ▪ Bilateral posterior column
    - ▪ Bilateral loss of position and vibration with ataxic gait
    - ▪ Rarely, peripheral sensory neuropathy
  - – Reflexes
    - ▪ Ankle reflexes absent
    - ▪ Knee reflexes either absent, or exaggerated
      - – Dementia
      - – Optic atrophy

Abbreviations: UMN, upper motor neuron

Adapted from: Mangione S. *Hanley & Belfus* 2000, page 418; Filate W, et al. *The Medical Society, Faculty of Medicine, University of Toronto* 2005, page 175; Talley NJ, et al. *Maclennan & Petty Pty Limited* 2003, pages 422-423, and McGee SR. *Saunders/Elsevier* 2007, pages 175 and 749.

- o Typical sequence
  - – Peripheral neuropathy = peripheral paresthesia
    ↓
  - – Column loss = sensory ataxia
    ↓
  - – Posterior Corticospinal tract damage = paraplegia

  - – No ankle reflexes

- o Hematological abnormality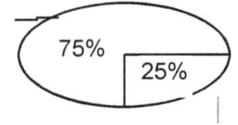

  75%   25%

No hematological abnormalities

- o Cognitive impairment

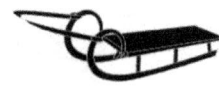

- Cervical myelopathy

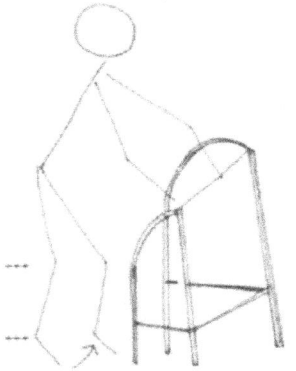

  - ○ Spastic tetraparesis progressive over several years
  - ○ Sensory symptoms less common
  - ○ Often asymmetrical

- Transverse myelitis

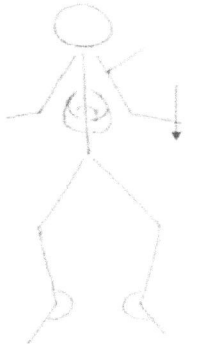

  - ○ Acute onset
    - – May relate to recent infection-'para-infectious'
    - – Commonly due to multiple sclerosis
    - – Occasionally 'band of pain' at affected level', flaccid paralysis

- Anterior spinal artery thrombosis

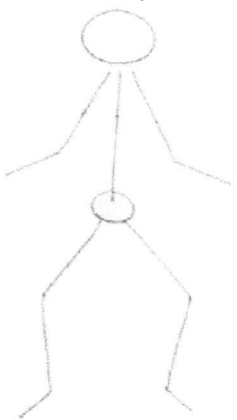

  - ○ Sensory level
  - ○ Flaccid paralysis
  - ○ Urine retention
  - ○ Acute onset
    - – Flaccid paraplegia
    - – Normal dorsal column sensation
    - – Spinal shock
    - – Spasticity develops later
  - ○ Causes/associations
    - – Emboli (e.g., atrial fibrillation)
    - – 'In-situ' thrombosis (e.g., sickle cell disease, hypercoagulable states)
    - – Decompression sickness 'the bends'

Adapted from: Davey P. *Wiley-Blackwell* 2006, page 380.

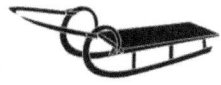

Spinal Cord Compression
- o Neurologic emergency
- o Diagnosis with MRI of spinal cord
  - – If MRI contraindicated (e.g., implantable devices) or unavailable, do CT myelopathy

➤ Causes/associations
- o Vertebral
  - – Spondylosis
  - – Trauma
  - – Prolapse of a disc
  - – Tumour
  - – Infection
- o Outside the dura
  - – Lymphoma, metastases
  - – Infection – e.g., abscess
- o Within the dura but extramedullary
  - – Tumour – e.g., meningioma, neurofibroma
  - – Metastatic
    - ▪ Breast
    - ▪ Lung
    - ▪ Prostate

➤ Clinical
- o Pain
- o Leg weakness
- o Features of primary Tumour

- Give the motor and reflex changes of spinal cord compression
  - o Upper cervical
    - – Upper motor neurone signs in the upper and lower limbs
    - – C5:
      - ▪ LMN- weakness and wasting of rhomboids, deltoids, biceps and brachioradialis
      - ▪ UMN- signs affect the rest of the upper and all the lower limbs.
      - ▪ Reflexes- Biceps reflex is lost, brachioradialis is inverted.
    - – C8:
      - ▪ LMN weakness and wasting of the intrinsic muscles of the hand.
      - ▪ Rflexes- UMN signs in the lower limbs.

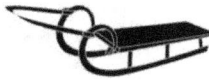

- o Midthoracic
  - – Intercostal paralysis
  - – UMN signs in the lower limbs
  - – Reflexes – loss of upper abdominal reflexes at T7 and T8
  - – T10-T11:
    - ▪ Loss of the lower abdominal reflexes and upward displacement of the umbilicus
    - ▪ UMN – signs in the lower limbs
  - – L1:
    - ▪ Reflexes – cremasteric is lost, normal abdominal reflexes
    - ▪ UMN signs in the lower limbs
  - – L4:
    - ▪ LMN weakness and wasting of the quadriceps
    - ▪ Reflexes – knee reflexes lost
    - ▪ Ankle reflexes may be hyperreflexic with extensor plantar response (up-going toes), but more often there is a lower motor neurone lesion
  - – L5-S1
    - ▪ LMN weakness of knee flexion and hip extension (S1), and abduction (L5) plus calf and foot muscles
    - ▪ Knee present
    - ▪ No ankle reflexes or plantar responses
  - – S3-S4:
    - ▪ Saddle sensory loss
    - ▪ Normal lower limbs
    - ▪ No anal reflex

*Lower motor neurone (LMN) signs may extend for several segments, and spastic paralysis occurs late, unlike the situation with extramedullary lesions.

- • Perform a focused physical examination to determine the site of a spinal cord and nerve root lesions

Site	Signs and symptoms of disorders
o Supratentorial – Cerebral hemispheres – Intracranial portions of CN I and CN II	▪ Defects in vision, olfaction, language, cognition, memory, emotions, autonomic control ▪ Motor and/or sensory deficits on contralateral side of head and body ▪ Symptoms of increased intracranial pressure

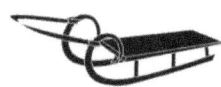

Site	Signs and symptoms of disorders
o Infratentorial – Midbrain – Pons – Medulla – Cerebellum – Intracranial portions of CN III and CN XII	▪ Ipsilateral head signs ▪ Contralateral signs below neck
o Spinal cord or Intraspinal portions of spinal nerves	▪ Frequently bilateral motor, sensory, and autonomic defects at and below the level of the lesion
o Cranial, autonomic, and spinal nerves outside cranium and vertebral canal	▪ Motor, sensory, and autonomic defects in the innervated segments ▪ Asymmetric lesions confined to one or a few segments

Adapted from: Filate W., et al. *The Medical Society, Faculty of Medicine, University of Toronto, 2005*, page 154.

- Perform a focused physical examination to distinguish between total spinal cord transaction or incomplete cord compression.

Physical finding	Total cord transection	Incomplete cord compression
o Paraplegia in flexion	+	+
o Paralysis	Symmetric	Asymmetrical
o Flexor – withdrawal reflex	Withdrawal phase without return)	+ with return to original position
o Other	Vasomotor and sphincter changes	Variable area of anaesthesia which is not consistent with motor loss

Source: Baliga RR. *Saunders/Elsevier* 2007, page 17.

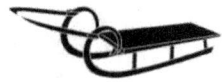

Mastering the Boards: Neurology   A.B.R. Thomson

- Give the triad of symptoms which suggest spinal cord disease.
    - Sensory level, a band of sensory change around the chest or abdomen
        - or a sharp level below which sensation is lost
    - Distal
        - usually symmetric weakness
    - Bowel and bladder changes

Source: Mangione S. *Hanley & Belfus* 2000, page 418.

- Give the lesions involving various sensory modalities.

Location of lesion	Distribution of Sensory Loss
○ Cortical (parietal)	– Able to recognize all primary modalities but localizes them poorly; loss of secondary modalities
○ Thalamic sensory pathway loss	– Contralateral hemisensory loss all modalities (face,body) and pain – Dysesthesia (e.g., burning feeling)
○ Brainstem	– Ipsilateral face – Pain and temperature – Contralateral body
○ Spinal cord	– Depends on level of lesion and complete vs.. partial lesion
○ Root or roots	– Confined to single root or roots in close proximity – Commonly C5,6,7 in arm and L4,5, S1 in leg
○ Peripheral nerve	– Distal "glove and stocking" deficit
○ Single nerve	– Within distribution of single nerve; commonly median, ulnar, peroneal, lateral cutaneous nerve

Adapted from: Filate W, et al. *The Medical Society, Faculty of Medicine, University of Toronto* 2005, Table 16, page 168.

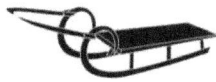

SO YOU WANT TO BE A NEUROLOGIST!

- In the context of a crossed hemiplegia, give the meaning of the Weber, Millard and Foville syndrome.

  o Weber syndrome: ipsilateral lower motor neurone lesion of the oculomotor nerve with contralateral hemiplegia.

  o Millard Gubler syndrome: lower motor neurone lesion of the abducens nerve which supplies the lateral rectus and contralteral hemiplegia.

  o Foville syndrome: in which there is a hemiplegia with paralysis of conjugate deviation towards the side of the lesion, i.e., the eyes are fixed towards the weak side; in a hemiplegia due to a lesion in the internal capsule, the eyes tend to be fixed away from the weak side.

  o Hemiplegia on one side with weakness of muscles supplied by the lower cranial nerves (IX-XII) on the opposite side.

Source: Davey P, *Wiley-Blackwell* 2006, page 246.

- Perform a focused physical examination to **localize** a spinal cord lesion to a specific lumbar or sacral nerve root level.
  - o 5th lumbar root level (L5)
    - Muscular weakness: hamstring, peroneus longus, extensors of all the toes
    - Deep tendon reflexes affected: none
    - Radicular pain/paraesthesia: buttock, posteolateral thigh, anterolaeral leg, dorsum of foot
    - Superficial sensory deficit: dorsum of the foot and anterolateral aspect of the leg
  - o 1st sacral root level (S1)
    - Muscular weakness: plantar flexors, extensor digitorum bevis, peroneus longus, hamstrings
    - Deep tendon reflexes affected: ankle jerk
    - Radicular pain/paraesthesia: buttock, back of thigh, calf and lateral border of the foot
    - Superficial sensory deficit: lateral border of the foot
  - o Lower sacral root level
    - Muscular weakness: none
    - Deep tendon reflexes affected: none (but anal reflex impaired)
    - Radicular pain/paraesthesia: buttock and back of thigh
    - Superficial sensory deficit: saddle and perianal areas

Adapted from: Mangione S. *Hanley & Belfus* 2000, page 418; Filate W, et al. *The Medical Society, Faculty of Medicine, University of Toronto* 2005 , page 175; Talley NJ, et al. *Maclennan & Petty Pty Limited*2003 pages 422-423.

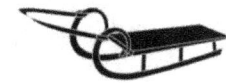

- Give the causes of dissociated sensory loss of only the spinothalamic tract or the dorsal column.

Only spinothalamic tract loss	Only Dorsal Column Loss
o Brown-Séquard syndrome (contralateral leg)	– Brown-Séquard syndrome (ipsilateral leg)
o Syringomyelia	– Subacute combined degeneration
o Anterior spinal artery thrombosis	– Spinocerebellor degeneration (Friedreich's ataxia)
o Diabetes	– Multiple sclerosis
o Amyloid	– Tabes dorsalis
o Lateral medullary syndrome (contra-lateral signs)	– Diabetes – Hypothyroidism – Dorsal root ganglion opathy (cancer, Sjögren syndrome, diabetes mellitus)

Adapted from: Talley NJ, et al. *Maclennan & Petty Pty Limited* 2003, page 424.

- Give the cervical spine movements and their respective myotomes.

Movement	Myotome
o Neck flexion	
– Forward	C1-C2
– Sideways	C3
o Shoulder	
– Elevation	C4
– Abduction	C5
o Elbow	
– Flexion and/or wrist extension	C5
– Extension and/or wrist flexion	C7
o Thumb	
– Extension and/or ulnar deviation	C8
– Abduction and/or adduction of hand intrinsics	T1

Adapted from: Filate W, et al. *The Medical Society, Faculty of Medicine, University of Toronto* 2005, page138.

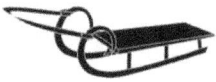

Spinal Cord Syndromes (Myelopathies; aka Spinal Cord Dysfunction)

➢ Types
- o Consider as
  - – Compressive or non-compressive, and so
  - – Intrinsic or extrinsic (intra- or extramedullary)

➢ Causes/associations
- o Compression
  - – Tumour/mass
- o Noncompression
  - – Inflamamation/immune
    - • Multiple sclerosis
    - • Neuromyelitis optica (aka "Devic disease)
  - – Infection
    - • Obstruction of anterior spinal artery
  - – Insufficiency
    - • Cobalamin (vitamin Ba)
    - • Copper
  - – Idiopathic
    - • Idiopathic transverse myelitis

➢ Clinical
- o Symmetric or asymmetric - ↓ motor/ ↓ sensory function
- o Motor
  - – Spastic
  - – Hyperreflexia
  - – Positive Babinski (extensor plantar response)
- o Sensory
  - – Loss
  - – Neuropathic discomfort
- o Cord myelopathy-UMN (upper motor neuron)
  - – Spastic paralysis
  - – ↑ DTRs (deep tendon reflexes)
  - – Exterior plantar responses

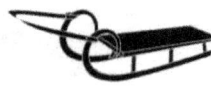

- o Cauda equine
  - – LMN (lower motor neuron)
    - ▪ Flaccid paralysis
    - ▪ No reflexes
- o Sensory loss below level of lesion (UMN and LMN motor loss is at or below lesion)
- o Incontinence occurs with severe myelopathies
- o Gait may be abnormal e.g.,
  - – Spastic gait
  - – Ataxia
  - – Paralysis

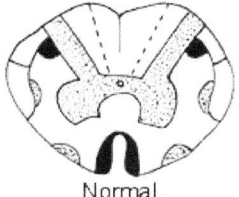

Normal

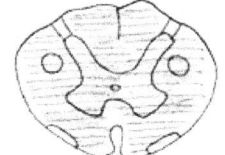

Complete cord transection

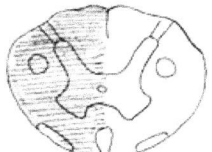

Brown-Sequard syndrome

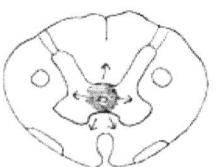

Central lesion
(Syringomyelia)

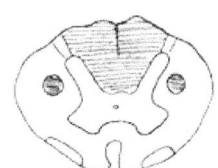

Posterolateral column syndrome
(Subacute combined degeneration)

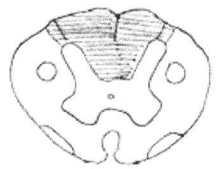

Posterior columns syndrome
(Tabes dorsalis)

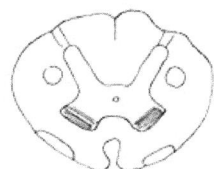

Anterior cell syndrome

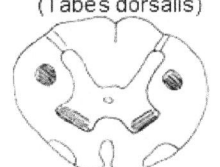

Combined anterior horn cell
pyramidal tract syndrome
(amyotrophic lateral sclerosis)

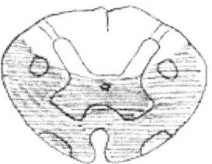

Anterior spinal artery
occlusion

Adapted from: Talley NJ, et al. *Maclennan & Petty Pty Limited* 2003, Figure. 10-52, page 423.

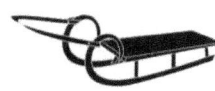

➤ Sensory syndromes
   o The gray shadding indicates hypalgesia (loss of pain temperature sensation).
   o The arrows indicate limbs with significant accompanying weakness.
   o In the Brown-Sequard syndrome (hemisection of the cord), there is often diminished tactile sensation on the side of weakness and opposite the side with hypalgesia.

• Perform a focused physical examination to detect the following sensory syndromes.

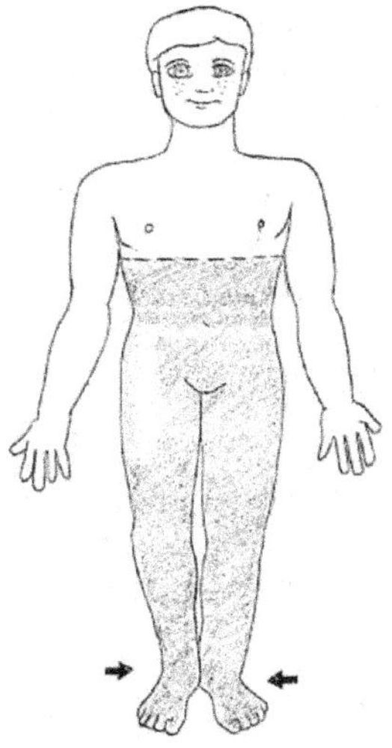

Complete spinal cord injury and anterior cord syndrome

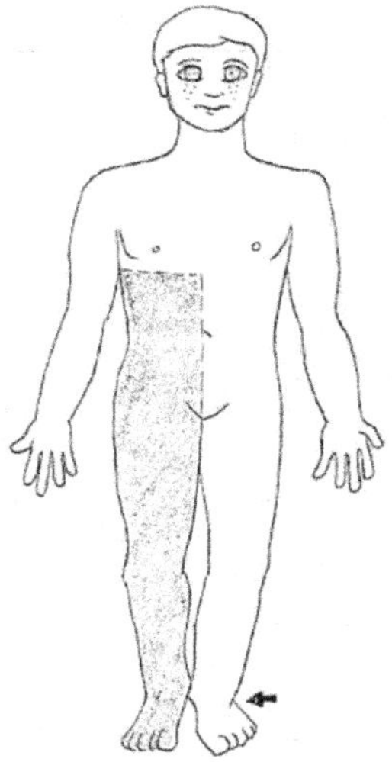

Brown-sequard syndrome

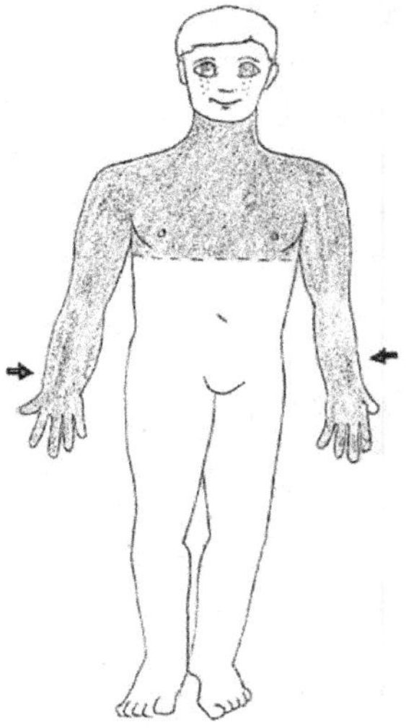

Central cord syndrome (syringomyelia)

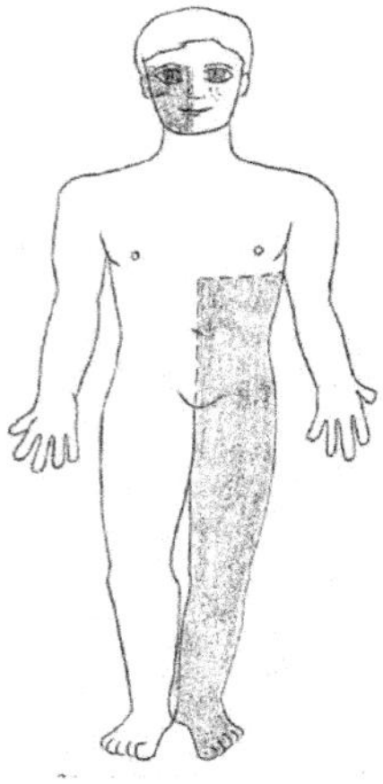

Brainstem injury

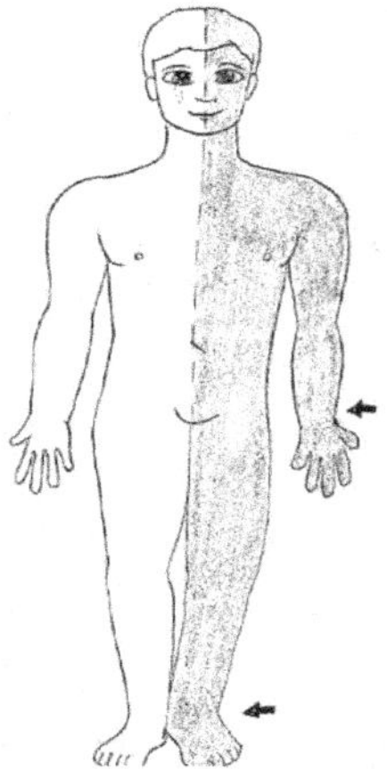

Thalamic or cerebral hemisphere injury

Adapted from: McGee SR. *Saunders/Elsevier* 2007, Figure 58-2, pages 746 to 747.

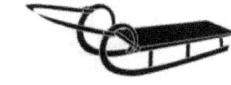

Mastering the Boards: Neurology   A.B.R. Thomson

- Perform a focused physical examination for the causes and site of spinal cord compression.

  o Intra-medullary
    - Neoplasm
    - Cyst
    - Hematomyelia

  o Intra-dural extra-medullary
    - Arachnoiditis
    - Cyst

  o Meninges, dura
    - Neoplasm (Meningioma, neurofibroma, metastatic Ca)
    - Hodgkin leukemic infiltrate
    - Abscess
    - Cyst
    - Epidural abscess
    - Arachnoiditis
    - Leptomeningitis
    - Meningioma
    - Neurofibroma
    - Lymphoma
    - Leukemia

  o Vertebral column
    - Congenital bone anomaly
    - Trauma
    - Vertebral collapse
    - Disc prolapse, spondylollisthesis, spondylosis
    - Neoplasm (primary or secondary) –glioma, ependymoma, 2°
    - Infection – TB or pyogenic
    - Crush fracture
    - Disc protrusion
    - Tumour
    - Myeloma
    - TB
    - Cervical spondylosis
    - Paget disease

Adapted from: Burton JL. *Churchill Livingstone* 1971, page 83.

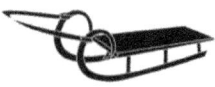

- Perform a focused physical examination of site in the spinal cord for loss of sensation.

Tracts	Sensation
o Posterior column	– Position (proprioception) – ataxia (with eyes closed, aka "Rombergism") – Vibration – Deep pain – Some light touch
o Anterior spinothalamic	– Light touch
o Lateral spinothalamic	– Superficial pain – Temperature – Tickle – "sex"
o Spinocerebellar	– Tone and co-ordination of muscle - ↓ deep tendon reflexes [DTR]*

* The stretch reflex is a proprioceptive reflex, so when the stretch sensory stimulus is reduced in posterior column disease, the DTRs are reduced.

Source: Davies IJT. *Lloyd-Luke (medical books) LTD* 1972, Figure 12, page 243.

SO YOU WANT TO BE A NEUROLOGIST!

- In the context of spinal cord, give the meaning of paragia-in-flexion.

  o Paraplesia-flexion is seen in partial transaction of the cord where the limbs are involuntarily flexed at the hips and kees because the extensors are more paralysed than the flexors.
  o In complete transaction of the spinal cord, the extrapyramidal tracts are also affected and hence no voluntary movement of the limb is possible, resulting in paraplegia-in-extension.

Source: Baliga RR. *Saunders/Elsevier* 2007, page 116.

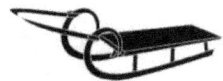

➢ Laboratory

    o Lumbar puncture immune/inflammatory causes

    o Blood   serum B$_{12}$ plus
         – Methylmaloric acid   If serum B$_{12}$
         – Hemocysteine   normal/borderline low

• Give the clinical situation in which the patient may develop cobalamine/copper deficiency leading to myelopathy.

    o Bariotric surgery may lead to malabsorption of cobalamin +/- copper, which leads to myelopathy

    o The patient with Wilson disease (WD) who is treated with high does of zinc to reduce the copper absoption in WD may develop sufficient deficiency to lead to myelopathy.

➢ Differential

Buzz Words Suggestive of Cause of Myelopathy

    o Cobalamin/copper deficiency
        – ↓ position/ vibration sensation, sensory ataxia, gait instability, leg weakness, parestesias/paraparesis
        – ↓methylmalonic acid/homocystein concentrations in blood

    o Idiopathic transverse myelitis
        – Viral infection followed by changes
        – Motor
            ▪ weakness
        – Sensation
        – Bowel/bladder
            ▪ dysfunction

    o Infarction
        – Sudden weakness and
            ▪ Loss of pinprick sensation
            ▪ No loss of position/vibration

    o Neuromyelitis optica
        – Recurrent myelitis and optica plus NMO-IgG autoantibody positive but no avoid white matter lesions on MRI of brain/spinal cord

---

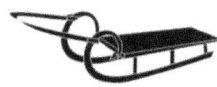

- ➢ Diagnosis
  - o CT / MRI of spinal cord

- ➢ Treatment
  - o Compressive
    - – Decompression
      - ▪ Urgent surgical
      - ▪ Corticosteroids
      - ▪ Radiotherapy
  - o Non-compression
  - o Treat associated conditions
    - – Cobalamine/copper deficiency
  - o Transverse myelitis
    - – IV methylprednisolone ___poor response_____➤
      - ▪ Cyclophosphamide, or
      - ▪ Plasmapharesis
  - o Multiple sclerosis (MS)

  - o IV dexamethasone 20 mg bolus, plus lower dose maintenance
  - o Emergency surgical decompression
  - o Chemoradiotherapy
  - o For Tumour
    - – Radiation
    - – Chemotherapy
  - o For pain
    - – Opioid

  - o Intramedullary*
    - – Tumour- e.g., glioma, ependymoma
    - – Syringomyelia
    - – Haematomyelia

Abbreviations: LMN, lower motor neuron; UMN, upper motor neuron

Adapted from: Talley NJ, et al. *Maclennan & Petty Pty Limited* 2003, Table 10.26, page 421.

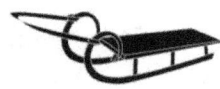

- ➢ Treatment (depends upon cause)
  - o Epidural abscess
    - – Antibiotics
    - – Surgical decompression
  - o Hematoma
    - – Surgical
    - – Decompression
  - o Trauma
    - – High-dose corticosteroids
    - – Stabilizattion of spine, including surgery
  - o Metastases
    - – High-dose corticosteroids
    - – Decompressive surgery, plus
    - – Radiotherapy
  - o Spinal degeneration/disk herniation/scarring (aka myelomalacia)/spinal stenosis plus impingement on nerve root (aka myelopadiculopathy)
    - – Remember that there may be signs of both UML / LMN
    - – Lumbar spinal stenosis
      - ▪ Neuroclaudication
      - ▪ Pain in groin, buttock, thigh, leg

Non-Compressive Myelopathies

- ➢ Causes/associations
  - o Infection
    - – HSV (Herpes simplex virus)
    - – VZ (varicella zoster)
    - – NV (West Nile virus)
    - – HTLV (human T-lymphotropic) virus
    - – Lyme disease
    - – Neurosyphillis
    - – Post-infectious ITM (idiopathic transverse myelitis; please see next page)
    - – HIV
      - ▪ At time of seroconversion, or
      - ▪ Degenerative vacuolar myelopathy
    - – Mycobacterium tuberculosis

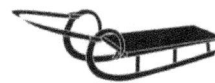

- o Nutritional deficiency
  - – Vitamin B12
  - – Copper

- o Vasculal
  - – Embolus
  - – Thrombus
  - – Hypotension
  - – AV fistulas of spinal blood supply

- o Inflammatory/autoimmune
  - – Rheumatoid arthritis
  - – Sarcoidosis

- o Genetic (aka Hereditary spastic paraplegia)
  - – One example is female carriers of X-linked adrenoleukodystrophy
  - – Results in a chronic progressive myelopathy (adrenomyeloneuropathy)

Ideopathic Transverse Myelitis

➢ Definition:

- o "……. a monophasic demyelinating myelopathy characterized by inflammation of a segment of the spinal cord" (Source: MKSAP 16 2012, Neurology, page 66)

➢ Clinical

- o Follows infection such as
  - – Viral gastroenteritis
  - – URTI (upper respiratory tract infection)

- o Partial myelopathic
  - – Signs of motor, sensory, or motor plus
  - – Sensory changes

- o Motor and/or sensory symptoms may be proceeded by
  - – Back pain
  - – Thoracis sensation of banding

➢ Treatment

- o Exclude other causes of transverse myelitis

- o High dose IV corticoids for 3-5 days

- o If steroid refractory
  - – Cyclophosphamide
  - – Plasmapheresis
  - – Both cyclophosphamide plus plasma pheresis

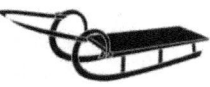

SO YOU WANT TO BE A NEUROLOGIST!

- A patient with Wilson disease is treated with oral zinc for maintenance therapy. In the hope that "more is better", he doubles the dose of zinc. The patient develops deficiencies in sensation of position and vibration. The serum vitamin B12 concentration is normal. Give the likely cause of the posterior column symptoms.
  - o Certainly neurosyphilis, MS and transverse myelitis need to be excluded, but the high dose zinc is likely causing posterior column toxicity.

SO YOU WANT TO BE A NEUROLOGIST!

- Give a clue from physical examination that a myelopathy is due to transverse myelitis rather than other disorders of the spinal cord

  - o In transverse myelitis, the myelopathy is partial, so there may be signs related to motor or sensory symptoms, or both; recall that with a complete transverse lesion, both motor and sensory will be involved.

- Give the clue from the history of the patient that suggests that in the patient with both motor plus sensory changes localized to the spinal cord, that the diagnosis is not idiopathic transverse myelitis (ITM).

  - o The clinical course of ITM is monophasic, so there should not be a recurrence of symptoms.

- In a patient with spinal cord-related symptoms and signs, MRI is performed and shows signal hyperintensity at the posterior aspect of the spinal cord. Give the cause of non-compressive myelopathy which have a predilection for the posterior aspect of the spinal cord.

  - o Predilection for posterior column aspect of spinal cord
    - – Vitamin B12 deficiency
    - – Copper deficiency
    - – Neurosyphilis
    - – MS (multiple sclerosis)
    - – Inflammatory causes of transverse myelitis

- In a woman with spinal cord disease plus a positive family history, give the blood test, which if positive should lead to genetic testing.

  - o In female carriers of X-linked adrenoleukodystrophy will have ↑ serum concentrations of VLCFA (very long chain fatty acids)

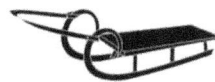

Mastering the Boards: Neurology   A.B.R. Thomson

Cauda Equina Syndrome

➢ Definition

    o Protrusion of disk posterior onto caudia equina, or Tumour, causing unilateral or bilateral pressure on nerve below L2

    o LMN signs

    o Pressure is more likely on the lower sacral nerves than on L3-L5

➢ Clinical

• Perform a focused physical examination for the cauda equina syndrome.

    o Paraplegia
      – Weak
      – Wasted
      – Flaccid

    o Numbness

    o Loss of reflexes
      – Ankle jerk loss, only with S1 lesions

    o Disorder of sphincter control
      – Hesitancy
      – Urgency
      – Retention of urine

    o Impotence

    o Pain in distribution of sciatic nerve

    o DRE patulus anal sphincter

    o Anesthesia
      – Sacral, anal, perianal regions

• Perform a focused physical examination to distinguish between the cauda equina syndrome (please see above), and the cauda equina claudication syndrome (see below).

➢ The features of the **cauda equina claudication syndrome** are

    o Exercise aggravated and rest relieved
      – Bilateral
        ▪ Pain
        ▪ Tingling

    o Weak foot dorsiflexors

    o Reflex changes

Source: Davies IJT. *Lloyd-Luke (medical books) LTD* 1972, page 292.

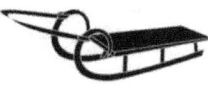

- Take a directed history and perform a focused physical examination for **tabes dorsalis**.
  - o   History
  - o   CNS
    - – Ataxia
  - o   Eyes
    - – Diplopia or ↓ vision
  - o   Voice – crisis: laryngeal
    - – Visceral crises
      - ▪ Gastric
      - ▪ Rectal
  - o   GI
    - – Loss of sphincter control
  - o   GU
    - – Impotence
  - o   MSK
    - – Paresthesia, especially in feet
    - – Lightning pains
  - o   Physical examination
  - o   Face
    - – Tabetic facies
  - o   Eyes
    - – Ptosis
    - – Argyll Robertson pupils
    - – Optic atrophy, etc.
  - o   Muscles
    - – Hypotonia
  - o   Sensation
    - – ↓ proprioception and vibration sense, with Romberginsm and ataxic gait
    - – ↓ superficial and deep pain sensation
  - o   Reflexes
    - – ↓ tendon reflexes (ankles affected first)
  - o   MSK
    - – Charcot joints
  - o   Skin
    - – Neuropathic ulcers

Adapted from: Burton JL. *Churchill Livingstone* 1971, page 89.

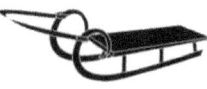

Posterior Column Tract

Cerebral cortex _____

Vibration and proprioception

o These fibres enter and
ascend ipsilaterally in the
posterior columns of the
spinal cord to the nucleus
gracilis and nucleus
cuneatus in the medulla,
where they decussate

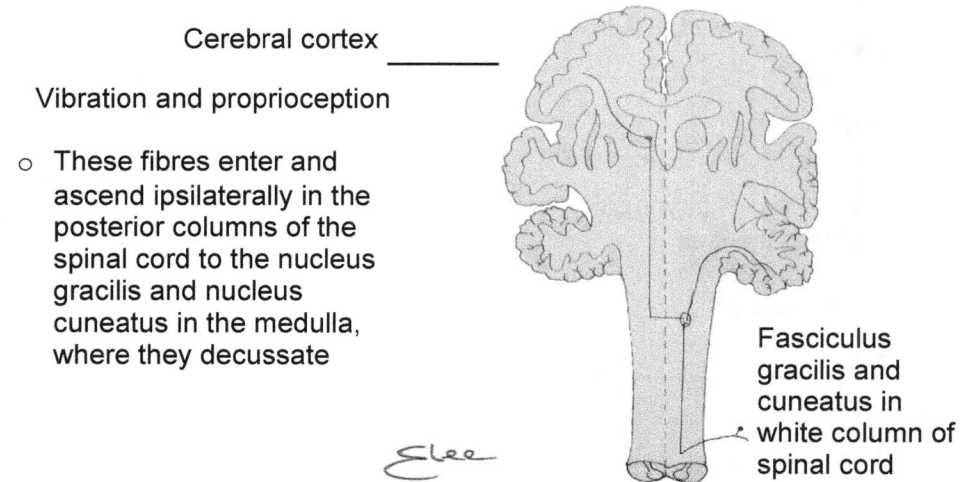

Fasciculus
gracilis and
cuneatus in
white column of
spinal cord

Adapted from: Talley NJ, et al. *Maclennan & Petty Pty Limited* 2003, Figure
10.35, page 399.

"A mind that is stretched by a new experience
can never go back to its old dimensions."

Oliver Wendell Holmes Jr

 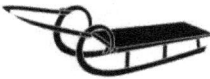

➢ Position/vibration

        Posterior nerve root
           ↓
        Posterior horn
           ↓
        Posterior column
           ↓
        Nucleus gracilis and cuneatus
           ↓
        Deep arcuate fibres   ⟶   Sensory decussation
                                    ↓
                              Open medulla
                                    ↓
        Lateral spinothalamic tract   ⟶   Medial lemniscus
                                    ↓
                          Pons medial lemniscus
                        Splits into R/L components, and
           is poned by the lateral spinothalamic tract
                                    ↓
                                Midbrain
                                    ↓
                      Internal capsule posterior limb
                                    ↓
                                Thalamus

- Perform a focused physical examination for a posterior column lesion.
  - o Sensation
    - – ↓ Position and vibration appreciation
  - o Reflexes
    - – ↓
  - o Tone
    - – Hypotonicity
  - o Balance
    - – Ataxia when eyes close
    - – Walking, looking at feet, to improve balance
    - – Rombergism
      - ▪ Steady with eyes open and feett together; becomes unsteady when eyes closed
  - o Astereognosis
    - – Inability to appreciate size or shape of objects held in their hand

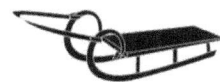

Guillain Barre Syndrome (GBS)

- Take a directed history and perform a focused physical examination for Guillain Barre syndrome (GBS).

➤ History
  o Weakness: difficultly in rising up from sitting position or climbing stair; legs usually affected before upper limbs
  o Dyspnea (late in the course of GBS, suggesting diaphragmatic and intercostals muscle weakness)
  o Cranial nerve involvement:
    – Diplopia
    – Drooling of saliva
    – Regurgitation of food
  o Paresthesias
  o Urinary symptoms
  o Systemic symptoms: (e.g fatigue)
  o Ascertain whether the onset was preceded by a trivial viral illness

➤ Physical
  o Palsy (weakness)
    – Legs, progressing proximally, including cranial nerves
    – Sphincters
    – Bulbar palsy
    – Respiratory muscles
  o Tender muscles
  o Sensory loss (paraesthesiae may occur as a symptom even though there are minimal signs of sensory loss)

- Perform a focused physical examination for subacute combined degeneration of the cord.
  o Posterior column loss symmetrically (vibration and joint position sense)
  o Ataxic gait
  o Upper motor neurone signs in the lower limbs symmetrically with absent ankle reflexes; knee reflexes may be absent or, more often, exaggerated
  o Peripheral sensory neuropathy (less common and mild);
  o Optic atrophy
  o Dementia

Source: Talley NJ, et al. *Maclennan & Petty Pty Limited* 2003, page 423.

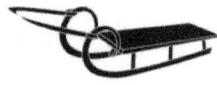

- Give the most common causes/associations of posterior root ganglial conditions.

    o Diabetes

    o Tabes dorsalis

    o Carcinomatous neuropathy

> **Spinal Cord: Spinothalamic (pain and temperature) pathways**

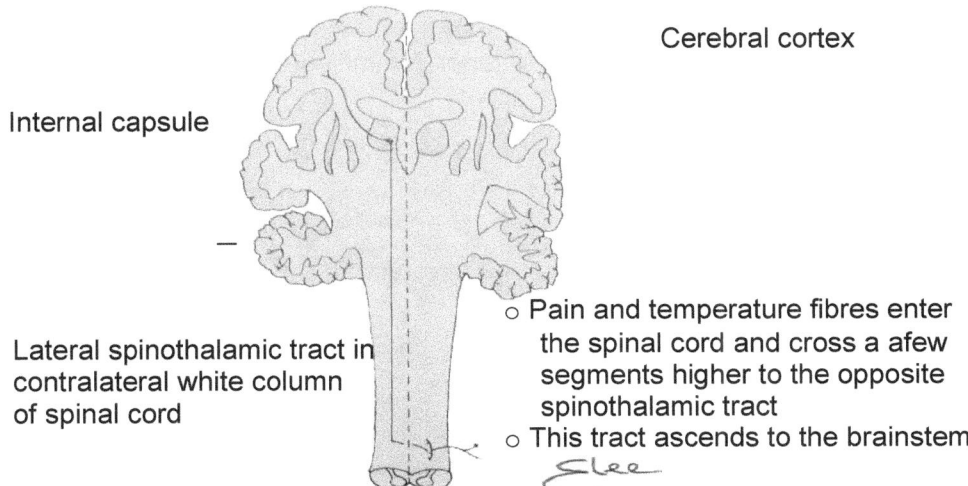

Cerebral cortex

Internal capsule

Lateral spinothalamic tract in contralateral white column of spinal cord

o Pain and temperature fibres enter the spinal cord and cross a afew segments higher to the opposite spinothalamic tract

o This tract ascends to the brainstem

Adapted from: Talley NJ, et al. *Maclennan & Petty Pty Limited* 2003, Figure 10.34, page 398.

Cobalamin and Posterior Column Disease

- Give the name of the mineral which mimics cobalamin deficiency, and may result from bariatric surgery, or the intake of large amounts of zinc.

    o Copper deficiency may damage posterior columns and be associated with sensory ataxia anemia.

Cobalamin deficiency is not always associated with anemia or reduced serum levels of the vitamin.

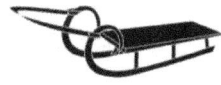

- Give the metabolites to measure to exclude cobalamin deficiency.

  o Serum vitamin B12 (cobalamin) concentrations will be low in late cobalaminedeficiency, and cells may be macrocystic or megaloblastic.

  o Methylmalonic acid and homocysteine concentrations in the blood will be elevated in early cobalamnin deficiency.

Lateral Spinothalamic Tract

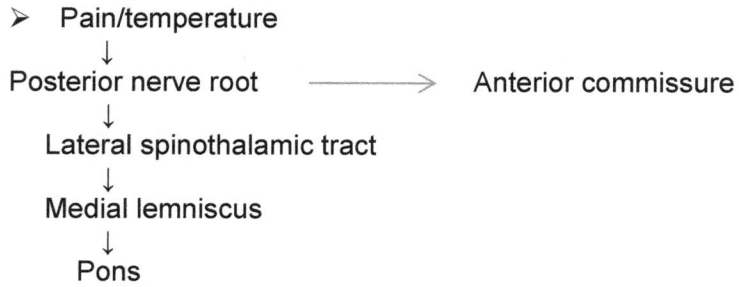

➢ Pain/temperature
↓
Posterior nerve root ⟶ Anterior commissure
↓
  Lateral spinothalamic tract
↓
  Medial lemniscus
↓
    Pons

Spina Bifida

➢ Definition
  o Incomplete closure of the bony vertebral canal
  o Is commonly associated with a similar anomaly of spinal cord
  o The commonest site is the lumbosacral reregion but the cervical spine can be involved
  o May be associated with hydrocephalus

➢ Clinical
  o The lateral cauda equina syndrome:
    – Pain in the anterior thigh
    – Wasting of the quadriceps muscle
    – Weakness of the foot invertors (due to L4 root lesion)
    – Absent knee jerk
    – Causes include neurofibroma, a high disc lesion

  o The midline cauda equina syndrome:
    – Bilateral lumbar and sacral root lesions
    – Causes include disc lesion, primary sacral bone tumours (chordomas), metastatic bone disease (from prostate) and leukemia

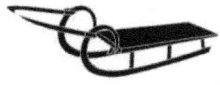

➤ Differentiate

  ○ UMN lesion of conus medullaris (lowest part of spinal cord)

  ○ Other causes of crossed hemiplegia (lesion is in the midbrain)
    – Weber syndrome: contralateral hemiplegia (lesion is in the midbrain) with ipsilateral LMN lesion of the oculomotor nerve.
    – Millare-Gubler syndrome: contralateral hemiplegia (lesion is in the pons) with LMN lesion of the abducens nerve.
    – Foville's syndrome: as Millard-Gubler syndrome, with gaze palsy

Adapted from: Baliga RR. *Saunders/Elsevier* 2007, pages 228,229,237 and 238.

• Perform a focused physical examination for a lesion in the spinal canal at any level below T10 (cauda equina syndrome).

  ○ Flaccid, asymmetrical paraparesis (LMN)

  ○ Knee and ankle jerks are diminished or absent

  ○ Saddle distribution of sensory loss up to the L1 level

  ○ Downgoing plantars

• Perform a focused physical examination for closed spina bifida.

  ○ Skin   – Lumbosacral lipoma
    – Hypertrichosis
    – Sinus or dimple above the sacrum
    – Nevus, or scarring

  ○ MSK   – Unilateral shortening of one leg and foot
    – Loss of muscles below the knee
    – Calcaneovalgus or equinovarus deformity
    – Sensory loss in L5/ S1

  ○ GU   – Neuropathic bladder
    – Enuresis

Adapted from: Baliga RR. *Saunders/Elsevier* 2007, page 174.

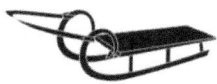

Prolapsed Vertebral Disc

➢ Anatomy

  o Distribution prevalence
    – L5-S1 disk (s1 nerve root), 60%
    – L4-5 disk (L5 nerve root), 30%
    – L4-5 plus L5-S1 disks combined, 10%

• In the context of a prolapsed intervertebral disc, give the nerve roots which supply the pain which radiates to

  o Lateral side of lower leg, and medial side of the foot

  o Lateral side of the foot, and sole of the foot

  o No, not L5 and S1!
    – Pain from a prolapsed intervertebral disc does not radiate in the cutaneous distribution of the nerve root
    – However, numbness and/or tingling (paraesthesiae) may occur along the appropriate cutaneous distribution of L5/S1

➢ Clinical

  o Source of pain from prolapsed vertebral disc
    – Acute
      ▪ Tear of annular fibrosis
      ▪ Protrusion of nucleus pulposus
    – Chronic
      ▪ Stretching of posterior longitudinal ligament of the spine
      ▪ Reflex protection spasm of erector spinae muscle
    – Acute/chronic
      ▪ Pressure on the nerve root
        –Pain along nerve
        –Tender nerve
        –Pain in muscles supplied by the nerve (myotome; e.g., biceps femoris, gastrocnemius, tibialis anterior)

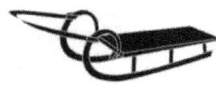

- Perform a focused physical examination for a prolapse intervertebral disc.

    o LMN weakness
        - L5-S1
        - Glutei
            ▪ Extension of thigh – gluteus (G) maximus
            ▪ Abductors of thigh – G. medius and G. minimus
        - Biceps femoris
            ▪ Flexion of knee
        - Peronei
            ▪ Eversion of foot
        - L4-L5
            ▪ Dorsiflexors of the foot
                –"extensor" muscles
                –Tibialis anterior
        - S1-S2
            ▪ Plentar flexors of foot
                –Gastroenemius
                –Soleus
            ▪ Small muscle of foot
                –Ask the patient shape the sole of the foot into a cup

    o Loss of deep tendon reflexes
        - Angle –S1

    o Lumbar spine
        - ↓ movement
        - Loss of normal lumbar lordosis
        - Scoliosis
        - Tenderness

    o Glutei
        - Unilateral drooping of buttock

    o Sciatic nerve
        - Tenderness with pressure over sciatic nerve

    o Leg
        - Reduced ability to raise a straightened leg

    o Cauda Equina syndrome

➤ Causes/associations

    o Centrally placed lumbosacral disc or spondylolisthesis at the lumbosacral junction

    o Tumours of the cauda equina (ependymoma, neurofibroma)

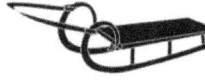

Dissociated Anesthesia

➢ Definition: dissociated anaesthesia is the loss of pain and temperature, but the retention of other sensory modalities.

➢ Neuroanatomy
  o Anterior half of cord
    – The dissociated anaesthesia is always a transient phenomenon
    – LMN at site, bilateral UMN below lesion, spinothalamic below
    – Only common cause is anterior spinal artery thrombosis

  o Lesions in lateral medulla-will affect whole of opposite side of body

➢ Types of dissociated anaesthesia

  o Lesion in centre of spinal cord
    – Bilateral, but not necessarily symmetrical dissociated anaesthesia
    – Upper and lower border to loss of pain and temperature
    – Affects posterior columns, but not the lateral spinothalamic fibres
    – May be associated with involvement of pyramidal tracts and anterior horn cells
    – Common causes
      ▪ Sphingomyelia
      ▪ Spontaneous hematomyelia
      ▪ Tumour

  o Hemisection of cord (Brown-Séquard syndrome)
    – Ipsilateral LMN and posterior column, UMN lesion below level of lesion
    – Contralateral spinothalamic below lesion
    – Causes include:
      ▪ Compression of spinal cord
      ▪ Intramedullary neoplasm (ependymoma)

➢ Clinical

• Perform a focused physical examination for hemisection of the spinal cord (Brown-Sequard syndrome).

  o Deficits at the level of the cord lesion:
    – Ipsilateral LMN paralysis
    – Ipsilateral zone of cutaneous anaesthesia and zone of hyperaesthesia just below the anaesthetic zone
    – Segmental signs are usually unilateral
      ▪ Muscular atrophy
      ▪ Radicular pain
      ▪ ↓ tendon reflexes

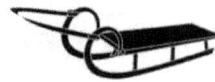

- o Deficits below the level of the cord lesion
    - – Ipsilateral monoplegia or hemiplegia
    - – Ipsilateral loss of joint position and vibration sense
    - – Contralateral loss of spinothalamic (pain and temperature) sensation

- ➢ Causes/associations
    - o Cord tumour
    - o Syringomyelia
    - o Trauma
    - o Degenerative disease of spine
    - o Multiple myeloma
    - o Hematomyelia

Adapted from: Baliga RR. *Saunders/Elsevier* 2007, pages 236 and 237.

- ➢ Differential diagnosis
    - o Multiple sclerosis (MS)
    - o Lesion of anterior half of cord
        - – Transient dissociated anaesthesia
        - – At level of lesion
            - ▪ LMN changes
        - – Below lesion
            - ▪ UMN changes
            - ▪ Spinothalmic sensory changes
        - – Common cause
            - ▪ Thrombosis of anterior spinal artery
    - o Lesion of lateral medulla
        - – Dissociated anaesthesia of all of the opposite side of the body
        - – Common causes

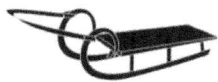

Spastic Paraperisis

- Perform a focused physical examination for causes of spastic paraperisis.

    o Inherited
      - Friedreich's ataxia
      - Familial spastic paraplegia

    o Infection
      - HIV
      - Tabes dorsalis
      - Transverse myelitis (involves all tracts of spinal cord; spastic or flaccid paralysis
        - May be incomplete cord compression
        - Total cord transaction

    o Infiltration
      - Spinal cord Tumour (meningioma, neuroma)
      - Metastatic carcinoma
      - Parasagittal falx meningioma

    o Degeneration
      - Motor neuron disease
      - Syringomyelia
      - Osteoarthritis of the cervical spine

    o Nutritional
      - Vitamin deficiency
      - Subacute combined degeneration of the cord

    o Vascular
      - Anterior spinal artery thrombosis
      - Atherosclerosis of spinal cord vasculature

    o Trauma

Adapted from: Baliga RR. *Saunders/Elsevier* 2007, page 116.

"We don't see things the way they are.
We see them the way WE are."

Talmud

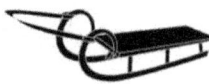

Mastering the Boards: Neurology   A.B.R. Thomson

Friedrich Ataxia

➤ Definition: spinocerebellar degeneration

  ○ Marked loss of cells in the posterior root ganglia

  ○ Degeneration of peripheral sensory fibres

  ○ Involvement of the posterior and lateral columns of the cord

➤ Clinical

• Take a directed history and perform a focused physical examination for Friedreich ataxia.

  ○ History
    – Age of onset (usually the same in each family, and ranges from 8 to 16 years of age)
    – High-arched foot in childhood in the family (Friedreich's foot).
    – Scoliosis developing in childhood
    – Cerebellar dysarthria and ataxia

  ○ CNS
    – Cerebellar signs (bilateral) including nystagmus
    – Optic atrophy (uncommon)
    – Normal mentation

  ○ Peripheral nerves
    – Peripheral neuropathy

  ○ Heart
    – Cardiomyopathy (ECG abnormalities occur in more than 50% of cases)

  ○ MSK
    – Spine
    – Kyphoscoliosis

  ○ Limbs
    – Pes cavus – cocking of the toes (other causes of pes cavus include hereditary motor and sensory neuropathy, spinocerebellar degeneration or neuropathies in childhood
    – Upper motor neurone signs in the limbs (although reflexes are absent)
    – Posterior column loss in the limbs

  ○ Signs of diabetes
    – Diabetes mellitus (common)

Abbreviations: CNS, central nervous system; ECG, electrocardiogram
Printed with permission: Talley NJ, et al. *Maclennan & Petty Pty Limited* 2003, Table 10.33, page 433.

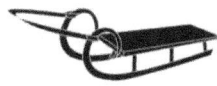

Mastering the Boards: Neurology   A.B.R. Thomson

➢ Diagnosis

● Give the **Harding criteria** for Friedreich ataxia

    ○ Essential criteria are onset before the age of 25 years
- Ataxia of limbs and gait
- Absent knee and ankle jerks
- Extensor plantars
- Autosomal recessive inheritance
- Motor conduction velocity greater than 40 ms
- Small or absent sensory nerve action potentials
- Dysarthria within 5 years of onset

    ○ Additional criteria (present in two thirds)
- Scoliosis
- Pyramidal weakness of lower limbs
- Absent upper limb reflexes
- Loss of vibration and joint position sense in the legs
- Abnormal ECG
- Pes cavus

    ○ Other features (present in less than 50% of cases)

    ○ Nystagmus

    ○ Optic atrophy

    ○ Deafness

    ○ Distal muscle wasting and diabetes

Source: Baliga RR. *Saunders/Elsevier* 2007, pages 191-193.

Syringomyelia and Syringobulbia

➢ Definition

    ○ Formation of a cavity in the inner portion of the cord

    ○ Destruction of the white and grey matter and an accompanying reactive gliosis

    ○ The process generally begins in the cervical cord, and with expansion of the cavity the brainstem and distal cord also become affected

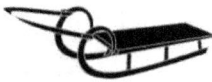

➤ Neuroanatomy

    o Involvement of
       – Cord
          ▪ Syringomyelia
       – Brainstem
          ▪ Syringobulbia

    o Gliosis and syrinx anterior to
       – The central canal
       – The docussation of the fibres of the lateral spinothalamic tract
       – Anterior horn cells
       – Pyramidal tracts

➤ Clinical

- Perform a focused physical examination for syringomyelia in a portion of the cervical cord.

    o In the affected cervical segment, or above
       – Lateral spinothalamic tract
       – Loss of pain, temperature, tickle, sex

    o In the affected segment
       – Anterior horn cells
       – LMN lesions in the corresponding motor nerve

    o Small muscles of the hands and forearm
       – ↓ tone
       – Weakness
       – Wasting
       – Fasciculation
       – ↓ DTR

    o Below the affected segment
       – Pyramidal tracts
       – UMN lesions

    o Sensory loss
       – ↓ pain and temperature sensation
       – Pain and temperature in lower face (descending tract of trigeminal nerve)
       – Intact vibration, light touch and joint position sense

      o Sympathetic pathway in cervical cord
        – Horner syndrome
        – Nystagmus (vestibular spinal tracts)

      o Charcot joints of the shoulder and elbow

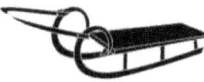

- o *At the level of the syrinx*
    - LMN lesion, causing anterior horn cell involvement
    - Involvement of the central decussating fibres of the spinothalamic tract producing
    - Dissociated sensory loss
    - Development of neuropathic arthropathy
    - Trophic changes
- o *Below the level of the syrinx:*
    - Involvement of pyramidal corticospinal tracts resulting in spastic paraparesis (sphincter function is usually well preserved)
- o *Involvement of cervical sympathetic*
    - Horner syndrome (miosis, enophthalmos, ptosis)
- o "la main succulente"
    - Ugly hand
    - Cold
    - Cyanosed
    - Swollen fingers and palms

➢ Differential

- o Anterior spinal artery occlusion (affecting the dorsal horn and lateral spinothalamic tract)
- o Diabetic small-fibre polyneuropathy
- o Hereditary amyloidotic polyneuropathy
- o Leprosy (the latter three conditions affect small peripheral nerve axons)

- o Other conditions with a similar picture
    - Intramedullary tumours of the spinal cord
    - Arachnoiditis around the foramen magnum obstructing the CSF pathway
    - Hematomyelia
    - Craniovertebral anomalies
    - Late sequelae of spinal cord injuries (manifest as a painful ascending myelopathy)
    - Rarely patients may have hypertrophy in limbs hand and feet
    - If fasciculation is seen, then the other diagnosis to consider is motor neuron disease

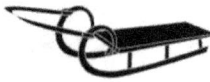

- In the context of cervical spondylosis, give the meaning of "inversion" of the biceps and triceps, deep tendon reflexes, and give the neuroanatomic explanation for this sign.
  - A lesion at C6 will cause a LMN lesion of the biceps muscle supplied by C5, 6, and an UMN lesion of the triceps muscle, supplied by C7. The biceps and triceps have one nerve in common, C6, stimulation of the triceps will contract briskly, in an "inverted" manner.

SO YOU WANT TO BE A NEUROLOGIST!

- In patients with syringomyelia affecting the middle of the cervical cord, give the neuroanatomical basis for the observation that the sensations of pain and, temperature are lost from only the upper part of the face, and not also from the lower face?
  - The sensory fibres of the trigeminal nerve (CN V) which carry pain and temperature enter the brainstem and descend to the level of CN III (third cervical segment)
  - From C3, the V1 fibres cross the midline, and then ascend in the lateral spinothalamic tract (LST)
  - The lowest fibres in LST supply the upper part of the face

V1 → brainstem → descend to C3 → decussate → ascend in the LST

- Give the clinical features of syringobulbia.

  - Dissociated sensory loss of the face of the 'onion-skin' pattern (extending from behind forwards, converging on the nose and upper lip).
  - Vertigo (common symptom).
  - Wasting of the small muscles of the tongue (important physical sign).
  - The process may be limited to the medullary region.
  - The main cranial nerve nuclei involved are those of the fifth, seventh, ninth and tenth cranial nerves.

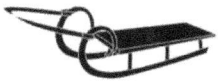

RADICULOPATHY AND NERVE ROOTS

Nerve Root Lesions

- Nerve root lesions are indicated by sharp, lancinating pain with a dermatomal or myotomal pattern.

- Pain is increased by sneezing and coughing.

- Pain often has a dermatomal pattern.

- Findings are weakness, sensory impairment, and decreased muscle stretch reflexes.

- Radiculopathies have many causes.

- Surgery is considered for increasing weakness, bowel or bladder dysfunction, or intractable pain with an appropriate lesion seen on MRI.

Source: Ghosh AK. *Mayo Clinic Scientific Press*, 2008, page 765.

- Give the performance characteristics of a focused physical examination for cervical radiculopathy.

Finding	PLR	NLR
o Motor examination		
- Weak elbow flexion (C5)	5.3	NS
- Weak wrist extension (C6)	2.3	NS
- Weak elbow extension (C7)	4.0	0.4
- Weak finger flexion [C8)	3.8	NS
o Sensory examination		
- Sensory loss thumb (C6)	8.5	NS
- Sensory loss affecting middle finger (C7)		
- Sensory loss affecting little finger (C8)	41.4	NS
o Reflex examination		
- ↓ biceps or deep tendon reflex (C6)	14.2	0.5
- ↓ triceps reflex (C7)	3.0	NS

NS, not significant; likelihood ratio (LR) if finding present= positive LR; LR if finding absent=negative LR. Findings shown in round ( ) brackets were not associated with a significant LR +/- , and the values of their sensitivity and specificity are not provided. The nerve involved in the radiculopathy is given in square [ ] brackets.

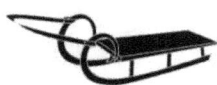

> Other tests

  o   Straight leg raising manoeuvre   1.3   0.3

  o   Crossed straight leg raising manoeuvre   3.4   0.8

Abbreviation: NLR, negative likelihood ratio; PLR, positive likelihood ratio

Adapted from: McGee SR. *Saunders/Elsevier* 2007, Box 60-2, pages 779 and 780, and Box 60-4, page 786.

Probability

	Decrease				Increase		
	-45%	-30%	-15%		+15%	+30%	+45%
NLR	0.1	0.2	0.5	1	2	5	10	PLR

> Sen N out – <u>Sen</u>sitive test; when negative, rules <u>out</u> disease

> Sp P in – <u>Sp</u>ecific test; when positive, rules <u>in</u> disease

---

- Give what are "the best"? The "best" clinical tests for lumbosacral radiculopathy.

  o Weak ankle extension and dorsiflexion

  o Ipsilateral calf wasting

  o Sensory loss in area of LSS

  o Asymmetric quadriceps reflex

  o Positive crossed straight leg-raising maneuver

Abbreviation: LSS, lumbar spinal stenosis

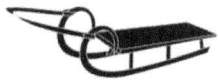

- Give the performance characteristics for diagnosing cervical radiculopathy in patients with neck and arm pain.

Finding	PLR	NLR
o Reflex examination		
– Reduced biceps reflex	9.1	NS
– Reduced biceps, triceps or brachioradialis reflex	3.6	0.8
o Other tests		
– Spurling test	3.6	0.7

Note that weakness of any arm muscle, reduced sensation in arm of , vibration or pinprick, reduced triceps reflex, ant rotation of neck to involved side are not included because than PLR was < 2.

Abbreviation: NS, not significant; likelihood ratio (LR) if finding present= positive LR (PLR); LR if finding absent=negative LR (NLR).

Adapted from: McGee SR. *Saunders/Elsevier* 2007, Box 60.1, page 778.

- Give the performance characteristics of test for lumbosacral radiculopathy in patients with sciatica.

Finding	PLR	NLR
o Motor examination		
– Weak ankle dorsiflexion	4.9	0.5
– Ipsilateral calf wasting	5.2	0.8
o Reflex examination		
– Abnormal ankle jerk	2.7	NS
o Other tests		
– Crossed straight-leg raising maneuver	3.4	0.8

Note that abnormal leg sensation and abnormal straight – leg raising have PLR < 2.
*Diagnostic standard: For lumbosacral radiculopathy, surgical findinds, electrodiagnostic, or magnetic resonance imaging or computed tomography indicating lumbosacral nerve root compression.

Abbreviation: NS, not significant; PLR, positive likelihood ratio, NLR, negative likelihood ratio

Adapted from: McGee SR. *Saunders/Elsevier* 2007, Box 60-4, page 786.

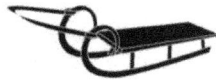

- Give the perform characteristics of tests for Lumbosacral Radiculopathy.

Finding	PLR	NLR
o Motor examination		
– Weak ankle extension (L3 or L4)	3.7	0.7
– Weak ankle dorsiflexion (L5)		
– Weak ankle plantarflexion (S1)		
– Ipsilateral calf wasting (S1)	2.4	0.7
– Weak ankle dorsiflexion	4.9	0.5
– Ipsilateral calf wasting	5.2	0.8
o Sensory examination		
– Sensory loss (L5)	3.1	0.8
– Sensory loss (S1; leg sensation abnormal)	2.4	0.7
o Reflex examination		
– Asymmetric quadriceps reflex (L3 or L4)	8.7	0.6
– Asymmetric Achilles reflex (S1)	2.9	0.4
– Abnormal ankle jerk	2.7	NS

Note that weak hallux extension (L3 or L4 lesion) is omitted because its PLR was < 2.

Abbreviation: NS, not significant; PLR, positive likelihood ratio, NLR, negative likelihood ratio The nerve involved in the radiculopathy is given in ( ) brackets.

Adapted from: McGee SR. *Saunders/Elsevier* 2007, Box 60-5, page 787.

"Our greatest glory is not in never failing, but in rising up everyt time we fall."

Ralph Waldo Emerson

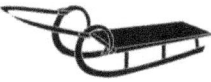

Upper and Lower Motor Neuron Lesions

➢ Neuroanatomy

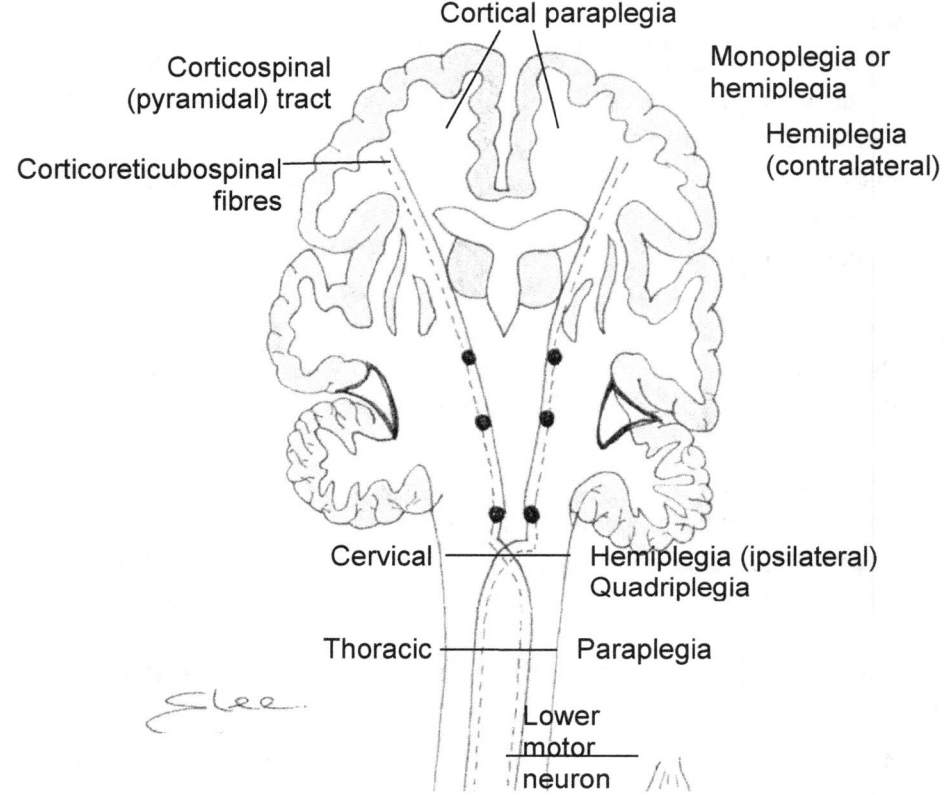

Adapted from: Talley NJ, et al. *Maclennan & Petty Pty Limited* 2003,page 416.

➢ Clinical
  o In the upper limbs, weakness is most marked in the abductors and extensors.
  o In the lower limbs, weakness is more marked in the flexor and abductor muscles.
  o Spasticity
    - Increased tone is present (may be clasp-knife) and often associated with clonus
  o The reflexes are increased except for the superficial reflexes (e.g., abdominal), which are absent.
  o There is an extensor (Babinksi) plantar response (uPageoing toe)
  o Weakness may be more obvious distally than proximally, and the flexor and extensor muscles are equally involved.

Adapted from: Talley NJ, et al*Maclennan & Petty Pty Limited* 2003, page 418.

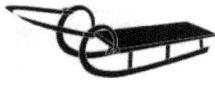

➤ Comparison of UMN versus LMN lesions

Site	Power
o Upper motor neuron	– Upper limbs - Flexors> extensors – Lower limbs - Extensors > Flexors
o Lower motor neuron	– Reduced power in specific motor neuron (or nerve root) distributions

   o Reinforcement can involve teeth clenching, hand grips, etc.
      – Remember to make side-to-side comparisons of tone, pattern of weakness and reflexes.

• Perform a focused physical examination to determine if a person has a UMN or an LMN lesion.

Loss	UMN lesion	LMN lesion
o Muscle wasting	-	++
o Fasciculations	-	+
o Power		
– Upper limbs	F > E	↓ (D > P)
– Lower limbs	E > F	↓ (E = F)
	Arms flexed, legs extended	Fasciculations
o Tone	Spastic	↓
o Co-ordination impaired due to weakness	+	+
o Reflexes		
– Superficial (e.g., abdominal)	Absent	Absent
– Deep	Increased/clonus	Decreased
– Barbinski	Up-going (present)	Downgoing (absent)

Abbreviations: D, distal; E, extensor muscles; F, flexor muscles; LMN, lower motor neuron; P, proximal; UMN, upper motor neuron

Adapted from: Filate W, et al. *The Medical Society, Faculty of Medicine, University of Toronto* 2005, Table 9, page 163.

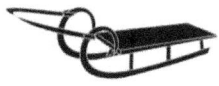

Mastering the Boards: Neurology   A.B.R. Thomson

- Perform a focused physical examination of the motor system of the upper limbs.

  - Drift of the arms:
    - Upper motor neuron (pyramidal) weakness
      - Muscle weakness
      - Drift of the extended arms, with the eyes closed, tends to be in a downward direction
      - The drifting starts distally with the fingers, and spreads proximally
      - There may be slow pronation of the wrist and flexion of the fingers and elbow
    - Cerebellar disease
      - The drift is usually upwards
      - Includes slow pronation of the wrist and elbow
    - Loss of proprioception
      - The drift here (pseudoathetosis) is really a searching movement
      - Usually affects only the fingers
      - Due to loss of joint position sense and can be in any direction

  - Ask the patient to relax the arms and rest them on his or her lap. Inspect the large muscle groups for

  - Fasciculations
    - Irregular spontaneous contractions of small areas of muscle which have no rhythmical pattern
    - May be coarse or fine present at rest, but not during voluntary movement
    - If present with weakness and wasting, fasciculation indicates degeneration of the lower motor neurone
    - Usually benign if unassociated with other signs of a motor lesion

Adapted from: Talley NJ, et al. *Maclennan & Petty Pty Limited* 2003, page 391.

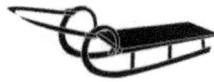

Mastering the Boards: Neurology   A.B.R. Thomson

- Perform a focused physical examination for **loss of corticospinal inhibition**.

  - Hoffman finger flexion reflexes: sudden stretching of finger flexors causes the other finger flexors to contract involuntarily (finding of hyprereflexia).

  - Jaw Jerk: sudden stretching of the masseter muscle causes the jaw to move upwards briskly.

  - Inverted knee reflex: tapping knee causes knee flexion, not extension, indicating L2-4 spinal cord disease.

  - Crossed adductor reflex: tapping on the medial femoral condyle, patella, or patellar tendon causes the contralateral adductor muscle to contract, moving the contralateral knee medially.[42]

Source: McGee SR. *Saunders/Elsevier* 2007, page 759.

- Give the root level for the major deep tendon reflex (DTRs).

  - Ankle   S1, 2
  - Knee   L3, 4
  - Biceps   C5, 6
  - Supinator   C5, 6
  - Triceps   C6, 7

Source: Burton JL. *Churchill Livingstone* 1971, page 83.

Extensor Plantars
  - Pyramidal lesion
  - Deep coma
  - 1st year of life
  - May not be present if there is complete paralysis of extensor hallucis longus (L4, 5),
  - Loss of sensation of sole of foot
  - Hallux rigidis

Source: Davey P. *Wiley-Blackwell* 2006,

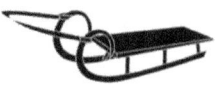

Clonus

➤ Definition

  ○ Sudden stretching of a muscle with continued stretch force applied causes continued oscillation of the muscle

  ○ Dorsiflex ankle, push down on patella, percuss lower jaw; with "true" clonus, sustained clonus increases with pressure

  ○ CNS disease with remissions-MS, infection, myasthenia

  ○ Failing memory-common initial intellectual failing

  ○ Delirium-abnormal perception and motor activity

  ○ Hallucination-sensory impression without sensory stimulus

  ○ Illusion-sensory impression which is inconsistently interpreted

Source: Davey P. *Wiley-Blackwell* 2006,

➤ Clinical

  ○ Motor changes

    − Upper motor neurone signs below the hemisection on the same side as the lesion

    − Lower motor neurone signs at the level of the hemisection on the same side

  ○ Sensory changes

    − Pain and temperature loss on the opposite side to the lesion - NB: the upper level of sensory loss is usually a few segments below the level of the lesion

    − Vibration and proprioception loss occur on the same side

    − Light touch is often normal

  ○ Causes

    − Multiple sclerosis

    − Angioma

    − Trauma

    − Myelitis

    − Post-radiation myelopathy

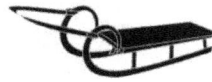

➤ Differential diagnosis

  o Causes of only spinothalamic loss
    - Cord Tumour
    - Hematomyelia
    - Bullet or stab wounds
    - Degenerative disease of spine
    - Multiple myeloma
    - Differentiate from MS
    - Syringomyelia
    - Brown-Séquard syndrome (contralateral leg)
    - Anterior spinal artery thrombosis
    - Lateral medullary syndrome (contralateral to the other signs)
    - Small fibre peripheral neuropathy (e.g., diabetes mellitus, amyloid)

  o Causes of dorsal column loss only
    - Subacute combined degeneration
    - Brown-Séquard syndrome (ipsilateral leg)
    - Spinocerebellar degeneration (e.g., Friedreich ataxia)
    - Multiple sclerosis
    - Tabes dorsalis
    - Peripheral neuropathy (e.g., diabetes mellitus, hypothyroidism)
    - Sensory neuronopathy (a dorsal root ganglionopathy which may be caused by carcinoma, diabetes mellitus or Sjögren syndrome)

Adapted form: Talley NJ, et al. *Maclennan & Petty Pty Limited* 2003, page 422, 425.

• Give the characteristics of abnormal **muscle tone**.

Characteristic	Possible Causes
o ↓ tone - Flaccid	• LMN lesion, cerebellar; rarely myopathies, 'spinal shock' (e.g., early response after a spinal cord trauma), chorea

o tone
  - spastic ('clasp knife')
  - rigidity ('lead pipe', cog wheeling')
	• UMN lesion; corticospinal tract (commonly late or chronic stage after a stroke)
	• Extrapyramidal tract lesion
	  - Parkinsonism
	  - phenothiazines

Adapted from: Filate W, et al. *The Medical Society, Faculty of Medicine, University of Toronto* 2005, page 164.

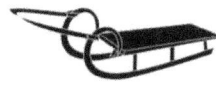

Mastering the Boards: Neurology   A.B.R. Thomson

- Give the muscle groups to test (myotomal distribution) for a specific spinal nerve root lesion.

Muscle	Movement	Nerve	Spinal Myotomes
o Biceps	– Elbow flexion	▪ Musculocutaneous	C5, 6
o Deltoid	– Arm abduction	▪ Axillary	C5, 6
o Triceps	– Elbow extension	▪ Radial	C6, 7, 8
o Flexor pollicis longus	– Thumb IP flexion	▪ Median	C6, 7
o Wrist extensors	– Wrist extension	▪ Radial	C7, 8
o Interossei of hand	– Fingers ab/adduction	▪ Ulnar	C8, T1
o Iliopsoas	– Hip flexion	▪ Femoral	L1, 2, 3
o Hip adductors	– Hip adduction	▪ Obturator	L2, 3, 4
o Quadriceps	– Knee extension	▪ Femoral	L2, 3, 4
o Tibialis anterior	– Ankle dorsiflexion	▪ Deep peroneal	L4, 5
o Tibialis	– Posterior foot inversion	▪ Posterior tibial	L4, L5
o Hip abductors	– Hip abduction	▪ Superior gluteal	L4, 5, S1
o Hamstrings	– Knee flexion	▪ Sciatic	L5, S1, 2
o Etensor hallucis longus	– Great toe dorsiflexion	▪ Deep peroneal	L5, S1
o Peroneus longus, brevis	– Foot eversion	▪ Superficial peroneal	L5, S1
o Gastrocnemius, soleus	– Ankle plantar flexion	▪ Tibial	S1, 2

Printed with permission: Filate W, et al. *The Medical Society, Faculty of Medicine, University of Toronto* 2005, page 164; Source: Davey P. *Wiley-Blackwell* 2006, page 250.

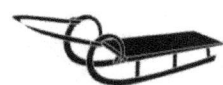

Dermatomes

- **Know the dermatomes!**

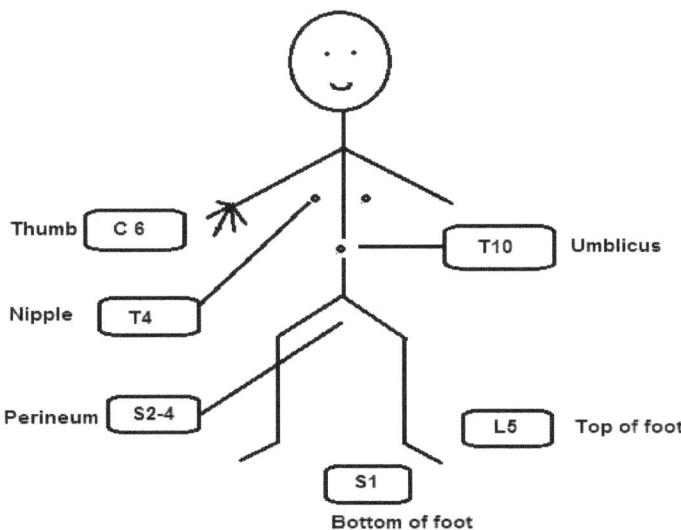

Source: Mangione S. *Hanley & Belfus* 2000,

Sensory dermatomes

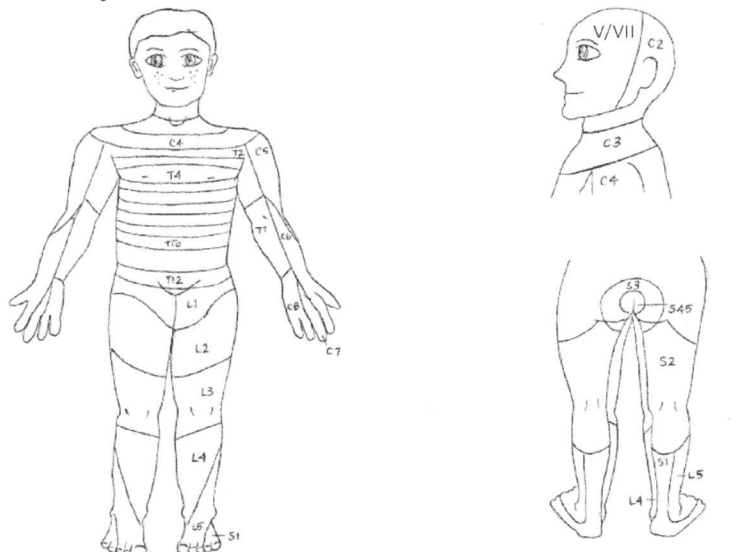

Adapted from: Filate W, et al. *The Medical Society, Faculty of Medicine, University of Toronto* 2005, Figure 1, page 155.

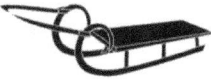

- Perform a focused physical examination to determine the nerve roots involved in spinal cord disease (sensory dermatomes).

  ➢ Dermatomes in the upper limb (Causes of wasting of small muscles of hand)
    - o Cord lesions at C8, T1 level
    - o Motor neurone disease tumour
    - o Syringomyelia
    - o Meningo-vascular Syphillis
    - o Cord compression
    - o Root lesions
    - o Cervical Spondylosis
    - o Neurofibroma, etc.
    - o Brachial plexus lesions
    - o Klumpke paralysis
    - o Cervical rib, etc.
    - o Ulnar or median nerve lesions
    - o Arthritis of hand or wrist, or disuse atrophy

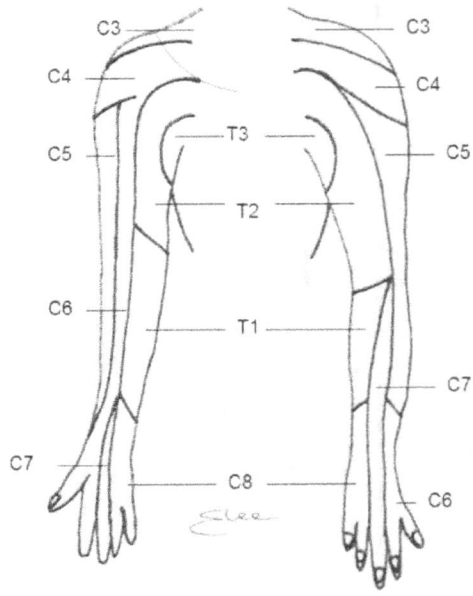

  ➢ Dermatomes of the lower limb

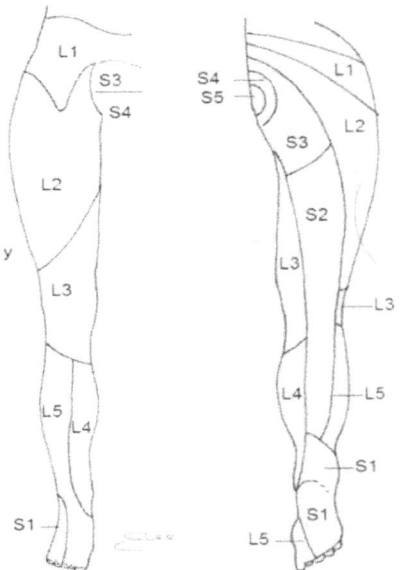

Adapted from: Burton JL. *Churchill Livingstone* 1971, page 86-87; McGee SR. *Saunders/Elsevier* 2007, page 743.

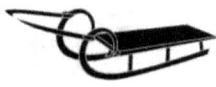

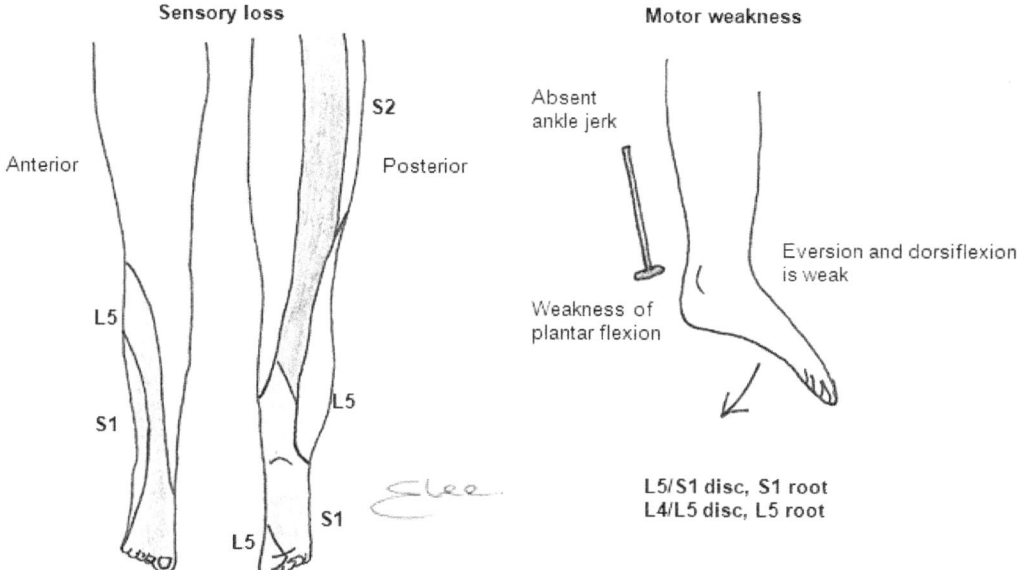

Damage to the fibres from a single nerve root (radiculopathy) will cause sensory loss to the cutaneous area supplied by this nerve (aka dermatome).

Nerve Entrapment Syndromes

Cervical Spondylosis

- o Disc protrusion – formation of osteophytes
- o Disc calcification – osteoarthritis

➤ Neuroanatomy

- o The intervertebral discs are anterior to the spinal cord
- o These discs herniate laterally where the herniate disc affects the roots (pyramidal tracts)
- o Usually a herniated disc affects motor roots more than sensory, except in the cerebral region
- o Cervical formation may narrow the canal carrying vertebra-basilar ischemia

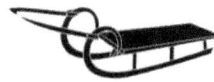

Mastering the Boards: Neurology   A.B.R. Thomson

Peripheral Nerves

Segmental innervation of muscles of the arm*

Spinal Segments — C5 C6 C7 C8 T1

- Proximal nerves
  - Rhomboids (dorsal scapular nerve)
  - Supraspinatus (supracapsular nerve)
  - Infraspinatus (suprascapular nerve)
  - Deltoid (axillary nerve)
  - Serratus anterior (long thoracic nerve)
- Musculocutaneous nerve
  - Biceps
- Radial nerve
  - Triceps
  - Brachioradialis
  - Extensor carpi radialis longus
  - Extensor carpi ulnaris
  - Finger extensors
- Median nerve
  - Pronator teres
  - Flexor carpi radialis
  - Flexor digitorum superficialis
  - Abductor pollicis brevis
- Ulnar nerve
  - Flexor carpi ulnaris
  - Hypothenar muscles
  - Interossei

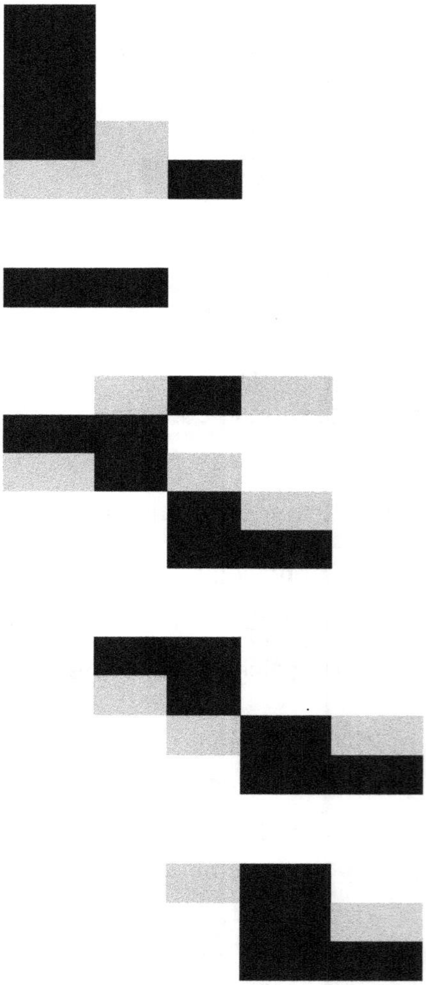

*Spinal levels that usually (black shade) and sometimes (gray shade) contribute to the corresponding muscle

Printed with permission: McGee SR. *Saunders/Elsevier* 2007, Table 60-1, page 773.

Useful background: Segmental innervation of the muscles of the leg*

Spinal segments	L2	L3	L4	L5	S1	S2

o Proximal nerves
  – Gluteus medius (gluteal nerves, internal rotation and abduction of hip)
  – Gluteus maximus (gluteal nerves; extension of hip)

o Femoral nerve
  – Iliopsoas
  – Quadriceps

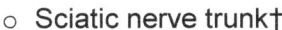

o Obturator nerve
  – Thigh adductors

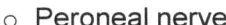

o Sciatic nerve trunk†
  – Hamstring (knee flexion)

o Peroneal nerve
  – Tibialis anterior (dorsiflexion of ankle)
  – Extensors of toes
  – Peroneal longus (eversion of ankle)

o Tibial nerve†
  – Tibialis posterior (inversion of ankle)
  – Gastrocnemius
  – Floxor digitorum (curl toes)

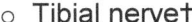
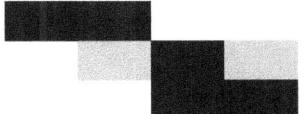

*Spinal levels that usually (black shade) and sometimes (gray shade) contribute to the corresponding muscles.

†The sciatic nerve trunk divides above the knee into theperoneal and tibial nerves. Therefore, lesions of the sciatic nerve affect muscles of all three branches.

Printed with permission: McGee SR. *Saunders/Elsevier* 2007, Table 60-3, page 783.

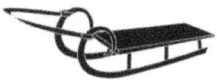

Mastering the Boards: Neurology

A.B.R. Thomson

- Give the segmental innervation of muscles (most muscles are innervated by nerves from more than one spinal root).

Spinal Level	Muscles
o Arm	
C5	Elbow flexors (biceps, brachialis)
C6	Wrist extensors (extensor carpi radialis longus and brevis)
C7	Elbow extensors (triceps)
C8	Finger flexors (flexor digitorum profundus of middle finger)
T1	Small finger abductors (abductor digiti minimi)
o Leg	
L2	Hip flexors (iliopsoas)
L3	Knee extensors (quadriceps)
L4	Ankle dorsiflexors (tibialis anterior)
L5	Long toe extensors (extensor hallucis longus)
S1	Ankle plantarflexors (gastrocnemius, soleus)

Source: McGee SR. *Saunders/ Elsevier* 2007, Table 57-6; Filate W, et al. *The Medical Society, Faculty of Medicine, University of Toronto* 2005, page 723.

- Perform a focused physical examination for muscle or UMN nerve root disease in the muscle groups of the upper and lower body.

Joint	Movement	Muscle	Nerve Roots
o Shoulder	– Abduction – Adduction	▪ Deltoid, supraspinatus ▪ Pectoralis major, latissmus dorsi	C5, C6 C6, C7, C8
o Elbow	– Flexion – Extension	▪ Biceps, brachialis ▪ Triceps brachii	C5, C6 C7, C8
o Wrist	– Flexion – Extension	▪ Flexor carpi ulnar, radialis ▪ Extensor carpi	C6, C7 C7, C8

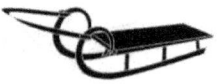

Joint	Movement	Muscle	Nerve Roots
o Fingers	– Flexion	▪ Flexor digitorum profundus and sublimis	C7, C8
	– Extension	▪ Extensor digitorum communis, extensor indicis, extensor digiti minimi	C7, C8
	– Abduction		C8, T1
	– Adduction	▪ Dorsal interossei ▪ Volar interossei	C8, T1
o Hamstrings	– Knee flexion	▪ Sciatic	L5, S1, 2
o Tibialis anterior	– Ankle dorsiflexion	▪ Deep peroneal	L4, 5
o Gastrocnemius soleus	– Ankle plantar flexion	▪ Tibial	S1, 2
o Extensor hallucis longus	– Great toe dorsiflexion	▪ Deep peroneal	L5, S1
o Tibialis	– Posterior foot inversion	▪ Posterior tibial	L4, L5
o Peroneus longus, brevis	– Foot eversion	▪ Superficial peroneal	L5, S1
o Hip	– Flexion	▪ Psoas; iliacas	L2, L3
	– Extension	▪ Gluteus maximus	L5, S1, S2
	– Abduction	▪ Gluteus medius and minimus	L4, L5, S1
	– Adduction	▪ Sartorius, tensor fasciae latae	L2, L3, L4
		▪ Adductors longus, brevis, magnus	
o Knee	– Flexion	▪ "Hamstrings" (biceps femoris, semimembranous, semitedninosis	L5, S1
	– Extension	▪ Quadriceps femoris	L3, L4

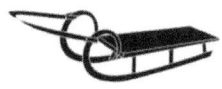

Joint	Movement	Muscle	Nerve roots
o Ankle	– Plantar flexion	▪ Gastrocnemius, plantaris, soleus	S1, S2
	– Dorsiflexion	▪ Tibialis anterior, extensor digitorum longus, extensor hallucis longus	L4, L5
o Tarsal joint	– Eversion	▪ Peroneus longus and brevis, extensor digitorum longus	L5, S1
	– Inversion	▪ Tibialis posterior, gastrocnemius, hallucis longus	L5, S1

Abbreviations: UMN, upper motor neuron

Adapted from: McGee SR. *Saunders/Elsevier* 2007, Table 57-6, page 723; Table 10.15, page 404; Table 10.16, page 406.

Sensory branches of peripheral nerves of the leg

Nerve	Sensory Branches
o Femoral nerve	– Anterior thigh
	– Medial calf
o Obturator nerve	– Medial thigh
o Sciatic nerve trunk*	– Posterior thigh
o Peroneal nerve*	– Lateral calf and dorsal foot
o Tibial nerve*	– Sole of foot

*The sciatic nerve trunk divides above the knee into the peroneal and tibial nerves. Therefore, lesions of the sciatic nerve trunk affect sensation from all three branches.

Source: McGee SR. *Saunders/Elsevier* 2007, Table 63-4, page 785.

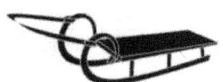

- Give the peripheral nerve and spinal level for common muscle stretch reflexes.

Name of Reflex	Peripheral Nerve	Spinal Level
o Brachioradialis	– Radial	C5-6
o Biceps	– Musculocutaneous	C5-6
o Triceps	– Radial	C7-8
o Quadriceps (patellar)	– Femoral	L2-L4
o Archilles (ankle)	– Tibial	S1

Source: McGee SR. *Saunders/Elsevier* 2007, page 756.

Useful background: Nerve innervations of the muscles of the hand and forearm radial nerve (C5-C8): triceps, brachioradialis, extensor muscles of hand

➢ Median nerve (C6-T1)

  o Muscles on front of forearm, except flexor

  o Carpi ulnaris and ulnar half of flexor digitorium profundus

  o Short muscle of hands ("LOAF" muscles: the two lateral lumbricals, opponens pollicis, abductor pollicis brevis, flexor pollicis brevis [in some persons])

➢ Ulnar nerve (C8-T1)

  o Small muscles of the hand except for "LOAF" muscles, flexor carpi ulnaris, ulnar half of flexor digitorum profundic

Adapted from: Mangione S. *Hanley & Belfus* 2000, page 462.

Peroneal Muscular Atrophy

  o Damage to peripheral nerve or cord, with some sensory loss

  o Hereditary, progressive wasting of distal parts of lower limbs (arms, face and trunk rarely affected)

  o Muscle wasting starts in legs, below the middle of the thigh or the middle of the calf

  o Wasting has a distinct upper border, with normal muscle above this area

  o Bilateral footdrop and inversion deformity

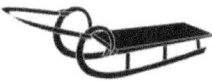

SO YOU WANT TO BE A NEUROLOGIST!

- You suspect that your patient has a disorder of the motor system of the upper limbs. What is the use of tapping the brachioradialis and biceps muscles to accentuate the finding of fasciculations?
    - None! Fasciculations are spontaneous; movements from a local stimulus is not spontaneous. Even if movement occurs, the movement may have nothing to do with fasciculations.

Source: Talley NJ, et al. *Maclennan & Petty Pty Limited* 2003, page 391.

CLINICAL PEARL

- Give the conditions which demonstrate an upgoing plantar reflex but absent knee reflexes.
    - Friedreich ataxia
    - Multiple sclerosis
    - Peripheral neuropathy in a stroke patient
    - Motor neuron disease
    - Conus medullaris-cauda equina lesion
    - Tabes dorsalis
    - Subacute combined degeneration of the spinal cord

CLINICAL GEM

Compression of lumbar discs and physical findings

- Perform a focused physical examination to distinguish a vertebral disc lesion at L4/5 affecting nerve root L5, and L5/S1 affecting S1.

Disc	Root	Motor weakness	Sensory loss	Reflex affected
L4/5	L5	Dorsiflexors, EDL, EHL	Lateral calf and dorsum of foot	Medial hamstring
L5/S1	S1	Plantar flexors	Lateral foot and sole	Ankle jerk

Legend: EDL=extensor digitorum longus, EHL= extensor hallucis longus

Source: Filate W, et al. *The Medical Society, Faculty of Medicine, University of Toronto* 2005, page 175.

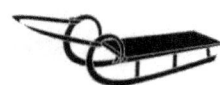

- Perform a focused physical examination for damage to C5 to T_1 motor nerve roots and brachial plexus trunks.

Nerve Roots	Trunks	Muscles Supplied
o C5 and 6	– Upper	▪ Shoulder (especially biceps and deltoid)
o C7	– Middle	▪ Triceps and some forearm muscles
o C8 & T1	– Lower	▪ Hand and some forearm muscles

Source: Talley NJ, et al. *Maclennan & Petty Pty Limited* 2003, Table 10.15, page 404.

- o Posterior columns
  - – Uncrossed fibres form the medial lemnisci
  - – The medial lemnisci decussate in the medulla
- o Lateral spinothalamic fibres
  - – Carry sensation of pain and temperature
  - – Continue through the medulla, and in the pons they join the medial lemniscus
  - – The medial lemniscus goes from the pons to the thalamus
- o Anterior spinothalamic fibres
  - – Carrying sensation of light touch
  - – These fibres form the reticular substance
  - – Reticular substance is in the medulla

- Note
  - o "The motor fibres of the spinal nerves (corticospinal or pyramidal fibres) decussate in the upper part of the medulla just below the pons.
  - o They continue on the opposite side to the spinal cord where they become the pyramidal or lateral corticospinal tract" (Davies IJT. *Lloyd-Luke (medical books) LTD* 1972, pg 246).

The basilar artery supplies the brainstem, and as well the midbrain (plus cerebral peduncles), pons and medulla are supplied by the y, plus brainstem basilar artery, plus posterior cerebral artery, anterior inferior cerebellar artery, and the posterior inferior cerebella artery, respectively.

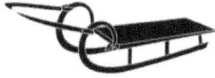

- Perform a focused physical examination for a **brainstem lesion** (crossed paralysis/hemiplegia).
  - o UMN lesion on one side
  - o LMN lesion of a cranial nerve on the opposite side

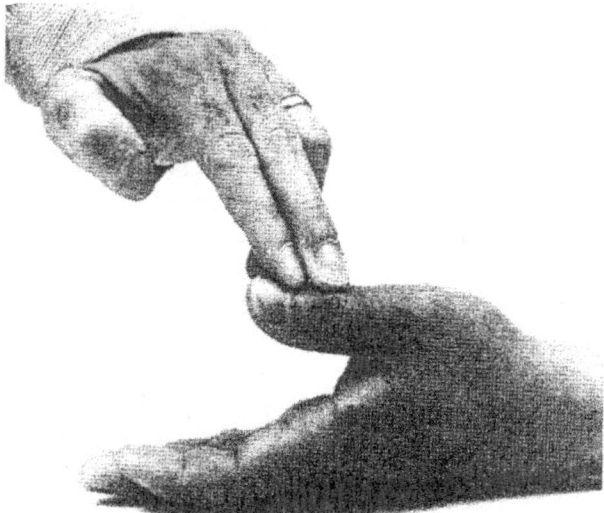

  - ➢ Testing thumb abduction

    - o Instruct patient to raise their thumb perpendicular to the palm.

    - o The examiner applies downward pressure on the distal phalanx.

    - o A defect in the thumb abduction test indicated weakness of the abductor pollicis brevis, which is innervated only by the median nerve.

Adapted from: Simel DL, et al. *JAMA* 2009, Figure 10-2, page 113.

- Perform a focused physical examination to establish the neurological cause of **wasting of the small muscles of the hand**.

  - o Spinal cord lesions (C8, T1)*
    - – Syringomyelia
    - – Cervical spondylosis
    - – Tumour
    - – Trauma
    - – Motor neuron disease
    - – Syphilis

  - o Anterior horn cell disease
    - – Motor neurone disease
    - – Poliomyelitis
    - – Spinal muscle atrophies

  - o Root lesion
    - – Spondylosis
    - – Neuro fibroma
    - – Tumour

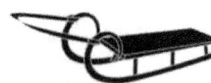

- o Lower trunk brachial plexus lesion
  - – Thoracic outlet syndromes
  - – Trauma, radiation, infiltration, inflammation
  - – Pancoast syndrome
  - – Cervical rib

- o Peripheral nerve lesions
  - – Median and ulnar nerve lesions
  - – Peripheral motor neuropathy

- o Myopathy
  - – Dystrophia myotonica (forearms are more affected than the hands)
  - – Distal myopathy

- o Trophic disorders
  - – Atrophy
  - – Ischemia
  - – Shoulder hand syndrome
  - – Arthritis of hand or wrist

* Rarely diabetes, lead poisoning or a carcinoma-associated neuropathy may display a similar cord lesion.

Adapted from: Talley NJ, et al. *Maclennan & Petty Pty Limited* 2003, Table 10.14, page 404.

- • Perform a focused physical examination of the cutaneous sensory innervation of the hand.

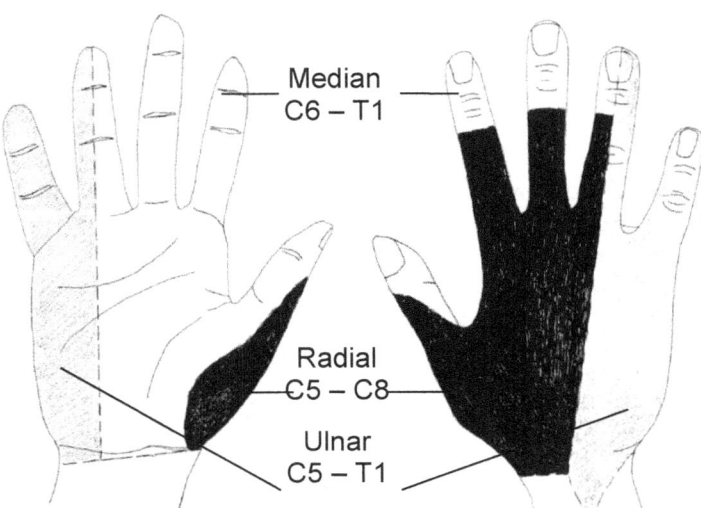

Adapted from: Talley NJ, et al. *Maclennan & Petty Pty Limited* 2003, Figure 10.37, page 401; Mangione S. *Hanley & Belfus* 2000, page 462.

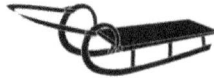

Mastering the Boards: Neurology   A.B.R. Thomson

- Perform a focused physical examination for ulnar nerve palsy (C8, T1).

  o Inspection
    - Generalized wasting of the small muscles of the hand.
    - Ulnar claw hand, (hyperextension at the metacarpophalangeal joints and flexion at the interphalangeal joints of the fourth and fifth fingers).
    - Ulnar paradox - the higher the lesion in the upper limb, the lesser is the deformity
    - A lesion at or above the elbow causes paralysis of the ulnar half of the flexor digitorum profundus, interossei and lumbricals.

  o Motor
    - Weakness of movement of the fingers, except that of the thenar eminence
    - *In the forearm* (lesions in the cubital fossa)
      - Flexor carpi ulnaris
      - Medial half of the flexor digitorum porfundus
    - Ulnar claw hand

  o Sensory
    - Sensory loss over the medial one and half fingers
    - Movers of the little finger – abductor digiti minimi, flexor digiti minimi and opponens digiti minimi
    - Adductor pollicis (oblique and transverse heads)
    - Dorsal and palmar interossei
    - Third and fourth lumbricals
    - Palmaris bevis
    - Inner head of flexor pollicis brevis

Adapted form: Baliga RR. *Saunders/Elsevier* 2007, pages 207 and 208.

- Take a directed history and perform a focused physical examination to distinguish between brachial plexus lesions and nerve root compression.

	Root	Plexus
o Previous trauma	– Occasionally	▪ Some types
o Insidious onset	– Usually	▪ Some types
o Neck pain	– Yes	▪ No
o Unilateral interscapular pain	– Yes	▪ No
o Weakness	– Mild-moderate	▪ Often severe
o Pattern of weakness	– Most commonly triceps C7 lesions	▪ Usually shoulder and biceps or hand

Printed with permission: Talley NJ, et al. *Maclennan & Petty Pty Limited* 2003, Tables 10.18a, b; Table 10.19, page 407.

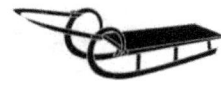

- Perform a focused physical examination for the cause of a **carcinomatous neuropathy.**

  - CNS
    - Dementia
    - Encephalomyelitis

  - Cerebellum and corticospinal

  - Cord – bone, meninges, cord itself

  - Post root ganglion

  - Nerve
    - Neuropathy
    - Mononeuritis multiplex

  - Muscle
    - Myopathy
    - Myasthenic syndrome

Adapted from: Burton JL. *Churchill Livingstone* 1971, page 87.

- Give the sensory branches of peripheral nerves of the arm

Nerve	Sensory branches
o Musculocutaneous nerve	– Radial aspect forearm
o Radial nerve	– Dorsal arm and forearm – Radial aspect dorsal hand
o Median nerve	– Radial palm – First three digits and radial aspect ring finger
o Ulnar nerve	– Ulnar aspect of hand and digits

Source: McGee SR. *Saunders/Elsevier* 2007, Table 60-2, page 776.

SO YOU WANT TO BE A NEUROLOGIST!

- Give the area of the skin (dermatome) which is supplied by the following nerve fibres originating from a single dorsal nerve root:

  C_6 - Thumb L_5 - Top of foot
  T_4 - Nipple lime S_1 - Bottom of foot
  T_{10} - Umbilicus S_{2-4} - Perineum

Source: Mangione S. *Hanley & Belfus* 2000, page 414.

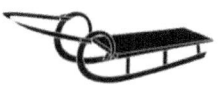

SO YOU WANT TO BE A NEUROLOGIST!

- Distinguish ulnar lesions from T1 root lesions (abductor pollicis brevis).

  o The thumb is moved vertically against resistance, with the hand supine.

- Give the way to distinguish between median and ulnar nerve defects affecting the hands.

The Median nerve supplies

  o Motor (mnemonic LOAF)
  - Lateral two lumbricals
  - Opponens pollicis
  - Abductor pollicis brevis
  - Flexor pollicis brevis

  o Sensory to the radial 3½ digits

  o Ulnar nerve supplies all the rest

Source: Burton JL. *Churchill Livingstone* 1971, page 84.

- In the context of cervical radiculopathy, give the meaning of the "Spurling test" or "neck compression test."?

  o In this test, the clinician turns and tilts the patient's head and neck toward the painful side and then adds a compressive force to the top of the head.
  o Aggravation of pain is a positive response!

Source: McGee SR. *Saunders/Elsevier* 2007, page 776.

Trick questions

- Give which deep tendon reflexes are affected in L5 lesions.

  o The knee jerk is innervated through nerve root L3 and L4, so this reflex remains normal with a L5 disc protrusion

- Give why protrusion of L4-L5 or L5-S1 never causes UMN signs.

  o The spinal cord ends at L2
  o Below L2 is the Cauda equina , which consists of all the nerve roots below L2
  o So, L4-L5 or L5-S1 prolapse cannot cause UMN signs.

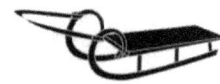

SO YOU WANT TO BE A NEUROLOGIST!

- From the history, give the way to distinguish radiculopathy from peripheral neuropathy.

    o Peripheral neuropathy – changes in motor and sensory function (denervation causing LMN lesion with weakness, atrophy, fasciculations)
    o Radiculopathy – motor and sensory loss, plus pain

- Give the causes of a claw hand (all fingers clawed).

    o Ulnar and median nerve lesion (ulnar nerve palsy alone causes a claw-like hand)
    o Brachial plexus lesion (C8-T1)
    o Other neurological disease – e.g., syringomyelia, polio
    o Ischaemic contracture (late and severe)
    o Rheumatoid arthritis (advanced, untreated disease)

Source: Talley NJ, et al. *Maclennan & Petty Pty Limited* 2003, Table 10.13, page 403; Baliga RR. *Saunders/Elsevier* 2007, page 209.

- Give the difference between neuropraxia, axonotmesis, and neurotmesis.
    o I don't really care. (Not a good response!)

    o Neurapraxia – concussion of the nerve after which a complete recovery occurs.
    o Axonotmesis the axon is severed, but the myelin sheath is intact and recovery may occur.
    o Neurotmesis – the nerve is completely severed, and the prognosis for recovery is poor.

Source: Baliga RR. *Saunders/Elsevier* 2007, page 211.

- In the patient with symptoms and signs suggestive of peripheral neuropathy, give the important symptom which suggests that the disease is at the nerve root?

    o Pain! Severe pain which may radiate down the arms or legs

Source: Mangione S. *Hanley & Belfus* 2000.

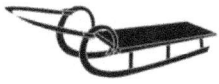

PERIPHERAL NEUROPATHY

➢ Definition

- o Bilateral and symmetrical weakness of muscle.

- o Bilateral symmetrical sensory loss for all modalities with all modalities with or without motor weakness.

- o Motor or sensory component, one or more peripheral or cranial nerves, as well as mononeuritis multiplex.

➢ Types

- o Mononeuropathy
  - – A disorder affecting a single peripheral nerve

- o Mononeuropathy multiplex
  - – A disorder affecting multiple noncontigious peripheral nerves

- o Polyneuropathy
  - – A disorder affecting multiple nerves

Types	Clinical	Causes
o Common mononeuropathies		nerve compression
o Median neuropathy (aka carpal tunnel syndrome)	Sensory-↓ over polmer surface, D1-3 motor- ↓ thumbs	
	Abduction opposition	
o Ulner neuropathy	Sensory- ↓ over D4-5	
	Motor - ↓ intraneseous muscles	
o Tarsol tunnel syndrome	Sensory- large toe medial aspect of foot	
o Bell palsy	Motor V1,V2 distribution of face	HSV infection
o Mono neuritis multiplex	Sensory	Simultaneous or sequented
	Motor	Multiple non contiguous peripheral nerves

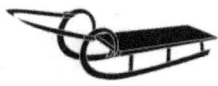

Mastering the Boards: Neurology   A.B.R. Thomson

- o Ischemia
  - – Vasculitis

- o Infection
  - – HIV
  - – Lyme disease
  - – Leprosy

- o Infiltration
  - – Lymphoma
  - – Amyloidosis
  - – Sarcoidosis

- o Idiopathic/immune
  - – Metabolic diabetes

- o Diabetic lumbosacral radicaloplexus neuropathy
  - – Sensory ⎤ Area supplied by lumbosacral radiculoplexus
  - – Motor ⎦

- **Polyneuropathies**

  - o Axonal
    - – Sensory
      - ▪ Distal ⎤ "Stocking-glove"
      - ▪ Symmetric ⎦
    - – Diabetes
    - – Alcohol
    - – Idiopathic- CMT disease
    - – Hematology
    - – Paraproteinemia
    - – B12 deficiency
    - – Paraneoplastic disease
    - – Endocrine hypothyroid
    - – Anal chronic renal failure
    - – Drugs/toxins antineoplastic drugs arsenix

  - o Chronic, inflammatory, demyelating polyneuropathy (CIDP)
    - – Sensory
    - – Motor

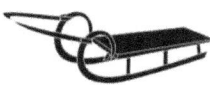

- o Critical illness polyneuropathy
  - – Sensory ⎤ often spares
  - – Motor ⎦ cranial nerves
- o Guillain-Barre syndrome
  - – Acute, ascending
  - – Motor and sensory
  - – No DTRS
- o Enton-Lambert syndrome
  - – Motor
    - Progressive
    - Proximal
    - ↓ DTRs

Abbreviations: DTRs, deep tendon reflexes

Buzzwords in Neuropathies

- o Difficulty moving thumb
  - – Carpal tunnel syndrome

- o Pain, tingling and numb big toe
  - – Tarsal tunnel syndrome

- o Weak face and ASV infection
  - – Bell palsy

- o Stocking-glove pain and tingling
  - – Axonal poly neuropathy

- o Acute, ascending numbness, weakness/paryhasis after gi infection of urinary tract infection

- o Patient MICU with flaccid paralysis and distal sensory loss, but normal cranial nerves
  - – Critical illness polyneuropathy

- o Patient with cancer in whom movement of muscle improves the proximal muscle weakness
  - – Eaton-Lambert syndrome

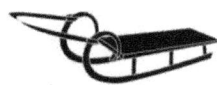

- Give the neuropathies which respond to

  - Corticosteroids
    - Local injection of corticosteroids, +/- decompression of entrapped/compressed nerve
      - Most mononeuropathies
    - Prednisome
      - Bell palsy (do not treat associated HSV infection)
      - Chronic inflammatory deydinating polyneuropathy (CIDP)

  - Plasma exchangem plus IV immune globulin
    - Guillain-Barre syndrome
    - Chronic inflammatory deydinating polyneuropathy (CIDP)

  - Antidepressants, neurogenic pain analgesics
    - Axonal polyneuropathies

➢ Classification

- Give the classification of peripheral neuropathy.
  - Number
    - Mononeuropathies
    - Polyneuropathies
      - Bell Palsy
      - Diabetes-associated
      - Hereditary
      - Inflammatory
        - Guillain-Barre syndrome
        - CIPD (chronic inflammatory demyelinating polyradiculoneuropathy)
      - Critical illness polyneuropathy

  - Distribution
    - Focal
      - Mononeuropathy
      - Multiple mononeuropathies
    - Widespread
      - Polyneuropathy

  - Pathology
    - Axonal
      - Affects axon, but not myelin
    - Demyelinating
      - Affects myelin, but not axon
    - Vasculitis (diseased small and medium blood vessels going to the nerve)
    - Mixed

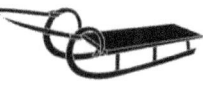

- o Symptoms/signs
  - – Motor
  - – Sensory
  - – Autonomic
  - – Combinations
  - – Small-fibre neuropathy

➢ Causes of peripheral neuropathy
  - o Drugs- e.g., isoniazid, vincristine, phenytoin, nitrofurantoin, cisplatinum, heavy metals (e.g., arsenic), amiodarone, thallium poisoning
  - o Alcohol abuse (with or without vitamin B1 deficiency)
  - o Metabolic – e.g., diabetes mellitus, chronic renal failure, porphyria, acromegaly
  - o Infection – HIV, sarcoidosis, diphtheria, leprosy, Lyme disease
  - o Guillain-Barre syndrome
  - o Malignancy- e.g., carcinoma of the lung (paraneoplastic neuropathy), leukemia, lymphoma
  - o Vitamin deficiency (e.g., B12) or excess (e.g., B6)
  - o Connective tissue disease - e.g., PAN, SLE, rheumatoid arthritis, amyloid
  - o Hereditary
  - o Multifocal conduction block neuropathy (MCBN)
  - o Compressive neuropathies
  - o Idiopathic

➢ Causes of a predominant motor neuropathy
  - o Guillain-Barre syndrome
  - o Chronic inflammatory polyradiculoneuropathy
  - o Perineal muscular atrophy
  - o Give **DAD** some **Rum** (mnemonic)
    - – **D**iabetes mellitus (diabetic chart, insulin injection sites, insulin pump)
    - – **A**lcoholic liver disease (palmar eryhtema, spider naevi, tender liver)
    - – **D**rug history
    - – **R**heumatoid arthritis
    - – **U**raemia
    - – **M**alignancy
  - o Hereditary motor and sensory neuropathy

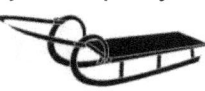

Mastering the Boards: Neurology   A.B.R. Thomson

- o Diabetes mellitus
- o Acute intermittent porphyria
- o Diphtheria
- o MCBN
- o Drugs/toxins e.g.,
  - – Lead
  - – Dapsone
  - – Organophosphorous poisoning

- ➢ Causes of a painful sensory peripheral neuropathy
  - o Diabetes mellitus
  - o Alcohol
  - o Vitamin B1, or B12 deficiency
  - o Carcinoma
  - o Porphyria
  - o Arsenic or thallium poisoning
  - o Chronic renal failure
  - o Leprosy

- ➢ Clinical
  - o Legs are affected more than the arms
  - o May be symptoms/signs of motor, sensory, or motor plus sensory loss (as in diabetic neuropathy)
  - o Rare to have disturbance of sphincters
  - o Recovery
    - – Fast
      - ▪ Demyelination (eg, diabetes, carcinoma, GBS)
    - – Slow
      - ▪ Loss of neuron

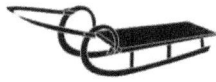

Diabetes, amyloid ⟶ Autonomic neuropathy
- Postural hypotension
- GI paresis, diarrhea
- Impotence
- Bladder disturbance

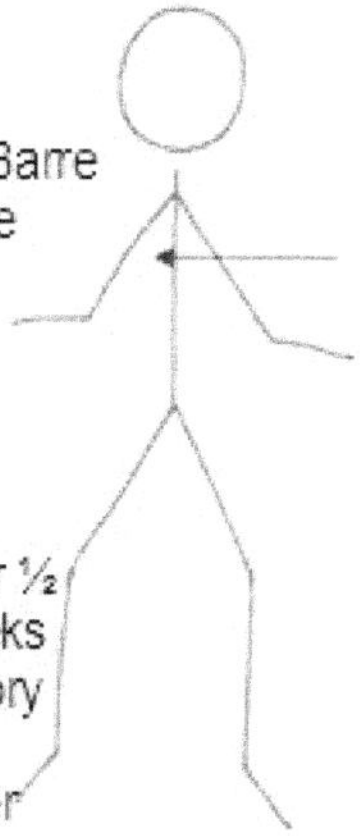

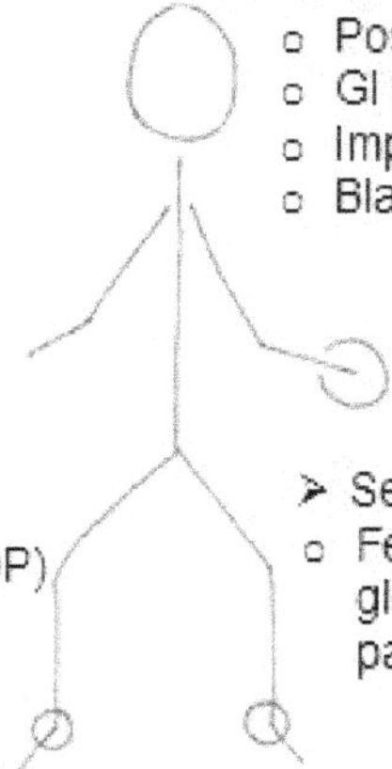

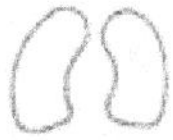

➤ Guillain-Barre syndrome

May cause respiratory failure

➤ Ascending paralysis over ½ hour to 3 weeks
- Mild/no sensory signs
- Recovery over months

➤ Cause of sensori-motor neuropathy
- Inflammatory (CIDP)
- Renal failure
- Alcohol
- Cancer
- Vasculitis e.g pain
- Genetic

➤ Sensory neuropathy
- Feet first then hands glove and stocking paraesthesia

- Diabetes
- Cancer
- Alcohol

➤ Charcot joints

Nerve lesions

➤ Carpal tunnel syndrome
- Nocturnal pain
- Weakness
- Thenar muscle wasting

➤ Plexus lesions 'plexopahty' e.g brachial plexus
- Trauma
- Tumors

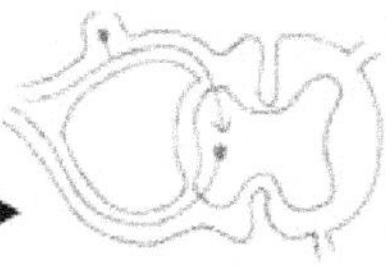

➤ Rediculopathy

➤ Compressive lesions
- Disc prolapsed
- Tumous

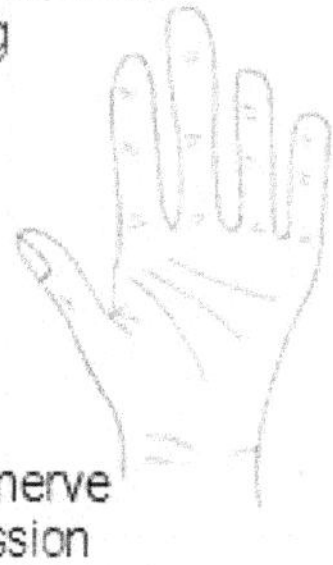

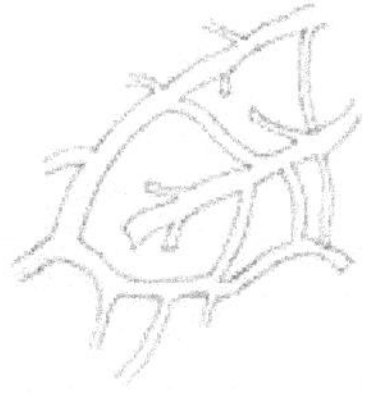

➤ Charcot joints
- Differential
  - Amyloidosis
  - Carcot-Marie-Tooth (CMT) disease
  - Leprosy
  - Refsum's disease (retinitis pigmentosa, deafness and cerebellar damage)
  - Dejerine-Sottas (hypertrophic peripheral neuropathy)

➤ Median nerve compression in carpal tunnel

➤ Individual nerve lesions 'Mononeuropathy'
- Palpate for thickened nerves

➤ If multiple peripheral nerves involved called 'mononeuritis multiplex'

➤ Causes:
- Diabetes
- Vasculitis
- Leprosy
- Sarcoid
- Cancer
- HIV

Adapted from: Davey P. *Wiley-Blackwell* 2006, page 387; Baliga RR. *Saunders/Elsevier* 2007, pages 164 and 165.

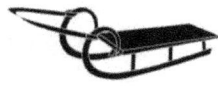

- Perform a focused **physical examination** for peripheral neuropathy.

  - Motor
    - Distal, asymmetrical weakness
    - Atrophy
    - Fasciculations
    - Tone – normal or ↓
    - Reflexes - ↓

  - Sensory
    - Numbness
    - Tingling
    - Burning
    - Paresthesias
    - Loss

  - Trophic changes
    - Loss of
      - Hair
      - Nails
    - Skin
      - Smooth
      - Shing

  - Autonomic
    - Heart
      - Dysrhythmias
      - Orthostatic hypotension
    - Skin
      - ↓ sweating
    - GI
      - Gastroparesis (early satiety)
      - Constipation
    - GU
      - ED (erectile dysfunction)
      - Impotence

"The teacher who is indeed wise does not bid you to enter
the house of his wisdom but rather leads you
to the threshold of your mind."

Khalil Gibran

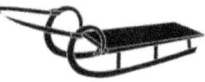

- Take a directed history and perform a focused physical examination to distinguish between dysfunction of the peripheral nervous system (PNS) from the central nervous system (CNS).

Features	PNS Origin	CNS Origin
o History		
– Onset	Slow	Slow gradual (space-occupying lesion) or sudden (CVA)
– Motor symptoms and sensory	Focal, unilateral, or generalized	Focal or unilateral
– Cramps and fasciculations	Yes	No
– Other CNS-related symptoms	No	Yes (such as headache, visual loss, or seizure)
o Physical		
– Atrophy	Yes	No
– Fasciculations	Yes	No
– Stretch reflexes	N / ↓	Hyperreflexia Pathologic (such as extensor plantar response)
– Sensory abnormality distribution	Dermatome, or stocking-glove	Entire limb
– Abnormal EMG	Yes	No

Abbreviations: CNS, central nervous system; EMG, electromyography; PNS, peripheral nervous system; N, normal

Modified from: MSKAP 16 2012, Neurology, Table 30, page 68.

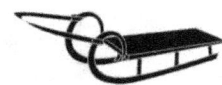

SO YOU WANT TO BE A NEUROLOGIST!

< From the characteristics of the abnormal findings on physical examination of motor and sensory function, give a differential diagnosis of the likely cause of the neuropathy.

Physical examination	DBP	EBS	LE-MG	MYO	Poly-rad	MG	ALS	IBM	RAD	MM	POLY	SFN	PNL	LFN
Muscle weakness														
o Distal	+													
o Ascending		+												
o Proximal			+	+	+									
o Fluctuation						+								
o Focal, asymmetric						+	+	+	+					
o Eye (extraocular)						+				+				
o Lips, palate, tongue (bulbar)						+	+	+						
Atrophy Yes							+							
No						+								
Fasciculation		+					+		+					
Numbness, burning, paresthesias	+	+												
Symmetric											+	+		
Dermatome									+				+	
Deep tendon reflexes												+		+

Note: Use this as a guide. Please don't try to memorize this!

Abbreviation: ALS, amyotrophic lateral sclerosis; DBP, dying-back polyneuropathy; GBS, Guillain-Barre' syndrome; IBM, inclusion body myositis; LE-MG, myasthenia gravis-like syndrome, Lambert-Eaton; LFN, large-fiber (poly) neuropathy; MG, myasthenia gravis; MM, mitochondrial myopathy; MYO, myopathy; PNL, peripheral nerve lesion; Poly, polyneuropathy; Polyrad, polyradiculopathy; RAD, radioculopathy; SFN, small-fiber neuropathy

A.B.R Thomson "Mastering The Boards and   Clinical Examinations" Part II

- Perform a focused physical examination for Charcot-Marie-Tooth disease (features of hereditary motor and sensory neuropathy due to peripheral nerve degeneration which does not usually extend above the elbows or above the middle third of the thighs).

  o Distal muscle atrophy

  o Pes cavus (short arched feet)

  o Sensation
    - Slight or no sensory loss in the limbs

  o Reflexes
    - Absent
  o Nerves
    - Thickened
  o Eyes
    - Optic atrophy
    - Argyll Robertson pupils

Adapted from: Talley NJ, et al. *Maclennan & Petty Pty Limited* 2003, Table 10.31, page 430.

SO YOU WANT TO BE A NEUROLOGIST!

- Give the clues on physical examination that the cause of a neuropathy is "small-fibre neuropathy".

  o In small-fibre neuropathy, there is no muscle weakness, but instead burning dysesthesia of the hands and feet, plus autonomic dysfunction.

- Give types of neuropathies associated with **autonomic dysfunction.**

  o Amyloid neuropathy small-fibre neuropathy

  o Diabetic polyneuropathy

  o Guillain-Barre syndrome

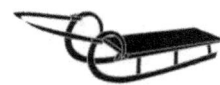

- Give the major nerves of the upper limbs in which a lesion will lead to loss of pain sensation (pinprick).
  - o A lesion of a peripheral nerve causes a characteristic motor and sensory loss
  - o The radial nerve (C5-C8)
    - – Motor supply the triceps and brachioradialis and the extensor muscles of the hand
    - – Characteristic deformity from radial nerve injury - wrist drop.
    - – Pin sensation over the area of the anatomical snuff box is lost with a radial nerve lesion before the bifurcation into posterior interosseous and superficial radial nerves at the elbow.
  - o The median nerve (C6-T1)
    - – Motor supply to all the muscles on the front of the forearm, except the flexor carpi ulnaris and the ulnar half of the flexor digitorum profundus.
    - – Also supplies the following short muscles of the hand (LOAF)
      - ▪ The lateral two Lumbricals
      - ▪ Opponens pollicis
      - ▪ Abductor pollicis brevis
      - ▪ In many people the Flexor pollicis brevis.
    - - Local causes, such trauma or compression, or may be part of a mononeuritis multiplex, where more than one nerve is affected by systemic disease.

Adapted from: Talley NJ, et al. *Maclennan & Petty Pty Limited* 2003, page 401.

- Perform a focused physical examination of the type and location of lesion causing abnormal sensation.

Location of Lesion	Abnormal Sensation
o Brainstem	
– Thalamus or upper brainstem (extensive lesion)	▪ Total unilateral loss of all forms of sensation
– Medulla involving descending nucleus of spinal tract of the fifth nerve	▪ Pain & temperature loss on one side of face & opposite side of body
– Ascending spinothalamic tract (lateral medullary lesion)	

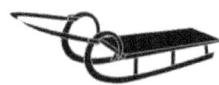

Location of Lesion	Abnormal Sensation
o Spinal cord	
– Spinal cord lesion (if only pain & temperature affected: anterior cord lesion)	▪ Bilateral loss of all forms of sensation below a definite level
– Partial unilateral spinal cord lesion on opposite side (Brown-Sequard syndrome)	▪ Unilateral loss of pain & temperature below a definite level
– Intrinsic spinal cord lesion near its centre anteriorly (involves the crossing fibres), e.g., syringomyelia, intrinsic cord tumour	▪ Loss of pain & temperature over several segments but normal sensation above & below
– More posterior lesions cause proprioceptive loss	
– Intrinsic cord compression more likely	▪ Loss of sensation over many segments with sacral sparing
– Cauda equina lesion (touch preserved in conus medullaris lesions)	▪ Saddle sensory loss (lowest sacral segments)
– Posterior column lesion	▪ Loss of position & vibration sense only
o Root	
– Posterior root lesion (purely sensory) or peripheral nerve (often motor abnormality associated	▪ Loss of all forms of sensation over a well-defined body part only
o Nerve	
– Peripheral neuropathy	▪ Glove & stocking loss (hands & feet)

Adapted from: Talley NJ, et al. *Maclennan & Petty Pty Limited* 2003, Table 10.27, page 426.

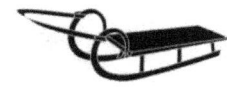

Mononeuropathy Multiplex

➤ Definition
- o Neuropathy of multiple, non-contiguous peripheral nerve
- o Involvement is simultaneous and sequential

➤ Causes/associations
- o Acute causes (usually vascular)
  - – Polyarteritis nodosa
  - – Diabetes mellitus
  - – Connective tissue disease – e.g., rheumatoid arthritis, SLE
- o Chronic causes
  - – Multiple compressive neuropathies
  - – Sarcoidosis
  - – Acromegaly
  - – HIV infection
  - – Leprosy
  - – Lyme disease
  - – Others- e.g., carcinoma (rare)
- o Diabetes mellitus
  - – Symmetrical, mainly sensory, polyneuropathy
  - – Asymmetrical, mainly motor, polyneuropathy (diabetic amyotrophy)
  - – Mononeuropathy
  - – Autonomic neuropathy

*separate involvement of more than one peripheral (or less often cranial) nerve by a single disease

Adapted from: Talley NJ, et al. *Maclennan & Petty Pty Limited* 2003, page 420.
- o Mnemonic: Go to the **WARDS**, **PLeaCe**
  - – **W**egener granulomatosis
  - – **A**myloidosis
  - – **R**heumatoid arthritis
  - – **D**iabetes mellitus
  - – **S**LE
  - – **P**olyarteritis nodosa
  - – **L**eprosy
  - – **C**arcinomatosis, Churg-Strauss syndrome

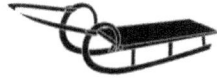

Source: Baliga RR. *Saunders/Elsevier* 2007, page 165.

- Give the conditions causing thickened nerve plus peripheral neuropathy or mononeuritis multiplex.

  - o Acromegaly
    - – Neurofibromatosis
  - o Amyloid
    - – Chronic inflammatory demyelinating polyradiculo neuropathy (CIDP)
  - o Sarcoid
    - – Autosomal dominant hereditary motor and sensory neuropathy
  - o Leprosy
  - o Diabetes
  - o Charcot-Marie-Tooth disease.
  - o Refsum disease (retinitis pigmentosa, deafness and cerebellar damage).
  - o Déjérine-Sottas disease (hypertrophic peripheral neuropathy)

Adapted from: Talley NJ, et al. *Maclennan & Petty Pty Limited* 2003, page 420.

Polyneuropathies

➢ Definition

  - o Dysfunction of multiple nerves at multiple sites, often affecting long nerves with initial damage peripherally, then ascending proximally.

➢ Types

o Axonal	-	Damage to nerve axons, but not the myelin sheath
o Demyelating	-	Damage to myelin sheath, but not to axon
o Vasculitis	-	Damage resulting from disease of small and medium sized blood vessels supplying the nerves

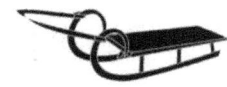

Asymmetrical Polyneuropathy

- The commonest causes of polyneuropathy are diabetes and alcohol abuse. When a polyneuropathy shows asymmetrical involvement, give the more likely causes

  - Radiculopathy
  - Plexopathy (e.g., brachial or lumbosacral plexopathies, from trauma, cancer infiltration, radiation, inflammation/autoimmunity [neurologic amyotrophy]
  - Mononeuritis multiplex
  - MND (motor neuron disease)
  - Compressive mononeuropathy

Critical Illness Neuropathy

A patient in the **ICU with sepsis** and multiple organ failure develops distal sensory loss and flaccid paralysis.

- ~50% of persons in ICU with sepsis and MOF (multiorgan failure) for > 7 to 14 days develop lower leg
  - Weakness → quadriplegia
  - Atrophy
  - Flaccid paralysis
- Distal sensory loss
- ↓↓ DTR (deep tendon reflexes)
- Difficulty weaning from mechanical ventilator
- ~1/3 of survivors will have major morbidity, including residual weakness → quadriplegia
- Differentiate from critical illness myopathy

- Give the diagnostic aspects of critical illness neuropathy.

  - Setting
    - ICU setting
    - Patient receiving corticosteroids and neuromuscular junction-blocking agents
  - Clinical
    - Inability to wean patients off mechanical ventilator
    - Severe, general weakness of arms and legs after recovery from critical illness
  - EMG

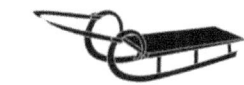

Mastering the Boards: Neurology   A.B.R. Thomson

╳╳╳

SO YOU WANT TO BE A NEUROLOGIST!

- Give the findings on EMG which suggest critical illness polyneuropathy.
  - o Axonal neuropathy
    - – Motor
    - – Sensory
  - o Absence of conduction block
  - o ↓ response on repeated stimulation of nerve (decremental response)

╳╳╳

Diabetes Mellitus, Impaired Glucose Tolerance

➢ Types

- o Multiple types of neuropathy may occur in the same patient
- o Commonest types of neuropathy
  - – Distal sensorimotor peripheral neuropathy
  - – Single mononeuropathies
    - ▪ Median nerve
    - ▪ Ulnar nerve
    - ▪ Cranial nerve

➢ Causes/associations

Diabetes may be associated with severe **types of peripheral neuropathy**, i.e.,
- o Mononeuritis multiplex
- o Stocking-glove axonal polyneuropathy
- o Amyotrophy

➢ Clinical

- Give the characteristic features of **diabetic amyotrophy** (diabetic lumbosacral radiculoplexus neuropathy)

  - o Unilateral leg
    - – Sensory
      - ▪ Pain
      - ▪ Numbness
    - – Muscle
      - ▪ Weakness
      - ▪ Atrophy

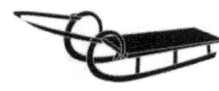

Mastering the Boards: Neurology   A.B.R. Thomson

- Give the less common types of neuropathy seen in diabetes.

    - Lumbosacral radiculopathy
        - L2-L4 involvement, causing
            - Pain
            - Numbness
            - Proximal weakness may develop
            - Sensory changes
            - Sensorimotor changes in other leg, or upper extremities

    - Small-fibre neuropathy
        - Severe pain in extremities
        - Burning, but no weakness

Hereditary Neuropathies

- Give when to suspect that a neuropathy has an inherited basis.

    - Few paresthesias
    - Slowly progressive distal weakness
    - Charcot-Marie-Tooth (CMT) disease is an example of an hereditary neuropathy

Charcot-Marie-Tooth Disease (CMT)

- Give the major distinctions between CMT1 and CMT2.

- Types

Name	Pathology	Age of onset	Palpable peripheral nerves	Prominent ↓ sensation	Foot ulcers
o CMT1	Demyelinating	10-20 yr	+	-	-
o CMT2	Exonal	20-30 yr	-	+	+

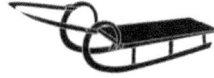

➤ Clinical
  - o PNS   – Numbness
                – Weakness, distal extremities
                – Gait, unsteady
                – ↓↓ DTR (deep tendon reflexes)

  - o Legs / feet   – Arches high
                – Toes "hammer"
                – Distal leg
                   Weakness   ⎤ "Stork leg" deformity
                   Atrophy   ⎦

➤ Diagnosis
  - o EMG (electromyelography)
  - o Genetic testing

Inflammatory Polyradiculoneuropathies

➤ Causes/associations of motor neuropathy
  - o Guillain-Barré syndrome
  - o Peroneal muscular atrophy
  - o Lead toxicity
  - o Porphyria
  - o Dapsone toxicity
  - o Organophosphorous poisoning

  - o To be considered
    - – Guillain-Barre syndrome (GBS)
    - – Chronic inflammatory demyelinating polyneuropathy (CIDP)
  - o Caused by " acquired immune-mediated inflammation of nerve roots and peripheral nerves" (MKSAP 16 2012, Neuropathy, page 71)
  - o Distinguish between the two by EMG, and by duration
    - – GBS – acute
    - – CIDP – chronic

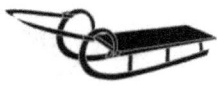

➢ Clinical

• Perform a focused physical examination for inflammatory polyradiculoneuropathy.

- o Guillain-Barré syndrome
    - – Flaccid paralysis in lower limbs progressing to upper limbs one week after an infective illness
    - – Sensory loss and wasting is minimal or absent
    - – Cranial nerves rarely affected, but may be confined there
    - – Sphincters never affected
- o Transverse myelitis
    - – As for Guillain-Barré syndrome (as above), with involvement of sphincters:
    - – HIV

Abbreviation: HIV, human immunodeficiency virus

Adapted from: Talley NJ, et al. *Maclennan & Petty Pty Limited* 2003, page 420.

Guillain-Barre Syndrome (GBS)

➢ Definition

- o Damage such as by infection by organisms with shared epitopes causes damage to peripheral nerve myelin or axons leading to rapid onset of symmetric weakness of upper and lower limbs

➢ Causes/associations

- o Campylobactor jejuni
- o Trauma
- o Surgery

➢ Clinical

o Muscles affected	– Oculomotor
	– Facial
	– Oropharyngeal
	– Diaphragm
o Sensory loss, if any, is minimal	– May be low back pain (inflammatory demyelination of spinal nerve root)
o ↓↓ DTR (deep tendon reflexes)	– Dysautonomia

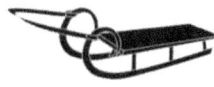

➢ Diagnosis

- o History and physical
- o CSF
  - ‑ ↑ protein (in > 80%)
  - ‑ ↑ albuminocytologic dissociation
- o EMG
  - ‑ Demyelation in 90%
  - ‑ Axonal changes in 10%
- o Because diaphragmatic muscles may be affected, causing respiratory failure) requiring mechanical ventilation in ~ 20%), 400 mg / Kg per day for 3-6 days

---

SO YOU WANT TO BE A NEUROLOGIST!

- In the context of GBS (Guillain-Barre syndrome), give the meaning of CSF albuminocytologic dissociation.
  - o In GBS, CSF shows ↑ protein but no ↑ WBC; absence of pleocytosis)

➢ Prognosis

About 80% of persons with GBS will do well with only mild disability.

- Give the factors which identify the patient with Guillain-Barre' Syndrome (GBS) who may have a poor prognosis.
  - o Patient   ‑ Older
    - ‑ Diarrhea at beginning of illness
  - o Disease   ‑ Rapid progression of weakness
  - o EMG   ‑ Early and major loss of axons (degeneration)

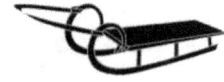

> Treatment

- o Early administration of either
  - – IVIG (intravenous, immunoglobulin), or
  - – Plasma exchange, 4-6 times over 8 to 10 days, for a total of 200-250 mL/kg
- o Repeat treatment for 10% who relapse
- o Pain management
- o Treatment of complications

Chronic Inflammatory Demyelanating Polyradiculoneuropathy (CIDP)

> Clinical

- Give the comparison of Guillain-Barre Syndrome (GBS) and Chronic inflammatory demyelinating polyradiculoneuropathy (CIDP).

	Finding	GBS	CIDP
o	Onset-peak, wk	4	8
o	Residual weakness - – Site predominantly	+	+
	– Proximal		
	– Distal		
o	Prominent pain	-	+
o	EMR		
	– Demyelination	+ (90%)	+
	– Degeneration	+ (10%)	+
o	Treatment	IV-IG Plasma exchange	Corticosteroids Immunosuppression IV-IG Plasma exchange

> Differential

- o GBS (Guillain-Barre syndrome)
- o Diabetes
- o Monoclonal paraproteinemia
- o Connective tissue disease

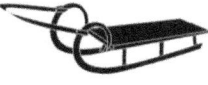

SO YOU WANT TO BE A NEUROLOGIST!

Both Guillain-Barre syndrome (GBS), CIDP (Chronic inflammatory demyelating polyneuropathy) are treated with IV immune globulin and plasma exchange, but CIPD is also treated with corticosteroids. Both ELS (Eaton-Lambert syndrome) and CID are associated with progressive proximal motor neuropathy.

- Give the difference in the clinical findings of the neuropathy of GBS, CIDP and ELS.
    - GBS
        - Progressive distal ascending motor and sensory neuropathy
        - Often proceeded by GI or upper respiratory infection
    - CIDP
        - Progressive proximal motor and sensory neuropathy
    - ELS
        - Progressive proximal motor weakness and ↓ DTR (deep tendon reflexes)
        - Look for associated malignancy
        - Repeated movement of affected proximal muscle improves the muscle
        - Positive antibodies voltage-gated calcium channels

Axonal Polyneuropathies

- Definition
    - Stocking-glove, i.e., distal and symmetric (hand and foot)

- Clinical
    - Pain
    - Paresthesias

- Causes/ associations
    - Endocrine
        - Diabetes
        - Hypothyroidism
        - Uremia
    - Drugs / toxins
        - Alcohol
        - Drugs (anti-neoplastic)
        - Arsenic
    - Deficiencies
        - Cobalamin (vitamin B12)
    - Cancer
        - Paraneoplastic disease
        - Paraproteinemia
    - CMT
        - Charcot-Marie-Tooth disease

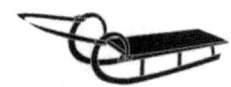

Autonomic Neuropathy

➤ Clinical

- Take a directed history and perform a focused physical examination for autonomc neuropathy.
  - o Symptoms
    - – Symptoms of damage to hypothalamus: disturbances of
      - ▪ Sleep
      - ▪ Apetite
      - ▪ Temperature
      - ▪ Diabetes insipidus
    - – Postural hypotension
    - – Loss of sweating
    - – Impotence
    - – Diarrhea
  - o Signs of
    - – Afferent side of autonomic nervous system (ANS)
      - ▪ Postural hypotension
    - – Central side of NAS
      - ▪ Increased blood pressure with mental arithmetric
      - ▪ Loss of sweating when in the heat
      - ▪ Signs of loss of spinal cord or medullary sympathetic pathways
    - – Efferent side of ANS
      - ▪ Failure of parasympathetic system to response to administration of atropine
      - ▪ Failure of sympathetic system to administration of noradrenalin

- Give the name of the MSK (musculoskeletal) condition which presents with fever, weight loss, abdominal pain and arthralgia, and is commonly associated with mononeuritis multiplex.
  - o Polyarteritis nodosa

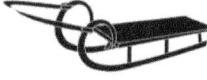

Hysterical Anaesthesia

➢ Clinical

- Perform a focused physical examination for hysterical anaesthesia.

  o May have usual motor or sensory symptoms/signs of peripheral neuropahthy, including
    - "glove and stocking" distribution of peripheral neuritis
    - Total anaesthesia of one side of the body, such as in thalamic and internal capsule lesions

  o Joint sensation is spared in hystorical anaesthesia

  o Sharp out-off for loss of sensation

  o Distribution of affected area
    - May change over time
    - May change in response to suggestion

Foot Drop

➢ Clinical

- Perform a focused physical examination for foot drop.

  o Nerve
    - Common peroneal nerve palsy
    - Peripheral motor neuropathy
    - Sciatic nerve palsy

  o Cord
    - Lumbosacral plexus lesion
    - L4, L5 root lesion

  o Muscle
    - Distal myopathy
    - Motor neurone disease

  o CNS
    - Stroke – anterior cerebral artery or lacunar syndrome ('ataxic hemiparesis')

Source: Talley NJ, et al. *Maclennan & Petty Pty Limited* 2003, Table 10.2, page 414.

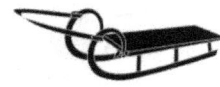

Common Peroneal Nerve Palsy

➢ Clinical

• Take a directed history and perform a focused physical examination for common peroneal nerve palsy (aka: lateral poplliteal nerve palsy [L4, 5]).

- o Motor
  - – Leg
    - ▪ Wasting of the muscles on the lateral aspect of the leg (namely the peronei and tibialis anterior muscle)
  - – Foot
    - ▪ Weakness of dorsiflexion
    - ▪ Eversion of the foot
    - ▪ Foot-drop
  - – Gait
    - ▪ High-stepping gait
    - ▪ Loss of sensation of the lateral aspect of the leg and dorsum of the foot
    - ▪ If the deep peroneal branch is affected, the sensory loss may be limited to the dorsum of the web between the first and second toes

➢ Differentiate from other causes of foot-drop

- o L4, L5 root lesion
- o Lumbosacral plexus lesion
- o Sciatic nerve palsy
- o Peripheral neuropathy
- o Motor neuron disease

Adapted from: Baliga RR. *Saunders/Elsevier* 2007, pages 210 and 211.

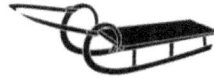

NEUROMUSCULAR DISEASE

- Perform a focused physical examination to determine a neuromuscular cause of weakness.
    - o Upper motor neuron disease ("pyramidal tract disease" or "central weakness")
        - – Cerebrovascular disease
        - – Multiple sclerosis
        - – Brain tumour
    - o Lower motor neuron disease ("denervation disease" or "peripheral weakness")
        - – Polyneuropathy (diabetes, alcoholism)
        - – Entrapment neuropathy
        - – Trauma
    - o Muscle disease in any patient with
        - – Symmetric weakness of the promixal muscles of the arms and legs
        - – Myasthenia gravis
        - – Drug-induced myopathy
        - – Thyroid disease
        - – Polymyositis
        - – Associated with
            - ▪ Muscle pain
            - ▪ Dysphagia
            - ▪ Weakness of the neck muscles
- ➤ Neuromuscular junction
    - o Consider in patients whose weakness varies during the day or who have ptosis or diplopia.
    - o Associated abnormalities of
        - – Sensation
        - – Tone
        - – Reflexes of the weak limb exclude muscle or neuromuscular junction disease, and argue for upper or lower motor neuron lesions.

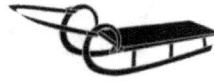

Mastering the Boards: Neurology   A.B.R. Thomson

Muscle Disease

- o Primary disease of muscle (myopathy) causes weakness.

- o There is no sensory loss with myopathy (an important clue).

- o The motor weakness is similar to that of the lower motor neurone (LMN) type.

- o There are two major patterns: proximal myopathy and distal myopathy.

- o Proximal myopathy is the more common form. On examination there is proximal muscle wasting and weakness.

- o Reflexes involving these muscles be reduced.

Adapted from: McGee SR. *Saunders/Elsevier* 2007, page 716; Talley NJ, et al. *Maclennan & Petty Pty Limited* 2003, page 426; Source: Filate W, et al. *The Medical Society, Faculty of Medicine, University of Toronto* 2005, page 719.

Proximal Myopathy and Spasticity

➤ Terminology

- o Myopathy
  - – Muscle disease

- o If myopathy is progressive and genetic → dystrophy.

- o Myotonic dystrophy
  - – Atrophy and weakness begin in the face and sternocleidomastoid muscles.

- o Myotonia
  - – Normal contraction but slow relaxation) of muscle (eg, the patient cannot let go quickly after a handshake).

- o Acquired myopathy: no underlying cause is found in many adults.

Source: Ghosh AK. *Mayo Clinic Scientific Press* 2008, page 771.

➤ Distribution of muscle wasting or weakness

Pattern	Possible causes
o Focal (one limb)	– Nerve root or peripheral nerve pathology
o Proximal (bilateral)	– Myopathy (no sensory loss)
o Distal (bilateral)	– Peripheral neuropathy (distal sensory loss)

Source: Filate W., et al. *The Medical Society, Faculty of Medicine, University of Toronto* 2005, page 163.

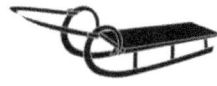

➢ Clinical

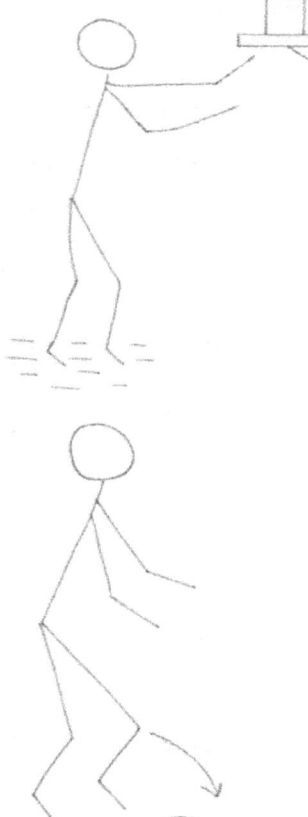

➢ Proximal myopathy
  o Causes
    - Metabolic (K$^+$, Ca^{2+} excess/deficiency)
    - Alcoholism
    - Steroids
    - Thyroid disease
    - Inherited disease
    - Inflammatory (myositis)
    - Myasthenia
  o Clinical
    - Difficulty reaching up

➢ Spasticity
  o Causes
    - Spinal cord disease
    - Cervical myelopathy
    - Multiple sclerosis
    - Stroke (legs held in adduction at the hip, thighs rub together, knees slide over each other)
  o Clinical
    - Easy tripping
    - Falls

• Perform a focused physical examination to distinguish between rigidity and spasticity of muscle.

  o Rigidity
    - ↑ tone of muscles around a joint
    - Causes by degenerative diseases, such as Parkinson's disease

  o Spasticity

    - Definition: "Spasticity is an involuntary velocity-dependent increase in muscle tone resulting from injury to the motor pathways in the brain or spinal cord" (Devonshire V, et al. Chapter 20. In: Therapeutic Choices. Grey J, Ed. 6th Edition, *Canadian Pharmacists Association*: Otttawa, ON, 2011, page 264).

    - Usually occurs as part of the UMN (upper motor neuron) complex

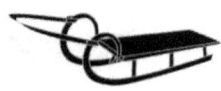

- Characterized by
  - Spasticity, and
  - Weakness of affected limb
  - Slow co-ordination
  - ↑ DTR (deep tendon reflexes)
  - Babinski sign
- ↑ tone of muscles around a joint
- Slowly and progressively increasing muscle tone as the joint is moved from muscle stretch
- At the end of muscle stretch, there may be a sudden loss of the increased tone ("clasp-knife" protective relaxation of muscle)
- Associated with damage to corticospinal (pyramidal) tract

- Give the clinical features of common neuromuscular diseases.

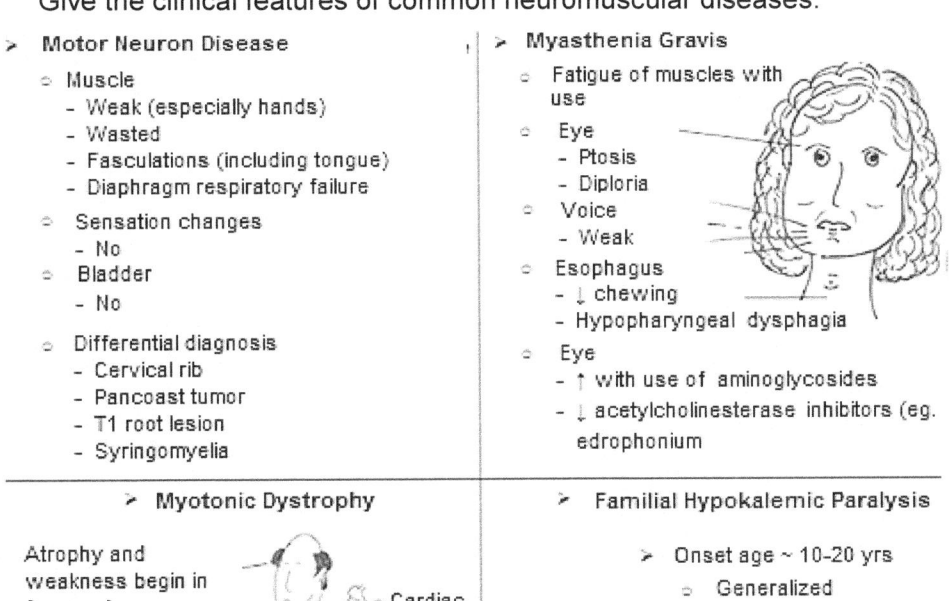

➤ Motor Neuron Disease
- Muscle
  - Weak (especially hands)
  - Wasted
  - Fasculations (including tongue)
  - Diaphragm respiratory failure
- Sensation changes
  - No
- Bladder
  - No
- Differential diagnosis
  - Cervical rib
  - Pancoast tumor
  - T1 root lesion
  - Syringomyelia

➤ Myasthenia Gravis
- Fatigue of muscles with use
- Eye
  - Ptosis
  - Diploria
- Voice
  - Weak
- Esophagus
  - ↓ chewing
  - Hypopharyngeal dysphagia
- Eye
  - ↑ with use of aminoglycosides
  - ↓ acetylcholinesterase inhibitors (eg. edrophonium)

➤ Myotonic Dystrophy
- Atrophy and weakness begin in face and sternocleidomastoid muscles
- Difficulty relaxing grip
- Frontal balding
- Cardiac disease
- Gynecomastia
- Testicular atrophy
- 0 / ↓ DTR

➤ Familial Hypokalemic Paralysis
- Onset age ~ 10-20 yrs
  - Generalized weakness
  - Association
    - Asian people
    - Thyrotoxicosis
    - Food provokes symptoms

Adapted from Davey P. *Wiley-Blackwell* 2006, page 382.

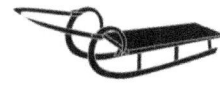

➢ Classification/causes

• Give a classification and causes/associations of muscle disease (myopathy).

• Primary

➢ Inherited myopathies
  o Many disorders
  o Muscular dystrophies
    – Symmetricular asymmetric weakness of
      ▪ Proximal, as well as
      ▪ Other muscles, such as
        - Shoulders
        - Hips
        - Face muscles
      ▪ Cardiomyopathy
      ▪ Conduction defects
  o Myotonia
    – Failure of muscles to relax
  o Congenital
    – Abnormalities of appearance of
      ▪ Face
      ▪ Skeleton
  o Channel opathies
    – Malignant hyperthermia
    – Periodic paralysis
  o May become unmasked by
    – Exertion
    – Anesthesia
    – High carbohydrate diet
  o Mitochondrial myopathies
    – May mimic myasthenia gravis
    – Mitochondria are seen at periphery of mitochondria
    – Trichrome-positive "ragged red fibres"
    – Immunohistochemical staining may show ↑ cytochrome oxidase

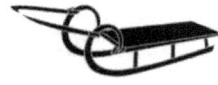

- Duchene (pseudohypertrophic)
  - Affects only males (sex [X] linked recessive)
  - Calves and deltoids: hypertrophied early, weak later
  - Proximal weakness: early
  - Compatible muscle biopsy
    - ↓↓ dystropin
  - Dilated cardiomyopathy
- Becker
  - Affects only males (sex linked recessive)
  - Similar clinical features to Duchenne's except for less heart disease, a later onset and less rapid progression
- Limb girdle
  - Males or females (autosomal recessive), onset in the third decade
  - Shoulder or pelvic girdle affected
  - Face and heart usually spared
- Facioscapulohumeral (Landouzy-Dejcrine)
  - Males or females (autosomal dominant)
  - Facial and pectoral weakness with hypertrophy of deltoids
- Dystrophia myotonica (autosomal dominant)
- Myasthenia
  - Myasthenia gravis
  - Carcinomatosis myasthenic syndrome
- Myositis
  - Infection
    - Staph. Aureus
    - Streptococcus
    - TB
    - Clostridium welchii
    - Granulomatous
    - Sarcoidosis
    - Trichiniasis
    - Cysticercosis

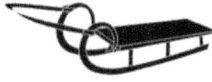

- o Collagen/vascular
  - – Polymyalgia rheumatica
  - – Dermatomyositis
- o Idiopathic
  - – Myositis ossificans
  - – Progressive myositis fibrosa
- Secondary myopathy
  - o Inherited
    - – Glycogen storage disease
    - – Paroxysmal myoglobinuria
    - – Mitrochondrial disorders
  - o Drugs/toxic
    - – Chloroquine
    - – Alcoholism
    - – Corticosteroids
  - o Endocrine/metabolic
    - – Hyper' and hypothyroidism
    - – Diabetes mellitus
    - – Cushing's syndrome
    - – Hyper' and hypo kalemia (including familial periodic paralysis)
    - – Osteomalacia
  - o Infiltrative
    - – Carcinomatous myopathy
    - – Amyloidosis
  - o Atrophy
    - – Secondary to disuse, neurological deficit etc.
  - o Ocular myopathy (Hutchinson)
  - o Distal myopathy (Gowers)

Adapted from: Burton JL. *Churchill Livingstone* 1971, pages 91 and 92; Hauser SC, et al. *Mayo Clinic Gastroenterology and Hepatology Board Review*, 3rd Review, page 771.

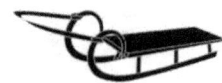

- Give the causes of proximal weakness and myopathy

  - Myopathy
    - Congenital myopathies (rare)
    - Acquired myopathy (mnemonic, PACE, PODS)
      Polymyositis or dermatomyositis
      Alcohol, AIDS (HIV infection)
      Carcinoma
      Endocrine - e.g., hypopituitarism, hyperthyroidism, hypothyroidism, Cushing's syndrome, acromegaly,

      Periodic paralysis (hyperkalaemic, hypokalaemic or normokalaemic)
      Osteomalacia
      Drugs - e.g., clofibrate, chloroquine, steroids, Zidovudine
      Sarcoidosis
    - Hereditary muscular dystrophy
      - Duchenne (pseudohypertrophic)
        - Affects only males (sex-linked recessive)
        - Calves and deltoids: hypertrophied early, weak later
        - Proximal weakness: early
        - Dilated cardiomyopathy
      - Becker (muscular dystrophy)
        - Affects only males (sex-linked recessive)
        - Similar clinical features to Duchenne's except for less heart disease, a later onset and less rapid progression

      - Face
        - No facial muscle weakness

      - Calves
        - Pseudohypertrophy of calves.

      - Back
        - Proximal weakness of the lower extremities
        - In later stages more generalized muscle involvement
        - Kyphoscoliosis
      - Limb girdle
        - Males or females (autosomal recessive), onset in the third decade
        - Shoulder or pelvic girdle affected
        - Face and heart usually spared
      - Facioscapulohumeral
        - Males or females (autosomal dominant)
        - Facial and pectoral weakness with hypertrophy of deltoids
      - Dystrophia myotonica (autosomal dominant)

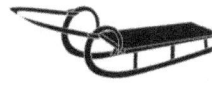

- o Neuromuscular junction disease, e.g., myasthenia gravis

- o Neurogenic, e.g., motor neurone disease, polyradiculopathy, Kufelberg-Welander disease (proximal muscle wasting and fasciculation due to anterior horn cell disease—autosomal recessive)

Adapted form: Davies, IJT. *Lloyd-Luke (medical books) LTD* 1972, page 300; Talley NJ, et al. *Maclennan & Petty Pty Limited* 2003, Table 10.29, page 428.

Thyroid-Myopathy

- Patients with thyroid disease may develop a myopathy, with normal serum CK and EMG. Give the typical clinical findings of myopathy in persons with hyper-and hypothyroidism.

  - o Symmetrical proximal muscle weakness plus
    - Hyperthyroidism
      - Muscle therapy
      - Fasciculations
    - Hypothyroidism
      - Muscle hypertrophy

Vitamin D Deficiency-Associated Myopathy

➢ Clinical

  - o Proximal weakness of arms and legs, plus
    - Bone pain
    - Muscle pain
    - Fatigue

Critical Illness Myopathy

➢ Clinical

- Give clinical distinction between critical illness myopathy and polyneuropathy.

Finding	Critical Illness Myopathy	Polyneuropathy
o Unable to wean patient from mechanical ventilator	+	+
o Associated with use of:	– Corticosteroids – Neuromuscular blocking agents	

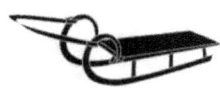

Finding		Critical Illness Myopathy	Polyneuropathy
o	Muscles affected	– Proximal arm and leg – Face, neck – Diaphragm	– Distal arm and leg – Atrophy – Flaccid paralysis
o	Sensation	– Normal	– ↓ distal sensation
o	Serum CK	↑	N
o	EMG findings	– Not typical	– Typical – Loss of motor axon

Drugs and Toxins-Associated Myopathy

➢ Classification

• Give a classification of drugs which may cause myopathy.

o	Heart	– Statins
o	MSK	– Chloroquine
		– Hydrochloroquine
		– Colchicine
o	GI	– Emetics
o	Antineoplastic	– Vincristine

o	Infectious
	disease
		– Anti-HIV
		  ▪ HAART
		  ▪ Zidovudine
		– Antiviral
		  ▪ Interferon

➢ Clinical

• Perform a focused physical examination for muscle disease.

    o Early   – Proximal and symmetrical (bilateral) muscle weakness
                     – Sensory loss – none

    o Late   – Mild loss of muscle tone, reflexes and bulk (atrophy)

• Perform a focused physical examination for disease of the neuromuscular junctions.

  o Weakness of proximal muscles of face
    – Eyelids – ptosis
    – Eyes – double vision
    – Face – weakness
    – Speech – slurred
    – Chewing/swallowing dysphagia

  o Weakness worsens with exercise (fatigability) and improves with rest

  o Tone, reflexes, muscle bulk – normal

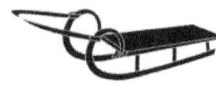

- Take a directed history for the causes of muscle weakness.
    - o Cerebral disease
        - Hemipararesis
        - Paraparesis-anterior cerebral artery

    - o Spinal cord disease
        - Transverse myelitis
        - Epidural abcess
        - Extradural Tumour
        - Epidural hematoma
        - Herniated intervertebral disk
        - Spinal cord Tumour

    - o Peripheral nerve disease
        - Guillain Barre syndrome
        - Acute intermittent porphyria
        - Arsenic poisoning
        - Toxic neuropathies
        - Tick paralysis
        - Neuromuscular junction disease
        - Myasthenia gravis
        - Botulism
        - Organophosphate poisoning
    - o Neuromuscular junction disease
        - Myasthenia gravis
        - Organophosphate poisoning
    - o Muscle disease (no sensory loss; access tone, atrophy, fasciculations)
        - Polymyosistis
        - Rhabdomyolysis-myoglobinuria
        - Acute alcoholic myopathy
        - Electrolyte imbalances
        - Endocrine disease
        - Myopathy
        - Non progressive or relatively non progressive congenital myopathies
        - Inflammatory myopathies
            - Toxoplasmosis, trichinosis, polio
            - Idiopathic-polymyositis, dermatomyositis
            - Collagen vascular disease
                - Metabolic myopathies
            - Glycogenoses

Modified from: Karkal SS. *Updates Neurology* 1991, pages 31 to 39.

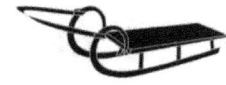

- Perform a focused physical examination for **dystrophia myotonica**.

o Continued contraction of muscle after voluntary contraction ceases, followed by impaired relaxation (combination of muscular dystrophy and myotonia)

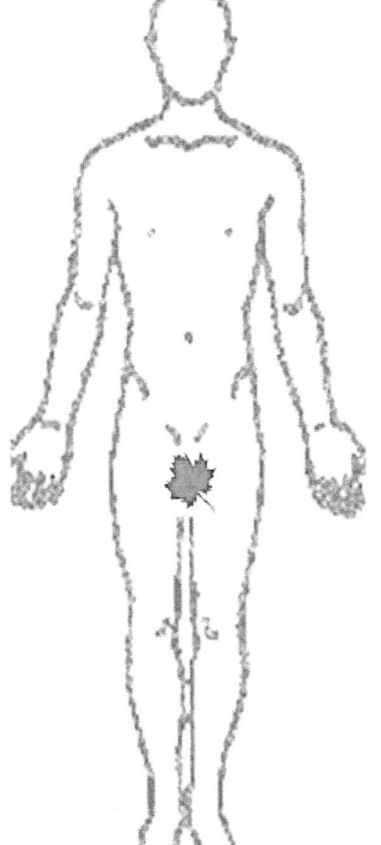

o Eye
  - Partial ptosis
  - Cataracts
  - Subcapsular fine deposits
  - Diplopia

o Proximal muscle
  - Wasting
  - Weakness

o Breast
  - Gynecomastia

o Proximal weakness
  - Myopathy
  - Neuromuscular junction disease e.g., myasthenia gravis
  - Neurogenic eg motor neurone disease, polyradiculopathy

o Proximal myopathy with peripheral neuropathy:
  - Paraneoplastic syndromes
  - Alcohol
  - Hypothyroidism
  - Connective tissue diseases

o Face
  - Baldness
  - Temporalis atrophy
  - Triangular facies

o Neck
  - Sternomastoid atrophy
  - Weak neck flexion

o Heart
  - Cardiac failure (cardiomyopathy)

o Muscle
  - Myotonia

o GU
  - Atrophy of ovaries/testicles

Adapted from: Talley NJ, et al. *Maclennan & Petty Pty Limited* 2003, Table 10.30, page 428; Table 10.59, page 429.

Adapted from: Ghosh AK. *Mayo Clinic Scientific Press* 2008, Table 19-16, page 771; Table 19-17, page 773; Talley NJ, et al. *Maclennan & Petty Pty Limited*, 2003, Table 10.29, page 428; Hauser SC, et al. *Mayo Clinic Gastroenterology and Hepatology Board Review*, 3rd Review, page 773.

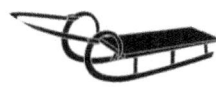

- Perform a focused physical examination for the causes of **fasciculations**.
  - o Motor root compression
  - o Peripheral neuropathy
  - o Motor neuron disease
  - o Primary myopathy
  - o Thyrotoxicosis

Source: Talley NJ, et al. *Maclennan & Petty Pty Limited* 2003, page 392.

- Perform a focused physical examination for a **hereditary peroneal muscular neuropathy.**
  - o Motor
    - – Calves/thighs
      - ▪ Wasting
      - ▪ Stops abruptly, usually in the lower third of the thigh
    - – Toes
      - ▪ Pes cavus (clawing of toes)
      - ▪ Contractures of the Achilles tendon
      - ▪ Weakness of dorsiflexion
    - – Ankle
      - ▪ Absent ankle jerks
      - ▪ Plantars are downing-going or equivocal
  - o Sensory
    - – Mild sensory impairment or no sensory loss (occasionally a response to pain in the stocking distribution).

Adapted from: Baliga RR. *Saunders/Elsevier* 2007, pages 165 and 166.

- A quick review: Give the common muscle stretch reflexes.

Name of Reflex	Peripheral Nerve	Spinal Level
o Brachioradialis	o Radial	– C5-6
o Biceps	o Musculocutaneous	– C5-6
o Triceps	o Radial	– C7-8
o Quadriceps (patellar)	o Femoral	– L2-L4
o Achilles (ankle)	o Tibial	– S1

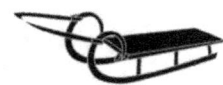

Name of Reflex	Peripheral Nerve	Spinal Level
o Abdominal	o Epigastric o Mid abdominal o Lower abdomen	– T6-T9 – T9-T11 – T1-L1
o Cremasteric reflexes		– L1, L2
o Saddle sensation		– S3, S4, S5
o Anal reflex		– S3, S4, S5

Adapted from: Filate W, et al. *The Medical Society, Faculty of Medicine, University of Toronto* 2005, Table 13, page 164; and McGee SR. *Saunders/Elsevier* 2007, Table 59-1, page 756.

- Give the grades of assessment of the power of deep tendon reflexes.

Grade		Assessment
0	Absent	No contraction detected
1	Trace	Slight contraction detected but cannot move joint
2	Weak	Movement with gravity eliminated only
3	Fair	Movement against gravity only
4	Good	Movement against gravity with some resistance
5	Normal	Movement againt gravity with full resistance

*Note: since raing scale is skewed towards weakness many clinicians further sub classify their findings by adding a (+) or a (-), e.g., 5- or 3+.

Source: Filate W, et al. *The Medical Society, Faculty of Medicine, University of Toronto* 2005, page 164.

- Perform a focused physical examination for (Becker) **muscular dystrophy** (MD).
  - o Eyes
    - – Ptosis, bilateral or unilateral .Differentiate bilateral ptosis if myotonia from
      - Myasthenia gravis
      - Congenital muscular dystrophies
      - Ocular myopathy
      - Syphilis
    - – Cataracts
    - – Difficulty in opening the eye after firm closure.

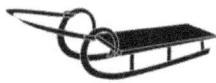

- o Face
    - Wasting of temporalis, masseters and sternomastoid mascles
    - Frontal baldness (is the patient maybe wearing a wig?).
- o Neck
    - "Swan neck"
- o Hands
    - Development of myotonia while shaking hands with the patient, note the myotonia (distal weakness)
- o Leg
    - Leg weakness (difficulty in kicking a ball)
    - "Pseudo-drop attacks" (weakness of quadriceps muscles)
        - Pharyngeal dyphagia (esophageal involvement)
- o Lung
    - Recurrent respiratory infection (weakness of muscles of bronchioles)
- o GU
    - Gonadal atrophy (impotence)

Adapted from: Baliga RR. *Saunders/Elsevier* 2007, pages 168 and 169.

- • Perform a focused physical examination **for limb girdle dystrophy**.
    - o Weakness and wasting of muscles of shoulder and/or pelvic girdle, but never the face occur
    - o Shoulder girdle
        - Biceps
        - Brachioradialis
        - Wrist extensors
        - Deltoids
    - o Pelvic girdle
        - In the early stages of the disease
            - Weak hip flexors and glutei
            - Wasting medial quadriceps and tibialis anterior
        - Hypertrophy of lateral quadriceps and calves

Adapted from: Baliga RR. *Saunders/Elsevier* 2007, page 185.

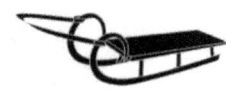

- Give the neuroanatomical sites where lesions result in muscle weakness.

  - Upper motor neuron (UMN)

  - Lower motor neuron (LMN)

  - Cerebellum

  - Extrapyramidal tract

  - Sensory disturbances, perceived as "weakness"

  - Malingering

  - LMN lesions, common causes (disorders involving motor pathways from the AHC [anterior horn cell] to the muscles)
    - Motor neuron disease
    - Polio
    - Peripheral neuropathy
    - Muscle disease
    - Unilateral LMN
      - Lesion unlikely to be in spinal cord

- Give the differences in the physical examination of upper (UMN) versus lower motor neuron (LMN) disorders.

Signs		LMN	UMN
o Weakness		+	+
o Wasting	– a few muscles	+	-
	– All muscles of one side of limb	-	+
o Fasciculations		+	-
o Tone		↓	
o Reflexes	– deep	↓	
	– superficial	-	↓
o Rigidity("clasp-knife")		-	+
o Extensor plantars		-	+
o Clonus, sustained		-	+

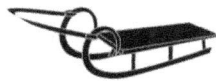

- Give the causes of lower motor neuron (LMN) signs in the legs.

  - o Peripheral neuropathy

  - o Prolapsed intervartebral disc

  - o Diabetic amytrophy

  - o Poliomyelitis

  - o Cauda equine lesions

  - o Motor neuron disease

Source: Baliga RR. *Saunders/Elsevier* 2007, pages 165 and 173.

- Give the causes of changes in muscle tone.

  - o ↓ tone
    - – UMN, extrapyramidal disorders
    - – LMN
    - – Cerebellum
    - – Posterior column
    - – Sensory nerve root (peripheral lesion)
    - – Transient after acute lesions of cerebral hemisphere or spinal cord

  - o Changes in DTR (deep tendon reflexes; "reflexes")
    - – DTRs
      - ▪ UMN lesion
      - ▪ Also DTRs with pain, strong emotion, anxiety, hysteria
    - – ↓ DTRs
      - ▪ LMN lesion
      - ▪ Lesion of posterior column, or posterior nerve root

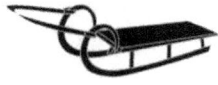

Neuropathic Pain

➢ Definition

   o Tingling, burning pain, usually of distal extremities and worse at night, caused by polyneuropathies of small fibres

➢ Treatment

   o Pregabalin

   o Long list of other drugs which may be useful. Please see standard textbook of Internal Medicine, UpToDate, or review such as MKSAP 16 2012, Neurology, page 73)

Carpal Tunnel Syndrome

➢ Definition

   o Compression of the median nerve at the wrist produces a mononeuropathy resulting in numbness / tingling of thumb, index finger and lateral aspect of third digit, although the entire hand and wrist may be involved.

➢ Clinical

• Perform a focused physical examination for carpal tunnel syndrome (median nerve compression).

Finding	PLR	NLR
o Hand diagram – 'Classic' or 'probable'	2.4	0.5
o Sensory examination (median distribution) – Hypalgesia	3.1	NS
o Other tests – Square wrist ratio	2.7	0.5

Note that a number of signs are not included because their PLR was < 2: Tinel's sign, Phalen's sign, pressure provocation test, Flick sign, weak thumb abduction, thenar atrophy, diminished 2-point discrimination, abnormal vibration sensation, diminished monofilament sensation.

Abbreviation: NS, not significant; likelihood ratio (LR) if finding present= positive LR (PLR); LR if finding absent=negative LR (NLR).

Adapted from: McGee SR. *Saunders/Elsevier* 2007, Box 60-3, page 781.

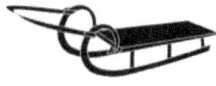

Mastering the Boards: Neurology　　　　　　　　　　A.B.R. Thomson

Probability

Decrease				Increase		

-45%	-30%	-15%		+15%	+30%	+45%
0.1	0.2	0.5	1	2	5	10

NLR ⟶ PLR

Sen N out – <u>Sen</u>sitive test; when negative, rules <u>out</u> disease

Sp P in – <u>Sp</u>ecific test; when positive, rules <u>in</u> disease

➢ Causes

  o Joint/ bone
- Arthritis of wrist (esp. rheumatoid arthritis)
- Previous scaphoid fracture
- Intermittent trauma

  o Metabolic
- Myxedema
- Acromegaly
- Mucopolysaccharidosis V (Scheie syndrome)
- Hyperparathyroidism

  o Sarcoidosis

  o Amyloid (such as in chronic renal failure or multiple myeloma)

  o Pregnancy, 'Pill', pre-menstrual

  o Idiopathic

Adapted form: Baliga RR. *Saunders/Elsevier* 2007, pages 212 to 213.

➢ Treatment

  o Avoidance of positions or wrist, or activities of wrist, which may precipitate symptoms

  o Treatment of underlying conditions, e.g., diabetes

  o No role for medical therapy, other than pain control

  o Progressive symptoms → surgery

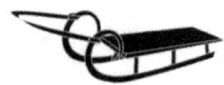

- Give an interpretation of deep tendon reflexes (DTR).

Characteristic of DTR	Possible causes
o Increased reflex or clonus	– UMN lesion above root at that level – Generalized ▪ Peripheral neuropathy – Isolated-peripheral nerve or root lesion
o Reduced (insensitive)	– Peripheral neuropathy – Cerebellar syndrome
o Inverted (reflex tested is absent e.g., biceps but there is spread to lower or higher level e.g., produces a triceps response)	– Spinal cord LMN involvement at the level of the absent reflex
o Pendular (reflex continues to swing for several beats)	– Cerebellar disease
o Slow relaxation (especially at ankle)	– Hypothyroidism

Cervical Rib (Scalenus Anterior) **Entrapment Syndrome**

➢ Cause / association

- o Compression of subclavian artery between first rib and clavicle

➢ Clinical

- o Rarely affects T1

- o Vascular symptoms, as in cervical rib syndrome, above

- o Signs in radial pulse
  - – Loss of radial pulse, especially when pulling clavical over subclavian artery, such as throwing shoulders backwards

- Perform a directed physical examination to establish the neurological cause of a brachial plexus lesion, and the cervical rib syndrome.

- **Brachial plexus lesions**
  - o Complete lesion (rare)
    - – Lower motor neurone signs affect the whole arm
    - – Sensory loss (whole limb)
    - – Horner syndrome (an important clue)
    - – NB: this is often painful

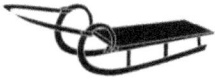

- o Upper lesion (C5, C6)
    - – Loss of shoulder movement and elbow flexion – the hand is held in the waiter's tip position
    - – Sensory loss over the lateral aspect of the arm and forearm
- o Lower lesion (C8, T1)
    - – True claw hand with paralysis of all the intrinsic muscles
    - – Sensory loss along the ulnar side of the hand and forearm
    - – Horner syndrome

- **Cervical rib syndrome**
    - o Weakness and wasting of the small muscles of the hand (claw hand)
    - o C8 and T1 sensory loss
    - o Unequal radial pulses and blood pressure
    - o Subclavian bruits on arm manoeuvring (may be present in normal persons)
    - o Palpable cervical rib in the neck (uncommon)

Adapted from: Filate W, et al. *The Medical Society, Faculty of Medicine, University of Toronto 2005*, page139; Talley NJ, et al. *Maclennan & Petty Pty Limited* 2003, Table 10.18(6), page 407.

"The function of education is to teach one to think intensively and to think critically. Intelligence plus character – that is the goal of true education."

Martin Luther King Jr.

 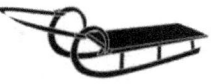

MUSCLE DISEASE

➢ Definition: "Muscle cramps are sudden, involuntary contractions of one or more muscle groups....caused by hyperexcitability of the anterior horn cells or peripheral nerves that subserve them" (Devonshire V, et al. Chapter 21. In: Therapeutic Choices. Grey J, Ed. 6th Edition, *Canadian Pharmacists Association*: Otttawa, ON, 2011, page 270).

➢ Causes/ associations
- o Idiopathic (commonest cause)
- o Inherited
- o Immune (antibodies against voltage-gated potassium channels)
- o Iatrogenic (medications)
- o Acute depletion of ECV
- o Metabolic
  - – Hypothyroidism
  - – Renal failure
  - – Cirrhosis
  - – Pregnancy

➢ Differential
- o Muscle
- o CNS
  - – Spasticity
  - – Myalgia
  - – Dystonia ("co-contraction of agonist/antagonist muscles during a movement or posture (Grey J, Therapeutic Choices. 6th Edition, *Canadian Pharmacists Association*: Otttawa, ON, 2011, page 270)
  - – Contractures
  - – Tetany
  - – RLS (restless legs syndrome); "....a neurological disorder characterized by an unpleasant sensation in the legs accompanied by an urge to move the legs, especially at bedtime" (Hafontaine A-L, et al. Chapter 22. In: Therapeutic Choices. Grey J, Ed. 6th Edition, *Canadian Pharmacists Association*: Otttawa, ON, 2011, page 274).

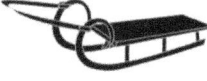

Lambert-Eaton Myasthenia Syndrome (LEMS)

Useful background

➢ Definition

- o Fluctuating and progressive weakness of voluntary muscles, including oculobulbar muscles, caused by autoantibodies against voltage-gated P/Q-type calcium channel in the presynaptic neuromuscular junction, resulting in proximal limb weakness.

- Give a comparison of LEMS (Lambert-Eaton Myasthenic Syndrome) with MG (myasthenia gravis).

		LEMS	MG
o	Autoantibody	P/Q-type calcium channel	Acetylcholine receptor muscle-specific tyrosine kinase
o	Affected neuromuscular junction	Presynaptic	Post-synaptic
o	Progressive proximal limb weakness	-	+
o	Oculobulbar muscle affected	++	+
o	Thymoma (paraneoplastic)	-	+
o	Associated with lung small cell cancer	+	+
o	Autonomic nerve dysfunction thyroid disease	+	+
o	Improvement (mDTR and weakness) with isometric exercise	Yes	No (worsen)

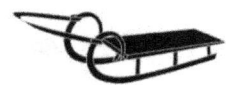

- Give the findings on nerve stimulation conduction studies which establishes the diagnosis of LEMS (Lambert-Eaton myasthenic syndrome).

  o > 100% increase of the amplitude of the action potential of the muscle after a 10 sec period of exercise

Motor Neuron Disease

➤ Definition: acquired degeneration of motoneurons in the frontal lobe and/or anterior horn cells in spinal cord

➤ Terms site of degeneration of motorneurons

  o Frontal lobe (cortical)
  - Primary lateral sclerosis

  o Anterior horn cells
  - Progressive muscular atrophy

  o Frontal lobe plus anterior horn cells
  - Amyotrophic lateral sclerosis (ALS)

➤ Clinical

  o Peripheral muscles
  - Weakness
    - Progressive
    - Asymmetrical
  - Atrophy
  - Fasciculations

  o Bulbar
  - Dysphagia
  - Dysphasia

- Perform a focused physical examination for motor neuron disease.

  o Anterior horn cells
  - Progressive muscular atrophy often starting in hands, from involvement of the LMN
  - Fasciculations decreased deep tendon reflexes (DTR)

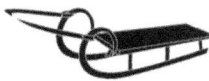

- o Pyramidal tracts
  - Amystrophic lateral sclerosis (ALS)
    - A progressive neurodegenerative syndrome with evidence of disease in both upper and lower motor neurons in one or several areas of the body, as well as abnormalities in behaviours and language (in ~ 50%), and bulbar dysfunction (in ~ 30%)
    - Treatment is supportive and symptomatic
  - UMN signs in legs
    - Weakness
    - No atrophy
    - Increased DTRs
    - Bobinski reflex positive
  - When LMN signs later develop in legs, DTRs are lost

- o Motor cranial nerve nuclei in pons and medulla
  - Progressive bulbar palsy
  - Pseudobulbar palsy
    - Muscles are stiff, spastic
    - Tongue is stiff but not wasted
    - Positive jaw jerk
  - Cranial nerve nuclei in pons and medulla

- Perform a focused physical examination for motor neuron disease in the adult.

- ➢ Definition
  - o Bulbar or pseudobulbar palsy
  - o Amyotrophic lateral sclerosis
    - Flaccid arms and spastic legs.
  - o Progressive muscular atrophy
    - Lesion in the anterior horn cells
    - Retention of deep tendon reflexes
    - Severe muscular atrophy of distal muscles
  - o Primary lateral sclerosis (rare): signs progress from an UMN to a LMN picture

  - o Upper limbs
    - Fasciculations
    - Reflexes
    - Painless weakness

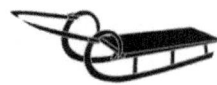

- o Lower limbs
  - Spasticity
  - ↑ reflexes
  - Up-going plantars

- o Cranial
  - Dysarthria and dysphagia.
  - Sluggish palatal movements, absent gag reflex, brisk jaw jerk.
  - Combination of the above signs
    - Presence of upper and lower motor neuron involvement of a single spinal segment, and motor dysfunction involving at least two limbs or one limb and bulbar muscles.
    - Sensory symptoms or signs are **not** seen.
    - Ocular movements are **not** affected.
    - Cerebellar or extrapyramidal systems are **not** affected.
    - Sphincters are involved late, if at all.
  - Emotional lability (if there is bulbar involvement).

Adapted from: Baliga RR. *Saunders/Elsevier* 2007, pages 193 and 194.

- o Dysmetria – inability to control one's range of motion

- o Dysdiadochokinesia – inability to perform rapid alternating movements

- o Ataxia – defective voluntary muscle co-ordination

- o Dysarthria – difficult or defective speech attributed to impairments of the tongue

- o Nystagmus – constant involuntary cyclical movements of the eyes

Source: Jugovic PJ, et al. *Saunders/ Elsevier* 2004, page 166.

CLINICAL TIPS

- o Muscle weakness, but
  - No fasciculations
  - Weakness of ocular muscles } not ALS

- o Fasciculations but no muscle weakness/atrophy

- o Pain, sensory loss cognitive decline

Abbreviation: ALS, amyotrophic lateral sclerosis

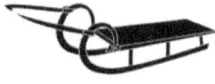

Clinical Curiosities and Buzzwords

- o Fatigue/neurological symptoms ↑ by heat
- o Sensory loss/paresthesia, ↑ by neck flexion
- o Internuclear opthalamohagia ↓↓ adduction of affected age

> **Power grading system** for weakness of the limbs

- o 0- Nil movement

- o 1 -Flicker of movement

- o 2 -Movement cannot overcome gravity

- o 3 -Movement cannot overcome any resistance

- o 4- Movement against resistance is weaker than "normal"

- o 5 –Normal

Adapted from: Filate W, et al. *The Medical Society, Faculty of Medicine, University of Toronto* 2005, page 164; and McGee SR. *Saunders/Elsevier* 2007, Table 57-1, page 709.

- Give a diagnostic approach to the major types of upper motor neuron weakness.

"STEP ONE"		"STEP TWO"	
Distribution of Weakness	Diagnostic Possibilities	Additional Finding	Location of Lesion
o Left monoparesis	– Right cerebral hemisphere – Right brainstem – Left spinal cord	▪ New seizures	- Right cerebral hemisphere
o Right hemiparesis	– Left cerebral hemisphere – Left brainstem – Right spinal cord	▪ Aphasia ▪ Right homonymous hemianopia ▪ Left sixth nerve palsy ▪ Loss of sensation left arm and leg; face spared	- Left cerebral hemisphere - Left cerebral hemisphere - Left brainstem - Right spinal cord

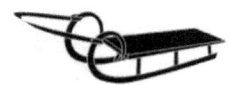

"STEP ONE"		"STEP TWO"	
Distribution of Weakness	Diagnostic Possibilities	Additional Finding	Location of Lesion
○ Paraparesis	– Bilateral lesion of thoracic cord or above	▪ Sensory level at midchest; normal arm strength and reflexes ▪ Spine tenderness between scapulae	- Bilateral lesion, thoracic cord
○ Tetraparesis	– Bilateral lesion of cervical cord or above	▪ Hyperactive jaw jerk ▪ Dementia ▪ Sensory level upper chest ▪ Absent biceps reflexes but hyperactive triceps reflexes	- Bilateral lesion, cerebral hemispheres - Bilateral lesion, cervical cord

Printed with permission: McGee SR. *Saunders/Elsevier*, 2007, Table 57-5, page 722.

SO YOU WANT TO BE A NEUROLOGIST!

- In the patient with corticosteroid-associated myopathy, give the significance of ↑ serum CK and/or abnormal EMG.
  - ○ In corticosteroids-induced myopathy, the serum CK is normal, as also is the EMG
  - ○ If CK or EMG abnormal, the diagnosis is likely to be wrong, with the correct diagnosis being
    Another myopathy
    Partially treated inflammatory myosistis, which has recurred

- A patient with inflammatory myopathy has proximal muscle weakness plus ↑ serum CK. Treatment with corticosteroids is associated with ↑ serum CK, but proximal muscle weakness increases. Give the likely explanation.
  - ○ Corticosteroid myopathy is associated with normal serum CK, whereas inflammatory myopathy is associated with ↑ serum CK
  - ○ As the inflammatory myopathy has improved with corticosteroids, the corticosteroids have induced a myopathy

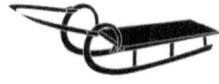

Mastering the Boards: Neurology   A.B.R. Thomson

➢ Diagnosis

   o EMG
- – Muscle functional degeneration

   o MRI
- – Site of degeneration
  - ▪ Complications
- – Dysphagia
  - ▪ Video fluoroscopy swallowing study (VFSS)
- – Respiration
  - ▪ Pulmonary function studies (PFTs)
  - ▪ Pulse oximetry

➢ Treatment

   o Psychosocial and physiotherapeutic support

   o Anticipate need for feeding tube (percutaneous and scopic gastrostomy [PGG] lube)

   o Riluzole- ↑ survival only- non invasive ventilator support 3 mon

   o Discuss end-of-life care

Myasthenia Gravis

➢ Definition

   o Weakness of the eye and facial muscles that worsens with repeated contraction

   o Fluctuating painless weakness of voluntary muscles, including ocular (~50%) and bulbar (~15%) muscles, caused by autoantibodies, against the post-synaptic acetylene receptor of the neuromuscular junctions, or against Mu SK (muscle-specific tyrosine kinase), which increases with exercise and in to evening.

   o "... an autoimmune disease caused by antibodies directed against the acethylclidine receptor, which results in impaired neuromuscular transmission"... and... symptoms... worsened by fatigue, exertion, [fever], stress, and intercurrent infections" (Board Basics, 2012, page 236).

- ➤ Clinical
  - ○ Eyes
    - − Ptosis
    - − Diplopia
  - ○ GI
    - − dysphagia
  - ○ Lung
    - − Dyspnea
  - ○ Thyroid associated hypothyroidism thymomia
  - ○ Note
    - − Normal
      - ▪ Sensory
      - ▪ DTRs
      - ▪ Pupils

Abbreviation: DTRs, deep tendon reflexes

- • Perform a focused physical examination for myasthenia gravis.
  - ○ Face
    - − Snarling face when the patient attempts to smile
  - ○ Eyes
    - − Worsening of ptosis after sustained upward gaze for at least 45 seconds
    - − Diplopia and variable squint

Myasthenia gravis

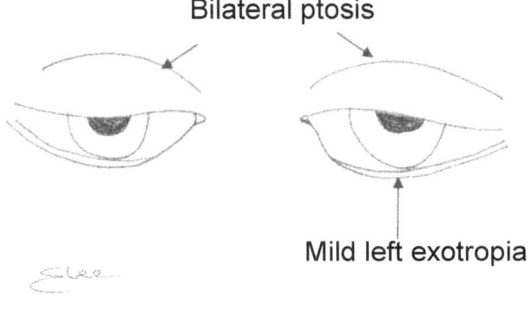

Bilateral ptosis

Mild left exotropia

- ○ Myasthenia gravis may mimic any ocular disorder causing diplopia
- ○ Most often it mimics weakness of the superior rectus muscle or medial rectus muscle (i.e., difficulty with sustained elevation or adduction of the eye, respectively)
- ○ Clues to the diagnosis of myasthenia gravis are associated ptosis, fluctuating course, and normal pupils

Source: McGee SR. *Saunders/Elsevier* 2007, Figure 55-3, page 699.

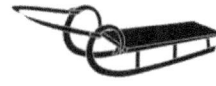

- o Speech
  - Nasal
- o Muscles
  - Weakness without loss of reflexes, or alteration of sensation or co-ordination.
  - The weakness may be generalized; it may affect the limb muscles, often proximal in distribution, as well as the diaphragm and neck extensors.
  - Muscle wasting is rare, and presents late in the disease.

Likelihood ratio for clinical history and physical findings in a person with symptoms for myasthenia gravis (MG)

		PLR
o	Abnormal sleep test	53
o	Peek sign	30
o	Abnormal ice test	24
o	Positive response to an anticholinesterase test	15
o	The history 'speech becoming unintelligible during prolonged speaking'	4.5

Abbreviations: PLR+, makes the diagnosis more likely

Source: Simel, DL, et al. *JAMA* 2009, Table 34-3, page 460.

- o Factors which increase the pretest probability of finding MG.
  - Patients with asymmetric fluctuating eyelid ptosis
  - Patients with extraocular dysmotility not referable to a single nerve
  - Patients with weakness of other specific muscles
  - Young women of child-bearing age, and men and women aged approximately 70 years

Source: Simel DL, et al. *JAMA* 2009, page 460.

- ➢ Causes/associations
  - o Endocrine
    - Thyrotoxicosis
    - Hypothyroidism
    - Diabetes mellitus

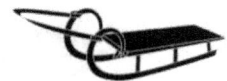

- o Tumour
  - – Thyrotoxicosis
  - – Thymoma (~75%)
  - – Associated cancer
    - ▪ Breast   – Cancer
    - ▪ Lung   – Small cell cancer
    - ▪ Blood   – Hodgkin lymphoma
- o MSK
  - – Rheumatoid arthritis (RA)
  - – Dermatomyositis
  - – SLE
  - – Sjogren disease
  - – Sarcoidosis
- o Skin
  - – Pemphigus
- o Autoimmune
  - – Pernicious anemia
- o Drugs

- Give the name of drugs which act on the neuromuscular junction and are therefore relatively contraindicated in MG (myasthenia gravis).

  - o Heart   – β-blockers
        – Calcium channel blockers
        – Anti-arrhythmic agents
  - o Antibiotics   – Aminoglycosides
  - o Analgesics   – Morphine
        – Barbiturates
  - o Neuromuscular blocking drugs

➢ Differentiate from
  - o Botulism
  - o Eaton-Lambert syndrome
    - – Myasthenic disorder, often associated with bronchial small cell carcinoma
    - – Commonly, weakness of truncal and proximal limb muscles

Adapted from: Baliga RR. *Saunders/Elsevier* 2007, pages 187 and 188.

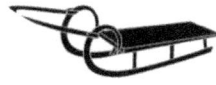

➢ Clinical
  ○ Fluctuation in muscle strength brought by
    – Activity
    – Stress
    – Fever
    – Infection

  ○ Thyroid disease associated in ~30%

➢ Differential

• Give the differentiation between MG (myasthenia gravis), botulism and ELMS (Eaton-Lambert myasthenia syndrome).

	MG	Botulism	ELMS
○ Muscle-weakness	With activity All muscles	+ Brainstem	↓ with activity Proximal
○ Autoantibodies	Against Acetylcholine Receptor	-	Against voltage-gated Calcium channel
○ Involvement of			
– Eye	Ptosis Diplopia	+	N
▪ Pupils	N	Slow non-reactive	N
– GI / Lung	Dysphagia Dyspnea	+	N

THIS IS FOR THE NEUROLOGY RESIDENT

• What is myasthenic crisis?
  ○ Exacerbation of MG, expecially bulbar and respiratory involvement, leading to need for ventilation.

• What is cholinergic crisis?
  ○ Excessive sensitivity to cholinergics in MG, such as in myasthenic crisis, with excessive salivation, confusion, lacrimation, miosis, pallor and collapse.

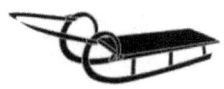

➤ Treatment
- o Pyridostimine $\xrightarrow[\text{Adverse effects}]{\text{poor response}}$ Immunosuppression
- o Pyrodostigmine
- o Immunosuppression
- o Thymectomy for thymoma
- o L-thyroxine for associated hypothyroidism
- o Respiratory for associated hypothyroidism
- o Respiratory failure
  - For VC (vital capacity) < 15 mL /kg
  - Intubation
  - Plasmapheresis
- o Screen for small cell lung cancer (in ~ 50%)
- o MuSK receptor antibody
  - Negative
    - Pyridostigmine (acetylcholinesterase inhibitor)
  - Positive
    - Plasma exchange
    - Immunosuppression
- o Severe / refractory MG
  - IV-IG (intravenous immune globulin)
  - Plasma exchange
- o Thymectomy, for thymoma

SO YOU WANT TO BE A NEUROLOGIST!

- Perform a focused physical examination to distinguish between LE-MS (Lambert-Eaton myasthenia syndrome) versus autoimmune myasthenia gravis associated with a thymoma.
  - o LE-MS has unique features
    - Dry mouth
    - ↓ DTR (deep tendon reflexes)
    - Proximal muscle weakness which improved with activity
- Give the name of the serum antibody found in mynethemia gravis, and in the Eaton-Lambert syndrome.
  - o Myasthenia gravis – anti-acetylcholine receptor antibody
  - o Eaton-Lambert syndrome – antibodies to voltage-gated calcium channels

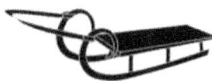

CNS INFECTIONS

Meningitis

➤ Clinical

Differentiate between four similar signs
1. Kernig   sign. To detect meningeal irritation

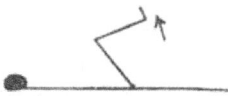

Straightening leg with hip flexed produces pain and sapsm of hamstrings

2. Brudzinski' sign. To detect meningeal irritation

Flexing neck produces flexion of lower limbs

3. Thomas   test. To detect fixed flexion deformity of the hip – joint

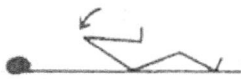

Eleminating lumbar lordosis produces flexion of the affected hip

4. Straight – leg raising test. To detect lesions of sciatic nerve or its spinal roots

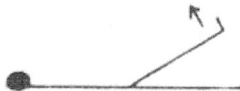

Straight – leg raising produces pain below the normal full excursion

Adapted from: Burton JL. *Churchill Livingstone* 1971, page 90; McGee SR. *Saunders/Elsevier* 2007, Figure 23.1, page 278.

What is "the best"? The two "best" clinical tests for the presence of a subarachnoid hemorrhage are: neck stiffness, and neurological findings which are not focal. Recall that neck stiffness is also common in persons with meningitis, and they will much more often have fever.

- Perform a focused physical examination to distinguish between meningeal irritation, versus lesion of the sciatic nerve or its spinal roots (Lasègue sign).

  o To detect meningeal irritation
    - Kernig sign
      ▪ Straightening leg with hip flexed produces pain and spasms of hamstrings

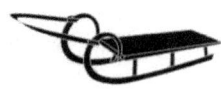

    o To detect lesions of sciatic nerve or its spinal roots

        – Straight-leg raising test produces pain below the normal full excursion

Source: McGee SR. *Saunders/Elsevier* 2007, Table 23-1, page 280.

SO YOU WANT TO BE A NEUROLOGIST!

- Give the typical neurological lesions associated with leptomeningeal lesions?
  - Cerebral
    - Headache
    - Seizures
    - Focal neurologic signs
  - Cranial nerve
  - Any cranial nerve can be affected, especially
    - CN III, IV, VI, and VII
  - CN VII is often affected in Lynne disease
  - Radicular (radiculoneuropathy or radiculomyelopathy) - neck and back pain as well as radicular pain and spinal cord signs

Source: Ghosh AK. *Mayo Clinic Scientific Press* 2008, page 762.

- We all know that meningitis will cause meningismus, symptoms of headache, photophobia and nuchal rigidity. Give two other non-neurological conditions may cause a stiff neck.
  - Intracerebral bleed
  - Posterior fossa tumour

- Perform a focused physical examination for meningitis (the numbers in brackets represent valves for sensivity)

  - General
    - Jolt accentuation of headache
    - Myalgia
    - Fever (87%)
    - Altered mental status (69%)

  - Eye
    - Papilledema

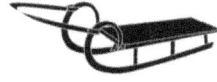

- o CNS
  - – Focal neurological signs (9%) (eg, cranial nerve palsy; 21%)
  - – Seizures (13%)
  - – Subarachnoid hemorrhage
  - – Acute bacterial meningitis
  - – Cervical fusion
  - – Spondylitis
  - – Parkinson disease
  - – Increased intracranial pressure (with impending tonsillar herniation)

- o Meningeal signs
  - – Stiff neck with passive motion (80%)
  - – Chin toward chest
  - – Kernig sign, Brudzinski sign (61%)

- o Skin
  - – Petechnal rash (13%)

- o CVS.
  - – ↓ PR
  - – SBP

- o *Note:
  - – The sensitivity is 46% for the classic triad (fever, neck stiffness, headache)
  - – Also note that fever and altered mental status are less frequent with subarachnoid hemorrhage than with acute bacterial meningitis.

Abbreviation: PR, pulse rate; SBP, systolic blood pressure
Adapted from: Jugovic PJ, et al. *Saunders/ Elsevier* 2004, pages 138 and 139; Simel D, et al. *JAMA* 2009, Table 30-5, 30-1, page 396; McGee SR. *Saunders/Elsevier* 2007, Table 23-1and Box 23-1, page 280 and 281; Talley NJ, et al. *Maclennan & Petty Pty Limited* 2003, page 349.

Aseptic Meningitis Syndrome

➤ Definition: ".....clinical and laboratory findings consistent with meningitis in a patient who has normal cerebrospinal fluid (CSF) stains and cultures on initial evaluation."

MKSAP 16, Infectious disease 2012, page 1

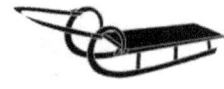

Bacterial Meningitis

➢ Demography

• Give the 3 groups of persons at highest risk for bacterial meningitis.

  o Young adults living closely together

  o Travel to endemic areas

  o Asplemic persons

➢ Bacteriology (common organisms)
  o Hysteria manocytogenes
    – Neonates, or > 50 yr
    – associations
  o Neisseria meningitides
    – Second most common (children, young adults)
    – Association
      ▪ Complement C5-C9, terminal component deficiency
  o Streptococcus pneumonia
    – Most common
    – Associations
      ▪ Endocarditis
      ▪ Otitis media
      ▪ Head trauma, with CSP leak
      ▪ Liver cirrhosis
        –Iron overload
        –Alcoholism
      ▪ Kidney
        –Chronic renal disease
      ▪ MSK
        –Collagen vascular disease
      ▪ Malignancy
      ▪ Infection
        –HIV
      ▪ Drugs
        –Immunosuppression

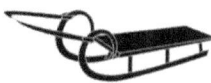

Haemophilus Influenza-associated bacterial meningitis occurs in only ~7% of cases.

- Give the clinical features which provide ↑ risk for H. influenzae meningitis.

  o Alcoholism

  o Diabetes

  o Splenectomy

  o Head injury / CSF leak

  o Hypogammaglobulinemia

- Give the factors which ↑ risk for nosocromial (health care-associated) bacterial meningitis.

  o Similar to those for gram-negative bacterial meningitis
    - Head injury
    - Neurosurgical procedure, or
    - Ventricular drains

  o However the major pathogens for in hospital bacterial meningitis differ from those responsible for bacterial meningitis contracted during hospitalization.

- Give the likely pathogens for in hospital-acquired bacterial pneumonia.

  o Staphylococcus aureus

  o P. aeruginosa

  o Propionibacterium acnes

- Dexamethasone is sometimes given as adjunctive therapy. Give with which antibiotic dexamethasone not given, and the reason why.

  o When dexamethasone is given with vancomycin, the ability of vancomycin to enter the CSF may be reduced.

  o The dexamethasone-associated entry of vancomycin into the CSF may be overcome by ↑ dose of vancomycin.

  o If dexamethasone is used with vancomycin plus a third generation cephalosporin (such as ceftaxime or ceftriaxone) with a MIC (minimal inhibitory concentration) > 2 microgram / mL, repeat the CSF aspirate (lumbar puncture) 36 to 48 hr after starting therapy to ensure that the antibiotics combination has penetrated the CSF and is therapeutically successful (i.e., CSF is sterile).

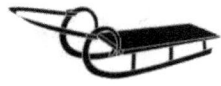

- Give the clinical associations with bacterial meningitis (especially S. pneumonia).

    o Otitis media

    o Pneumonia

    o CSF leak (basilar skull fracture)

    o Sinusitis

o Neisseria meningitides	– ↓ properdin
	– ↓ complement (C_5, C_6, C_7, C_8)
o Listeria monocytogenes	– Contaminated food
o Streptococcus agalactide	– Screening for rectovaginal colonization at 35 to 37 wk gestation to determine carrier status
	– Anti-microbial prophylaxis for carriers

➢ Gram negative

o Organisms	– Escherichia coli
	– Klebsiella
	– Pseudomonas aeruginosa
	– Serratia marcescers

- Give the predisposing associations for gram-negative causes of bacterial meningitis.

    o Gram-negative bacteremia

    o Head trauma

    o Neurosurgery

    o Ventricular drains

    o Immunodeficiency

    o Disseminated strongyloid

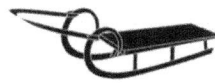

➢ Laboratory

• Give the measurements on CSF that helps to distinguish between meningitis of bacterial, viral, tuberculous and cryptococcal causes, or encephalitis.

Diagnosis	WBC (cells / µL)	Glucose (mg/dL)	Protein (mg/dL)
○ Encephalitis	Lymph pleocytosis	?	↑
○ Meningitis			
– Bacterial	> 1000 PMN	< 40	> 100
– Viral	< 500 lymph	> 40	< 300
– TB	< 300 lymph	< 40	
– Cryptococcus	< 500 lymph	< 40	

Abbreviations: CSF, cerebral spinal fluid; PMNs, polymorphonuclear cells (aka neutrophils); TB, tuberculosis; WBC, white blood cell

  ○ Note

RBCs in CSF occur in encephalitis, but not in meningitis unless the lumbar top as traumatic.
Meningitis plus encephalitis may coexist (meningencephalitis)
When to do a Gram stain on CSF ↑ PMN (>1000) ↓ glucose (<40) protein >100 mg/dL.

| If bacterial meningitis suggested
↓

Gramstain

| If Gram stain negative despite CSF
↓ findings suggesting bacterial meningitis

Latex agglutination test

➢ Gram positive

  ○ 90% of community acquired bacterial meningitis is caused by 3 organisms Streptococcus pneumonia (58%), Strept. agalactiae (18%); group B Strept. and Neisseria meningitides

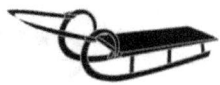

Mastering the Boards: Neurology   A.B.R. Thomson

- Give the performance characteristics for PCR as well as the rapid immunochromatographic test for S. pneumonia.

Characteristics	Rapid test	PCR
o Sensitivity	95-100%	92%-100%
o Specificity	100%	100%

➢ Treatment

- Give the empiric antibiotic treatment of bacterial meningitis.

  - o Age < 50   VC ± A   ⎫
  -         >50   VCA   ⎬ add dexamethasone if
  - o Trauma   pneumococcal infection
    - – fracture, base of skull   VC   ⎭ suspected/diagnosed
    - – post-op neurosurgery, or   VC, or, V plus cefepine or meropenem
    - – CSF shunt

Abbreviations: A, ampicillin; C, cefotaxime, or ceftriaxone; V, vancomycin

- Give the empiric anti-microbial treatment of nosocomial bacterial meningitis, and the likely organism against for which treatment is selected.

  - o Likely micro-organisms
    - – Gram-positive
      - ▪ Staphylococcus aureua
      - ▪ MRSA (methicillin-resistant S. aureus)
    - – Gram-negative
      - ▪ Pseudomonas aeruginosa
      - ▪ Acinetobacter
  - o Recommended antibodies
    - – Vancomycin plus meropenem

- Give the recommended antimicrobial therapy is as follows.

	Third-generation Cephalosporin, e.g., Cefotaxime or Ceftriaxone	Vancomycin plus Possible Rifampin	Ampicillin or Penicillin G plus Aminoglyco-side
o Streptococcus pneumonia	√	√	
o Neisseria meningitides	√		
o Haemophilus influenza	√		
o Listeria monocytogens			√

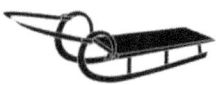

Mastering the Boards: Neurology   A.B.R. Thomson

Note: Vancomycin plus meropenem in place of either cefotaxime or ceftriaxone may be used empirically for bacterial meningitis after head trauma, neurosurgery or ventricular shunts (catheters).

For further details, please refer to a standard medical textbook, or to a review such as UptoDate or MKSAP 16, Infectious disease 2012, Table 5, page 6.

- Give the serotype of meningococci which is not included in the quadrivalent meningoccal conjugate vaccine.
    - Serotype B meningococci is not included in the quadrivalent meningococcal conjugate vaccine.

Brain Abscess
➢ Causes/associations
- Give risk factors for the development of a brain abscess.

    - Direct extension
        - Trauma
        - ENT
    - Hematogenous extension
        - Lung
          Pyogenic abscess
        - Heart
            ▪ Infective endocarditis
        - Abdomen
        - Bone
            ▪ Osteomyelitis
        - Skin
    - HHT (hereditary hemorrhagic telangiectasia)
    - Congenital heart disease

➢ Diagnosis
    - MRI, diffusion
    - Cerebritis not seen, but purulent stage
    - Differentiated from tumour

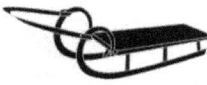

➢ Treatment   o Aspiration stereotactic

    o Surgical

    o IV antibiotics (empiric choice based on predisposing conditions) for 4-6 wks, followed by oral antibiotics

    o Corticosteroids for
       – Mass effect
       – Brain edema

    o Treat predisposing condition

Note: For full information on empiric antimicrobial therapy for various predisposing conditions, please see standard textbooks or reviews such as UptoDate or MKSAP 16, Infectious disease 2012, Table 6, page 7.

Cranial Subdural Empyema

- Give the common organisms associated with cranial subdural empyema, and a recommended treatment.

  o Often from paranasal sinuses

  o Common organisms

  o Diagnosis
     – Neural MRI

  o Treatment
     – Emergency condition, team approach
     – Craniectomy and drainage
     – Empiric antibiotics
       ▪ Vancomycin
       ▪ Metronidazole
       ▪ Ceftaxime, Ceftriaxone, Cefepime (4th generation cephalosporine)

Spinal Epidural Abscess

➢ Microbiology   o Usually is hematogenous spread of Staphylococcus aureus

    o May be gram-negative (GI, GU) or IVDU (IV drug use)

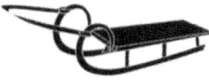

Mastering the Boards: Neurology   A.B.R. Thomson

- ➤ Clinical

- • Give the clinical presentations and treatment for spinal epidural abscess.

  - o Vertebra   – Pain in back
  - o Nerve root   – Radiculopathy
                 – Peresthesias
  - o Spinal cord   – Dysfunction
                 – Paraplegia

- ➤ Diagnosis
  - o MRI with gadolinium

- ➤ Treatment
  - o Emergency decompression and drainage (to prevent paralysis)
  - o Initially empiric antibiotics
    - Anti-staphylococcal
      - Vancomycin
    - Anti-pseudomonal
      - Cephalosporin, or
      - Carbapenem
  - o Follow treatment response with serial MRI studies

Viral Meningitis

- ➤ Clinical

- • Give the proportion of patients with mumps meningitis with enlargement of the salivary glands.

  - o Only about ½ of patients with mumps as a course of their aseptic meningitis will have enlarged salivary glands on physical examination.

- • Give the typical clinical picture of benign recurrent lymphocytic meningitis, and the associated virus shown on PCR (polymerase chain reaction).

  - o Clinical
    - About 10 episodes of aseptic meningitis, lasting 2 to 5 days, and then followed by spontaneous recovery
  - o Laboratory
    - PCR demonstrates HSV-2

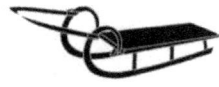

- Give the CSF findings which may help distinguish viral from bacterial meningitis.

CSF Parameter	Viral Meningitis	Bacterial Meningitis
o Opening pressure	≤ 250 mm H_2O	200-500 mm H_2O
o Leukocyte count	50-1000 / μL	1000-5000 / μL
	(50-1000 x 10^6 / L)	(1000-5000 x 10^6 / L)
o Leukocyte differential	Lymphocyte	Neutrophils
o Glucose	> 45 mg / dL (2.5 mmol / L)	< 40 mg / dL (2.2 mmol/L)
o Protein	< 200 mg / dL (2000 mg / L)	100-500 mg / dL (1000-5000 mg / L)
o Gram stain	Negative	Positive in 60%-90%
o Culture	Negative	Positive in 70%-85%

MKSAP 16, Infectious disease 2012, Table 1, page 1

Viral Encephalitis

➤ Definition

  o "…. infection of the brain parenchyma with associated neurologic dysfunction", including ↓ LOC (level of consciousness) or seizure

Source: MKSAP 16, Infectious disease 2012, page 8.

  o The word "meningoencephalitis" is often used because of frequent infection of both meninges as well as parenchyma of brain

  o Over 100 infectious causes, but
      – Common   ▪ HSV1, HSV2
                        ▪ West Nile virus
      – After animal bite ▪ Rabies virus
      – Mosquito bite   ▪ St. Louis encephalitis virus
      – Immunosuppression ▪ HSV2
                        ▪ JC virus

Note: JC virus may cause PMC (progressive multifocal leucoencephalopathy).

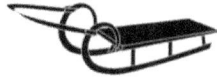

Mastering the Boards: Neurology   A.B.R. Thomson

- ➢ Common causes
  - ○ Infection
    - – NSV
    - – Enterovirus
    - – WNV (West Nile Virus)
  - ○ Idiopathic

- ➢ Clinical
  - ○ The acute onset of a febrile illness with headache and ↓LOC (level of consciousness) occurs in both meningitis and in encephalitis. Meningtis is usually not associated with focal neurological signs, whereas encephalitis is usually not associated with meningism.

- ➢ Diagnostic imaging
  - ○ In meningitis, the MRI head is not helpful, whereas in encephalitis, MRI shows enhancement of the temporal lobe.

- ➢ Treatment
  - ○ If HSV encephalitis is suspected, perform a lumbar puncture, and give IV ocyclain before obtaining the results of CSF IgM antibodies for WNV, or HSV or PCR.

$$\text{Encephalitis acyclovir} \xrightarrow[\text{Poor response}]{\text{CSF positive for HSV}} \text{brain biopsy}$$

Herpes Simplex Encephalitis

  - ○ HSV-1 (herpes simplex virus 1) → encephalitis
  - ○ HSV-2 → meningitis
    - – May be proceeded or accompanied by genital herpes
    - – Most persons with serological evidence for HSV-2 do not have a history of genital ulcer disease
    - – Some HSV-2 infected persons may have a fissure rather than anHSV-2 ulcer
    - – Perform PCR on CSF for diagnosis
    - – For non-CVS. HSV, perform viral culture or HSV PCR

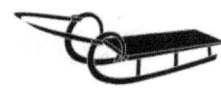

- Give the diagnostic findings for HSV-1 encephalitis.

    o Orolabial herpatic lesion (< 10%)

    o CSF
      - In 95%   Pleocytosis
                     ↑ Lymphocytes
      - In 5%   Normal cell counts

    o PCR
      - 95% sensitive
      - 100% specific

    o MRI
      - Temporal lobe inflammation → necrosis → MR ~ 20%

    o EEG (Electroencephalogram)
      - Temporal lobe periodic seizure-like discharge

    o Treatment
      - IV acyclovir (use early if high clinical suspicion)

West Nile Virus (WNV) **Encephalitis**

  ➢ Clinical   o Asymptomatic

                                o Symptomatic
                                      - 19%, fever
                                          ▪ Rash
                                    - 1% neuroinvasion (WNND, West Nile neuroinvasive disease)
                                      Meningitis ± Encephalitis ± Myelitis

- Give the signs of WNV, and the means of making the diagnosis.

    o Focal weakness

    o Acute flaccid paralysis

    o Respiratory failure (paralysis of diaphragm)

    o Extrapyramidal
      - Tremor
      - Bradycardia

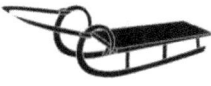

➤ Diagnosis o CSF
    – Pleocytosis
    – Lymphocytosis
    – ↑ Neutrophils
    – IgM antibody to West Nile virus

    o MMRI with gadolinium may see bilateral enhancement on T2-weighting of thalamus / basal ganglia

---

Clinical Skill

A patient develops encephalomeningitis and asymmetric flaccid paralysis. WNW (West Nile Virus) infection is suspected, but the WNV IgM serum test was negative.
- Give the next diagnostic test.
  - o A negative serum antibody test does not exclude WNV since the duration of uremia is short.
  - o The next test should be vial culture of CSF (cerebrospinal fluid) obtained from a LP (lumbar puncture)

PCR has 86% to 100% sensitivity and 92% to 100% specificity for diagnosing enteroviral meningitis, but the performance characteristics for nucleic acid amplification tests are poor for WNV.
- Give the findings in CSF which is most helpful to make WNV diagnosis.
  - o IgM antibiotics to the virus press in CSF is the best diagnostic test for WNV.

➤ Treatment o General support
    o Specific anti-viral therapy
      - None

SO YOU WANT TO BE A NEUROLOGIST / ID EXPERT!
- Give the flavavirus which may give a false-positive IgM-antibody to West Nile virus in CSF.
  - o St. Louis encephalitis virus
  - o Japanese encephalitis virus
  - o Dengue virus
  - o Yellow fever virus

Abbreviations: CSF, cerebrospinal fluid; UTI, urinary tract infection

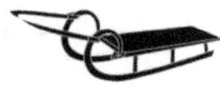

Limbic Encephalitis

- Give a definition of limbic encephalitis, give the name of 2 associated antibodies found in CSF or serum which point to the incriminated Tumour causing the encephalitis paraneoplastic syndromes.

  - ➢ Clinical

    - o CNS
      - - Memory, subacute loss
      - - Personality change
      - - Encephalopathy
      - - Seizure
      - - Psychosis

    - o Mouth
      - - Involuntary movements of mouth (oral dyskinesia)

  - ➢ Diagnosis

    - o Flair-MRI (fluid-attenuated inversion recovery MRI)
      - - Memory, subacute loss
      - - Personality change
      - - Encephalopathy
      - - Seizure
      - - Psychosis

    - o Antibodies
      - - Anti-NMDA
      - - Anti-ANNA-1
        - ▪ These anti-Hu antibodies are often associated with SCC (small cell cancer) of lung

- Give the primary causes of rapid deterioration of cognition and behaviour, associated with **myoclonus**.

  - o Limbic encephalitis

  - o CJK (Creutzfeldth-Jarcob disease)
    - - A prion disease of the brain causing a spongiform encephalopathy
    - - Note: Natalizumab is a disease modifying biologic use to treat MS (multiple sclerosis), but carries a risk of 1:1,000 of the development of PML (progressive multifocal leukoencephalopathy) from CNS infection with CJ virus.

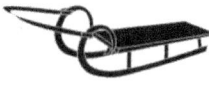

Prion Disease

➤ Definition: "…….. transmissible proteins that lack associated genetic material…….."

➤ Types

- o Sporadic Creutzfeldt-Jakob disease (sCJD; most common)
  - – Dementia (rapidly progressive)
  - – Myoclonus
  - – Extrapyramidal signs

- o Variant CJD (vCJD)
  - – Psychiatric symptoms
  - – Paresthesias
  - – Dementias

- o Eating meat contaminated with brain tissue from cows infected with BSE (bovine spongiform encephalopathy)
  - – Variant CJD
  - – Other forms of CJD
    - ▪ fCJD, familial CJD
    - ▪ iCJD, iatrogenic CJD

- o Rare
  - – Kuru (eating human in Papua New Guinea)
  - – PRNP gene mutation
    - ▪ Gerstmann-Straussler-Scheinker syndrome
    - ▪ Fatal familial insomnia

➤ Clinical

- o Use the WHO (World Health Organization) criteria for probable diagnosis of sCJD
  - – Progressive dementia
  - – ≥ 2 of the following (with duration < 2 years):
    - ▪ Myoclonus
    - ▪ Pyramidal or extrapyramidal dysfunction
    - ▪ Visual or cerebellar disturbance
    - ▪ Akinetic mutism

➤ Laboratory

- o CSF
  - – No inflammatory changes
  - – ↑ protein 14-3-3

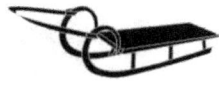

- o EEG
  - – Periodic sharp pattern
  - – 1- to 2-Hz period sharp waves
- ➢ Diagnostic imaging
  - o MRI
    - – sCJD
      - ▪ Use
        Diffusion-weighted imaging
        Fluid-attenuated immersion recovery (FLAIR) sequences
    - – vCJD
      - ▪ Pulvinar sign
- ➢ Pathology
  - o "spongiform changes"
  - o Positive tissue staining for Pr Psc (prion protein)
- ➢ Diagnosis
  - o Laboratory and EEG findings (at least one of the following):
    - – Cerebrospinal fluid positive for 14-3-3 protein
    - – No alternative diagnosis identified by routine investigation
    - – Characteristic EEG findings (1- to 2-Hz periodic sharp waves)

Source: MKSAP 16, Infectious disease 2012, Table 9, page 11.

- ➢ Treatment
  - o Supportive
  - o MR 100%; time to death depends on pathophysiology

Useful background: For an excellent outline of the clinical varieties of neuro-syphilis, please see: Burton J.L. *Churchill Livingstone* 1971, page 88.

- ➢ No mass effect (does not enhance with contrast)
  - o PML (Progressive multifocal leukoencephalopathy)
    - - Patchy areas of low attenuation on CT. MRI twice as sensitive. Not contrast enhanced and mass effect is absent. Lesions are bilateral, asymmetrical usually periventricular and subcortical. May have a normal CT or MRI.
    - - HIVE- HIV encephalopathy. Subcortical and cortical atrophy, non enhancing, symmetrical and bilateral. Usually associated with dementia but no focal motor or sensory deficit.

Useful background: For an excellent background on how to take a directed history of chronic disease, please see Jugovic P.J., et al. *Saunders/ Elsevier*, 2004, page 203.

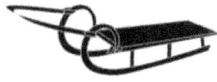

ONCOLOGY

- Give the Tumours for which adjuvant chemotherapy has been shown to be beneficial.

    o **Brain**

    o Breast

    o Lung

    o GI   - Esophagus
    - Stomach
    - Pancreas
    - Colon

Intracranial Tumours

Useful background

o Common presentations	- Seizures - Focal neurological deficits - Personality changes (frontal lobe) - Cognitive decline

- ➤ Pathology

    o Metastatic (commonest)   - Metastasis
    - Breast
    - Lung
    - Melanoma

    - Primary   - Glioma
    - Meningioma
    - Schwanoma
    - Medulloblastoma
    - Lymphoma (PCNSL, primary CNS lymphoma)

- ➤ Diagnosis   o MRI with contrast may show Distinction from other mass lesions
    o Brain biopsy may be necessary

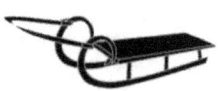

> ## SO YOU WANT TO BE A NEUROLOGIST!
>
> - Give the name of the primary tumour of the brain that may be diagnosed by examining the eyes.
>   - Slit-lamp examination of the eyes may allow identification of lymphomastous cells from PCNSL (primary CNS lymphoma)
>
> - Corticosteroids are often given to the patient with a brain tumour to ↓ ICP (intracranial pressure). Give the reason why corticosteroids are not given to patients with primary CNS lymphoma (PCNSL) until the diagnosis is made.
>   - Corticosteroids are effective to treat PCNSL, and when given before a brain biopsy, may make it difficult to establish the diagnosis.

Paraneoplastic Syndromes

➢ Definition

  - Benign or malignant Tumour from outside the nervous system (NS) produce antibodies which cross-react with epitopes in the NS to result in subacute progressive neurological paraneoplastic syndromes.

- Give the paraneoplastic syndromes associated with benign or malignant extra-nervous system Tumours.

Tumour	Neuropathy	Cerebellum	Opsoclonus-myoclonus	Limbic Encephalitis	Stiff Syndrome
○ Small cell lung cancer	+	+	+	+	+
○ Breast cancer		+	+		+
○ Ovary / testicular Cancer		+			
Teratoma				+	+
○ Thymoma		+		+	+
○ Hodgkin lymphoma		+			

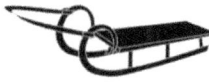

Mastering the Boards: Neurology   A.B.R. Thomson

➢ Treatment

  o Remove the causative and associated neoplasm

  o Symptomatic

    - IV-IG (IV immune globulin)
    - Plasma exchange
    - Corticosteroids

- Give the characteristics of **paraneoplastic** neurological degeneration associated tumours.

  o Tumours are often difficult to detect.

  o Tumours are histologically identical to tumours that develop in patients without paraneoplastic neurological degeneration (PND), except that many tumours have evidence of immune infiltration (immunogenic tumours).

  o Patients often have improved prognosis relative to those with comparable but non-immunogenic tumours (anti-Hu paraneoplastic syndrome, Lambert-Eaton myasthenic syndrome and some paraneoplastic cerebellar degeneration).

  o Spontaneous regression is rare.

  o Presence of antitumour immune response predicts improved prognosis (Hu syndrome)

  o Tumours are associated with circulating PND-antigen-specific killer T-cells (paraneoplastic cerebellar degeneration).

Source: Davey P. *Wiley-Blackwell* 2006, page 361.

Brain Metastases

➢ Common Primary Sites

  o Parenchyma

    - Lung
    - Breast   often metastasize to interface between
    - Mydoma   grey and white matter in parenchyma

  o Leptomeningeal

    - Leukemia

      ▪ Metastasize to
        - Brain surface
        - Spinal cord
        - Nerveroots

    - Lymphoma

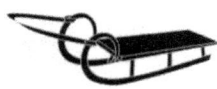

➢ Common causes

    o Primary

    o Secondary (metastatic)

       - CNS
       - Lung
       - Melanoma

➢ Clinical

    o ↑ ICP (intracranial pressure) → brainstem herniation → death

    o In the patient with systemic cancer plus new neurological symptoms/signs →

    o Suspect metastatic brain tumours to parenchyma or leptomeningitis, with proven otherwise by MRI Brain

➢ Diagnosis

    o CT or MRI of head

    o Do **not** perform LP (lumbar puncture) – risk of cloning

• Give the comparison of parenchymal versus leptomeningeal involvement of metastatic brain tumours

		Parenchymal	Leptomeningeal
o	Diagnostic imaging (CT / MRI)	– Multiple – Ring-shaped – Central necrosis	▪ Diffuse or patchy enhancement
o	Characteristics – Ring-enhancing – Central necrosis – Multiple nodules – Diffuse, patchy	+ –	– +
o	Site	– Junction of grey / white matter	▪ Brain ▪ Spinal cord ▪ Nerve roots
o	Source	– Lung – Breast – Melanoma	▪ Leukemia ▪ Lymphoma
o	Associations – Hydrocephalus (communicating)	–	+

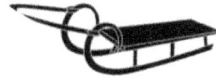

Mastering the Boards: Neurology   A.B.R. Thomson

	Parenchymal	Leptomeningeal
o CSF	– May be normal	■ ↑ protein ■ ↓ glucose ■ Positive cytology
o Treatment	– Corticosteroids – Whole brain radiation – Resection for single metastasis plus small primary Tumour with good prognosis	■ Corticosteroids ■ Methotrexate plus cytarabine

➤ Treatment
- o Parenchymal
  - known primary
  - – Corticosteroids ⟶ (whole-brain radiotherapy)
  - multiple nodules
- o Leptomeningeal
  - – Corticosteroids → treatment for causative leukemia/lymphoma (methorexate pluscytarabine)
- o Brain biopsy if lymphoma suspected (perform before giving corticosteroids)
- o Mannitol (osmotic diuretics
- o Obstructing hydrocephalus
  - – Surgical drainage
- o Brain metastases
  - – Isolated ■ Resection plus radiation
  - – Multiple ■ Whole brain radiation +/- chemotherapy

Clinical Skill

- o The auscultation of the lungs is normal in SVC syndrome.

- o Don't forget that examination of the chest is an important part of the pulmonary examination, and may be rewarding in the patient with SVC syndrome.

MCQ Therapeutic Heads-Up

- o Chemotherapy is not used for two types of brain tumours
  - – Metastatic parenchymal brain tumour from most solid organs (e.g., lung, breast)
  - – Meningioma

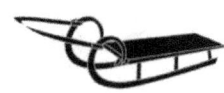

MULTIPLE SCLEROSIS

➢ Definition

- o "Multiple sclerosis (MS) is a chronic neurologic disorder characterized by targeted destruction of central nervous system (CNS) myelin, as well as exonal degeneration and loss. (Namaka M, et al. Chapter 25. In: Therapeutic Choices. Grey J, Ed. 6th Edition, *Canadian Pharmacists Association*: Otttawa, ON, 2011, page 308).

- o A chronic condition caused by immune-mediated injury over space and time to the brain, brainstem, spinal cord, and optic nerves and resulting in plaques of focal demyelination which acutely leads to functional disruption of white matter and chronically leads to degeneration in both white and grey matter.

- o Idiopathic demyelination of brain, brainstem and spiral cord in different areas and over different times.

➢ Demographics

- o Prevalence in CAN / USA is ~ 150/10^5

- o W (women) 2x > M (men)

- o M are more likely to have the more severe primary progressive form

➢ Pathogenesis

- o It is speculated that there is an autoimmune response to an unknown foreign molecule, (viral infection, dietary or hormonal risk factor) which has a structure similar to a component of myelin, leading to an initial focal inflammatory phase, followed by more diffuse inflammatory and immune-mediated destruction of myelin.

➢ Causes

- o Inherited factors
  - – Risk alleles in genes
    - ▪ Histocompatibility complex
    - ▪ IL-2 receptor
    - ▪ IL-7 receptor

- o Environmental
  - – Northern European descent
  - – Geographic location before adolescence

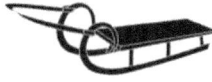

- ➢ Types
  - o Primary progressive
  - o Secondary progressive
  - o Relapsing
    - – Remitting
      - ▪ 50% move to a secondary progressive clinical course, especially in smokers

- ➢ Clinical
  - o Demyelation causing remissions and relapses of: weakness, inco-ordination, pain, paraesthesias, urinary urgency, impotence
  - o Steinberg's triad: history of incontinence of bladder, impotence and constipation
  - o There are four clinical presentations of MS
    - – RRMS (relapsing remitting; commonest form, ~90%)
      - ▪ RRMS (65% → SPMS)
    - – PPMS (primary progressive)
    - – SPMS (secondary progressive)
    - – PRMS (progressive relapsing)
    - – 80% present with a clinically isolated syndrome (are initial acute "attack"

  - o Clinical motor/sensory loss of areas of brain, brainstorm and spiral cord, depending upon area of plaques (demyelisation)

"The art of being wise is the art of knowing what to overlook."

William James

 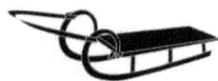

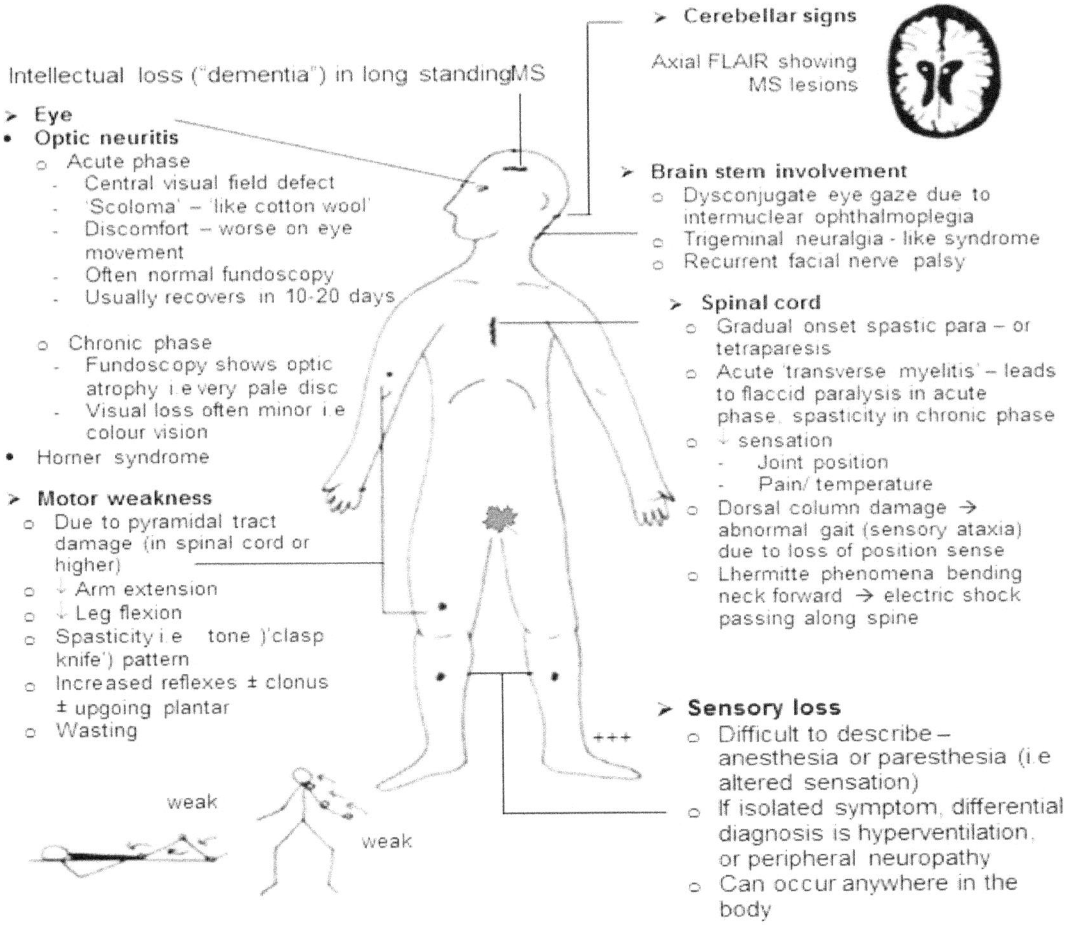

> Cerebellar signs

Axial FLAIR showing
MS lesions

Intellectual loss ("dementia") in long standingMS

> Eye
• Optic neuritis
  ○ Acute phase
    - Central visual field defect
    - 'Scoloma' – 'like cotton wool'
    - Discomfort – worse on eye movement
    - Often normal fundoscopy
    - Usually recovers in 10-20 days

  ○ Chronic phase
    - Fundoscopy shows optic atrophy i.e very pale disc
    - Visual loss often minor i.e colour vision
• Horner syndrome

> Motor weakness
  ○ Due to pyramidal tract damage (in spinal cord or higher)
  ○ ↓ Arm extension
  ○ ↓ Leg flexion
  ○ Spasticity i.e   tone)'clasp knife') pattern
  ○ Increased reflexes ± clonus ± upgoing plantar
  ○ Wasting

weak

weak

> Brain stem involvement
  ○ Dysconjugate eye gaze due to intermuclear ophthalmoplegia
  ○ Trigeminal neuralgia - like syndrome
  ○ Recurrent facial nerve palsy

  > Spinal cord
  ○ Gradual onset spastic para – or tetraparesis
  ○ Acute 'transverse myelitis' – leads to flaccid paralysis in acute phase, spasticity in chronic phase
  ○ ↓ sensation
    - Joint position
    - Pain/ temperature
  ○ Dorsal column damage → abnormal gait (sensory ataxia) due to loss of position sense
  ○ Lhermitte phenomena bending neck forward → electric shock passing along spine

> Sensory loss
  ○ Difficult to describe – anesthesia or paresthesia (i.e altered sensation)
  ○ If isolated symptom, differential diagnosis is hyperventilation, or peripheral neuropathy
  ○ Can occur anywhere in the body

Adapted from: Davey P. *Wiley-Blackwell* 2006, page 374.

> Clinical syndromes

Pseudorelapse (↑ symptoms associated with fever)

○ Optic neuritis

○ Myelitis, partial
  - Flaccid → spastic paralysis

○ Brainstem
  - Diplepsia, disconjugate eye movement
  - Jerking perception of objects (oscillopsia)
  - Nystagmus

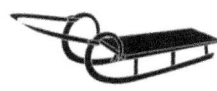

- o Vertibulo/cerebellar
  - – Vertigo
  - – Ataxia
- o Cortex
  - – ↓ cognition
  - – Fatigue

Note: Cortical syndromes do not occur

- o Symptoms which are often troublesome for patient
  - – CNS
    - ▪ Fatigue
    - ▪ Depression
    - ▪ Neuropathic pain

  - – MSK
    - ▪ Spasticity
    - ▪ ↓ mobility

  - – GU
    - ▪ Urinary urgency

SO YOU WANT TO BE A NEUROLOGIST!

In the context of the patient with MS (multiple sclerosis), who progresses to develop new sensory and motor symptoms below an area of pain in the neck as well as new dysfunction of the bowel and bladder, give the name of the syndrome and its pathogenesis.

- o Lhermitte syndrome is partial transverse cervical myelitis, causing shock-like pain in the neck, worsened by movement of the head and neck.

- o Note
  - - Fatigue is defined as "…. exhaustion that is unrelated to physical activity and may be exacerbated by hot weather" (Source: MSKAP 16 2013, Neurology page 132). In the patient with multiple sclerosis (MS), give the conditions which must be excluded before calling the fatigue idiopathic (MS-related fatigue).

- o Clinical course
  - – Relapsing-remitting (RR) intermittent attacks, with accumulation over time of
    - ▪ Residual disability

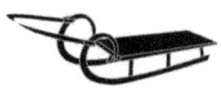

- Secondary progressive
  - May arise from RR-MS
  - ↑ by smoking
  - Only disease-modifying drug, mitoxantrone
- Primary progressive
  - Rapid worsening (25% needing gait-assist device within 7 yr)
- Incidental MRI findings (radiologically associated syndrome)
- Benign (debated)

o Relapsing-remitting: episodes of acute worsening with recovery and a stable course between relapses.

o Secondary progressive: gradual neurological deterioration with or without superimposed acute relapse in a patient who previously had relapsing-remitting multiple sclerosis.

o Primary progressive: gradual, almost continuous neurological deterioration from the onset of symptoms

o Progressive relapsing: gradual neurological deterioration from the onset symptoms but with subsequent superimposed relapses

o Variation of MS
  - Optic neuritis alone
  - Optic neuritis plus a single episode of transverse myelitis

Adapted from: Baliga RR. *Saunders/Elsevier* 2007, pages 175 to 178.

SO YOU WANT TO BE A NEUROLOGIST!

- Give the **prognostic markers** that predict more severe multiple sclerosis.
  o Progressive disease from the onset of symptoms.
  o Frequent relapses in the first two years.
  o Motor and cerebellar signs at presentation to neurologist.
  o Short interval between the first two relapses.
  o Male gender.
  o Poor recovery from relapse.
  o Multiple cranial lesions on T2-weighted MRI at presentation.

Source : Baliga RR. *Saunders/Elsevier* 2007, page 178.

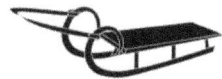

Mastering the Boards: Neurology   A.B.R. Thomson

➢ Curiosities to remember

    o Flexon of neck
- ↑ Paresthesias
- ↑ loss of sensation

    o Heat sensitivity
- ↑ fatigue
- ↑ neurological symptoms

    o Internuclear ophthalmoplegia
- Loss of adduction of affected eye

➢ Laboratory

    o CSF
- Oligoclonal bands in CSF but not serum
- ↑ IgG index
- ↑ rates of synthesis of CSF

➢ Diagnostic imaging

• Give the features on MRI of MS from sequelae of head injury.

    o Location
- Brainstem
- Spinal cord
- Cerebellum

    o Subcortical
- Contrast enhancement from active inflammation

    o MRI (fluid-attenuated inversion recovery MRI)
- Ovoid white plaques of demyelination
  ▪ In brain
  ▪ Brain stem
  ▪ Spinal cord
- Oval periventricular lesion
- Open ring perpendicular to the corpus callosum

    o MRI of brain/spinal cord
- Exclude compression
- Identify affected areas

    o Abnormal electrophysiological evoked potentials
- Visual
- Auditory
- Somatosensory

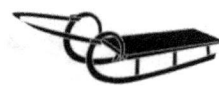

- o OCT (optical coherence tomography) of retina
  - – ↓ thickness

- In the context of multiple sclerosis, give the meaning of Devic disease.
  - o Devic disease is aka neuromyelitis optica (NMO)
  - o Clinically presents with recurrent
    - – Myelitis
    - – Optic neuritis
  - o No brain lesions
  - o NMO-IgG autoantibody may be positive

- ➢ Differential diagnosis
  - o Neuromyelitis optica (aka Devic disease)
  - o Acute disseminated encephalomyelitis
    - – Usually follows an infection, and results in ".... subacute.... profound, simultaneous demyelination in multiple regions of CNS" (Source: MKSAP 16 2012, Neurology, page 57)
    - – Encephalopathy associated with fever
    - – ↑ CSF lymphocytes
    - – ↑ brain (diffuse) involvement of brainstem on MRI

Please see full differential diagnosis in standard textbooks of Internal Medicine, or recent reviews such as UpToDate or MSKAP 16, 2012, Neurology, Table 27, page 60.

- ➢ Diagnosis
  - o Poser criteria: a history of two episodes of neurological deficit and objective clinical signs of lesions at more than one site within the central nervous system establishes the diagnosis of definite multiple sclerosis
  - o In the presence of only one clinical sign, the demonstration of an additional lesion by laboratory tests – such as evoked potentials, MRI, CT or urological studies – also fulfills the criteria
  - o A diagnosis of probable multiple sclerosis is defined as either two attacks with clinical evidence of one lesion, or one attack with clinical evidence of two lesions.
  - o Clinical suspicion from symptoms/signs of recurrent episodes of dysfunction

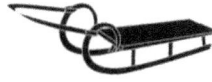

➢ Treatment
  o Treat fever and its cause
  o Stop smoking (↓ risk of developing progressive MS)
  o Life style
    – Exercise program
    – Dexascan (surveilance for osteoporosis)
    – Routine immunizations
    – Bladder care / UTI (urinary tract infection) antibiotic prophylaxis
    – Infections may cause "pseudorelapse"
    – Avoid over-heating and any other "triggers"

  o Acute exacerbations
    – Treat associated fever/infection
      ▪ ↓ symptoms of MS
    – IV methylprednisolone plus interferon or glatiramor acetate

                                              │   Poor response
      ▪ Natalizumab   │
      ▪ Mitoxantrone   ▼   ┌ ─ ─ ─ ─ ─ ─ ─ ─ ┐
                                                    ┊   **AE Alert**   ┊
                                                    └ ─ ─ ─ ─ ─ ─ ─ ─ ┘

  o Physiotherapy

  o Stop smoking

XXXXXXXXXXXXXXXXXXXXXXXXXXXXXXXXXXXXXXXXXXXXXXXXXXXXXXXXXXXXXXXXXXX
SO YOU WANT TO BE A NEUROLOGIST!
• In the context of MS (multiple sclerosis) and the management advise to
  avoid overheating (shower, sunshine), give the meaning of the **Uhthoff
  phenomenon**.
  o The Uhthoff phenomenon is the increase of disease symptoms
    when the person becomes hot (exercise-related ↑ body,
    temperature)

  o This exercise-associated ↑ symptoms is frequent in MS, and does
    not represent any suggestion of neurological damage

• Give the effect of pregnancy on the symptoms/severity of MS.
  o Risk of relapse
    – ↓ in T3 (third trimester)
    – ↑ 3 mon postpartum
XXXXXXXXXXXXXXXXXXXXXXXXXXXXXXXXXXXXXXXXXXXXXXXXXXXXXXXXXXXXXXXXXXX

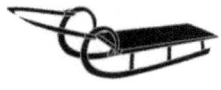

o Non-pharmacologic management for symptoms/complications

		Pharmacologic management	Drugs
o	CNS	– Fatigue*	▪ Amantadine
			▪ Modofinil
		– Neuropathic pain	▪ Gabapentin
			▪ Pregabalin
			▪ TCAs
		– Depression	▪ SSRIs
			▪ SNRIs
			▪ Anti-psychotics
o	MSK	– Spasticity	▪ Baclofen
			▪ Botulinum toxin
			▪ Benzodiazepines
		– ↓ mobility	▪ Dalfampridine
o	GU		▪ Oxybutynin
			▪ Tolteodine

Abbreviations: SNRIs, serotonin norepinephrine reuptake inhibitors; SSRI, selective serotonin reuptake inhibitors; TCAs, tricyclic anti-depressants

*Exclude other causes of fatigue
– Anemia
– Hypothyroidism
– Depression
– Sleep disorder

o Pharmacotherapy

– Corticosteroids	▪ Acute attack	Yes; IV methylprednisolone 1 g/d for 3-5 days, then 10 to 14 day prednisone taper
	▪ Maintenance of remission	No
	▪ Maintenance of remission in RR-MS	↓ number of relapses ↓ accumulation of new demyelinating plaques ↓ progression of disability

Name	Dosing / route / frequency	Mechanism of action	Benefit-↓rate of			FDA pregnancy category
			Relapse	Progression	MRI changes	
First line						
o IFN beta 1a	IM, 1/wk, or SC, 3/wk	Immune response Directed away from autoimmunity				C
beta 1b	SC, q 2 days	Protect BBB	+ (1/3)	+	+	
o Glatiramer acetate	SC, OD	Binds major histocompatibility complex molecules	+ (1/3)	+	+	B
Secondary line						
o Natalizumab	IV, 1/mon	Monoclonal antibody, binds α4 integrin on activated T cells Blocks active T cells binding to vascular endothelium				C
o Mitoxantrone	Anthrace- medione, which ↓ proliferation of lymphocytes	↓ BBM passage Only Rx useful for secondary MS	+ (2/3)	+ (40%)	-	D
o Fingolinod	PO	Sphingosime-1-phosphate modulator, blocking release of activated T cells from lymphoids	+	+	+	C

Abbreviation: BBM, brush border membrane

Modified from MKSAP 16 2012, Neurology, page 62.

- **Give the severe toxicities** of disease-modifying drugs in MS.

    - Natalizumab   – ↑ risk of PML (progressive multifocal leukoencephalopathy)
    - Fingolimod   – Serious HSV infection
                            – Cardiac
                                ▪ Hypertension
                                ▪ Bradycardia
                            – Eye
                                ▪ Macular edema

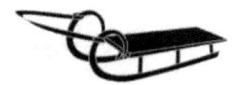

Clinical Gem

- When MS is associated with muscle spasms and cramps, the motorneuron spasticity, useful management includes.
  - Physiotherapy
  - Anti-spasticity drugs
    - Tizanidine
    - Centrally acting
    - α2-adrenergic agonist
    - Baclofen or cyclobenzaprine
    - Botulinum toxic injection
    - Intrathecal baclofen pump

  - Clinical syndrome (relapsing-remitting)
    - Interferon-β
    - Glatiramer acetate
  - Refractory to interferon-β or glatiramer
    - Natalizumab plus mitoxantrone
  - ↓ functional status
    - IV methylprednisolone

In relapse-remitting MS, interferon-B or glatiramer acetate is used to treat optic neuritis, or a syndrome such as spinal cord or brain stem-cerebellar syndrome.
- Give the name of the agents to use when these drugs are not effective, and give the adverse effects.
  - Natalizumab has the serious adverse effect (AE) of the development of PML progressive multifocal leukoencephalopathy)
  - Mitoxantrone has the AE of cardiotoxicity

Gems and Pearls

- Give the reason for the "AE alert" [Adverse Effect] of natalizumab/mitoxantrone for interferon/glatiramer poor responders in multiple sclerosis

  - Natalizumab is associated with ↑ risk of progressive multifocal leukoencephalopathy (PML)

  - Mitoxantrone is associated with ↑ risk of cardiotoxicity

- Give the reason to advise all MS patients to stop smoking.

  - Smoking in MS is associated with 300% risk of secondary progression

---

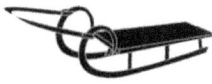

Mastering the Boards: Neurology   A.B.R. Thomson

Clinical Scenario

A young woman presents with a short history of ↓ vision and pain on moving her eyes. Examination showed an afferent pulpillary defect, and MRI of the optic nerve demonstrated contrast enhancement, compatible with optic neuritis, and there are also 3 periventricular lesions in the white matter. She improves with IV methylprednisolone, but she does not wish to take oral corticosteroids long-term.

- Give her optimum management in the long-term.

   o Corticosteroids are ineffective for maintenance therapy in this situation.

   o She requires disease-modifying therapy to reduce by half her likelihood of progressing to MS (multiple sclerosis).

   o In this patient with a clinical isolated syndrome, it is recommended to use
      - Glatiramer acetate, or
      - Interferon B

"Your present circumstances don't determine where you can go; they merely determine where you start."

Nido Qubein

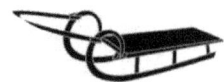

MISCELLANEOUS

Transplantation Candidates and Brain Death

A patient has prepared a living will, specifying she/he wishes to be considered as a transplantation donor at the time of their death.

- Give the clinical and laboratory means to establish brain death.

  - Clinical
    - Eyes
      - Pupils fixed and dilated
      - No corneal reflexes
      - No oculovestibular response
    - Responses to stimuli
      - Absent to
        - Visual
        - Auditory
        - Cutaneous
    - Throat
      - No gag reflex
    - Lung
      - No breathing
    - Sites of brain stem damage
      - Pons, midbrain
        - No corneal reflexes
      - Pons
        - No oculovestibular maneuvers
      - Medulla
        - No gag reflex
        - No breathing

  - Apnea test
    - No spontaneous breathing
    - Baseline P_{CO_2}
    - Spontaneous respiration
    - A 1 and 3 min, remeasure P_{CO_2} and observe for spontaneous breathing
    - Positive test
      - No spontaneous breathing
      - $\uparrow P_{CO_2} > 2$ mm Hg

  - Physical tests
    - EEG
      No activity
    - Cerebral blood flow study, no flow

    } brain dead

- Give the **neurological complications of diabetes mellitus.**
  - o Cerebellum
    - – Cerebral disturbance due to hyper- or hypo glycaemia
  - o Cranial nerves
    - – Isolated cranial nerve lesions
  - o Spinal column
    - – Diabetic pseudotabes
    - – Diabetic amyotrophy
  - o Peripheral nerves
    - – Asymptomatic loss of ankle jerks and vibration sense, with decreased motor conduction-velocity
    - – Painful subacute neuritis, usually in lower limbs
    - – Mononeuritis multiplex
    - – 'Insulin neuritis' during stabilization
  - o Autonomic
    - – Visceral disturbances due to autonomic involvement
  - o Miscellaneous/mixed
    - – Mixed syndromes

Adapted from: Burton JL. *Churchill Livingstone* 1971.

Sleep Disorders

➢ Clinical

Please see "A directed history of insomnia": Jugovic PJ, et al. *Saunders/ Elsevier* 2004, pages 51 to 53.

- Give a differential diagnosis of difficulty initiating or maintaining sleep.
  - o Transient stress reactions or adjustment reactions
  - o Psychiatric disorders (depression, anxiety)
  - o Restless leg syndrome
  - o Psychophysiologic insomnia
  - o Drug and/or alcohol abuse
  - o Disturbances of sleep wake cycle
  - o Sleep related respiratory disorders

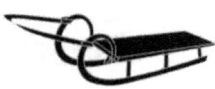

ONLINE RESOURCES:

MedEdPORTAL: https://www.mededportal.org/

Portal of online geriatric education: http://www.pogoe.org/

AGA educator resources: http://www.gastro.org/gi-fellowship/educator-resources

http://www.gastro.org/practive/medical-osition-statements

Home parenteral Nutrition: www.oley.org

Intestinal transplantation: http://www.intestinaltransplant.org

CCFA: http://www.ccfa.org

CCFC (Crohn's and Colitis Foundation of Canada): www.ccfc.ca

http://www.pathology.pitt.edu/lectures/gi

www.orl.cz/ehorroby/ustni/vestibulum/veozena

http://www.pathologyatlas.com

http://www.mayoclinic.org/gi-risk/mayomodel2.html

http://mayoclini.org/meld/mayomodel6.html

www.gastro.org/practice/meicacl-osition-statements

Natural Comprehensive Cancer Network (NCCN) guidelines: www.nccn.org

http://www.accessdata.fda.gov/drugsatfda_docs/label/2011/201917lbl.pdf

http://www.accessdata.fda.gov/drugsatfda_docs/label/2011/201917lbl.pdf

http://www.aidsinfo.nih.gov/guidelines/

http://www.fda.gov/Drugs/DrugSafety/ucm291119.htm

http://www.fda.gov/Drugs/DrugSafety/ucm291119.htm

http://www.fda.gov/NewsEvents/Newsroom/PressAnnouncements/ucm256299.htm

http://www.fda.gov/Safety/MedWatch/SafetyInformation/SafetyAlertsforHumanMedicalProducts/ucm291144.htm

http://www.fda.gov/Safety/MedWatch/SafetyInformation/SafetyAlertsforHumanMedicalProducts/ucm211796.htm

www.aasid.org/practiceguidelines/Page/default.aspx

http://www.accessdata.fda.gov/drugsatfda_does/label/2011/201917lbl.pdf

www.aasld.org/practiceguidelines/Page/default.aspx

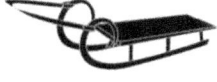

National Endoscopy Program : www.grs.nhs.uk

*MELD, Model for End-Stage Liver Disease, available online calculator: www.mayoclinic.org/meld/mayomodel7.html

www.motherisk.org/women/index.jsp

National Endoscopy Program : www.grs.nhs.uk

CAPstone: http://www.giandhepatology.com

MedicineNet: www.medicinenet.com/irritable_bowel_syndrome/article.htm

IBS Support group: www.ibsgroup.org

UpdateToDate: www.uptodate.com/patients/index

International Association for the Study of Obesity: http://www.iaso.org

Liver and intrahepatic bile ducts. www.PathologyOutlines.com

Medical council of Canada. Weight Gain/Obesity. http://mcc.ca/Objectives_Online/

Medical Council of Canada. Weight Loss/ Eating Disorders/ Anorexia http://mcc.ca/Objectives_Online/

Medical council of Canada. Weight loss/Eating Disorders/Anorexia. http://mcc.ca/Objectives_Online/

http://www.fda.gov/Drugs/DrugSafety/PostmarketDrugSafetyInformationf orPatientsandProviders/ucm213038.htm.

Medecins San Frontieres: http://www.msf.org

Recommendations about chemoprophylaxis for malaria. Also see http://www.nc.cdc.gov/travel/yellowbook/2012/chapter-3-infectious-disease-related-to-travel/malaria.htm

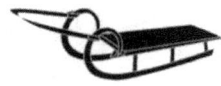

INDEX

Note: Locators followed by 'f' and 't' refer to figures and tables respectively.

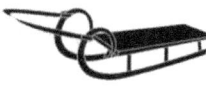

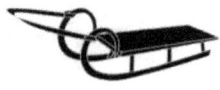

519

B
Bacterial meningitis
  bacteriology, 481–483
  demography, 481
  dexamethasone, 482
  gram negative, 483
  gram positive, 484–485
  H. influenzae, 482
  hospital-acquired bacterial pneumonia, pathogens for, 482
  laboratory, 484, 484t
  nosocromial, 482
  S. pneumonia, 482, 483
  treatment, 485–486, 485t
Bamford clinical classification of stroke
  lacunar syndrome, 45
  parietal anterior circulation syndrome, 44
  posterior circulation syndrome, 45
  total anterior circulation syndrome, 44
Basal ganglia calcification, 314
Bell palsy, 214–217, 240
Benedikt syndrome, 219, 281
Benign intracranial hypertension (BIH), 164, 259, 345–346
Benzodiazepines, 91, 132
Biernacki sign, 103
BIH. *See* Benign intracranial hypertension
Blindness
  amaurosis fugax, 148
  anterior ischemic optic neuropathy (AION), 146
  central scotoma, 149–150
  concentric diminution, 149
  Eale Disease, 148
  gradual, 147
  macula and, 148
  retinal vein *vs.* artery, physical examination, 147
  sudden, 145, 146
Blue slerae, 178
Body temperature disorders
  characteristics, 91t–93t
  neuroleptic malignant syndrome (NMS), 92t, 93–94
Botulism *vs.* myasthenia gravis, 476t
Bovine spongiform encephalopathy (BSE), 494
Brachial plexus lesions *vs.* nerve root compression, 414t
Bradycardias, 96
Bradykinesia, test for, 304, 306f
Brain
  abscess, 486–487

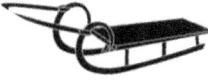

Mastering the Boards: Neurology   A.B.R. Thomson

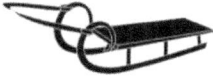

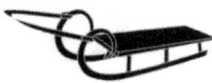

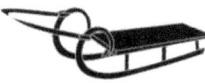

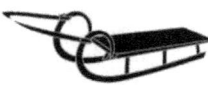

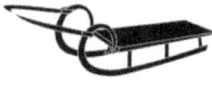

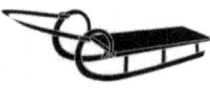

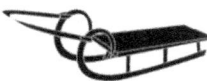

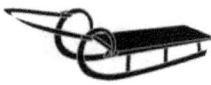

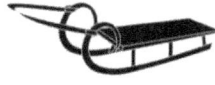

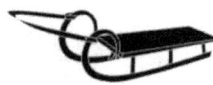

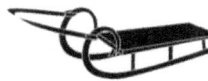

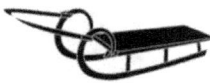

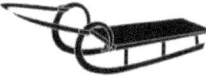

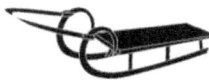

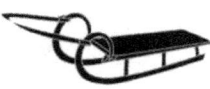

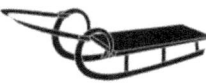

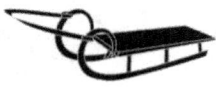

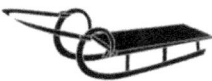

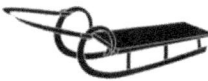

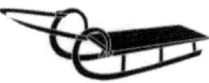

Mastering the Boards: Neurology A.B.R. Thomson

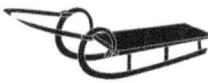

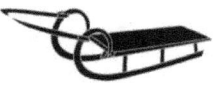

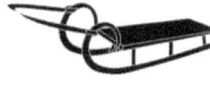

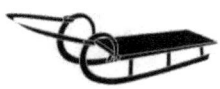

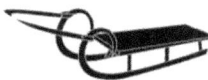

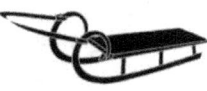

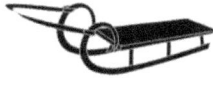

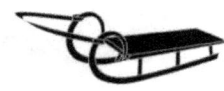

www.ingramcontent.com/pod-product-compliance
Lightning Source LLC
Chambersburg PA
CBHW080632180526
45168CB00008B/3146